Risk and Substance Use

This interdisciplinary collection examines the role that alcohol, tobacco and other drugs have played in framing certain groups and spaces as 'dangerous' and in influencing the nature of formal responses to the perceived threat.

Taking a historical and cross-national perspective, it explores how such groups and spaces are defined and bounded as well as the processes by which they come to be seen as 'risky'. It discusses how issues of perceived danger highlight questions of control and the management of behaviours, people and environments, and it pays attention to the way in which sanctions and regulations have been implemented in a variety of often inconsistent ways that frequently impact differently on different sections of the population.

Bringing together a range of case studies drawn from different countries and across different periods of time, the chapters collected here illustrate issues of marginalisation, stigmatisation, human rights and social expectations. It is of interest to a diverse audience of historians, philosophers, human geographers, anthropologists, sociologists and criminologists interested in substance use and misuse, deviance, risk and power among other topics.

Susanne MacGregor is Emeritus Professor at Middlesex University London and Honorary Professor at the London School of Hygiene and Tropical Medicine, UK.

Betsy Thom is Professor of Health Policy and Co-Director of the Drug and Alcohol Research Centre at Middlesex University, UK.

Routledge Studies in the Sociology of Health and Illness

For more information about this series, please visit: www.routledge.com/
Routledge-Studies-in-the-Sociology-of-Health-and-Illness/book-series/RSSHI

Risk and Substance Use

Framing Dangerous People
and Dangerous Places

**Edited by Susanne MacGregor
and Betsy Thom**

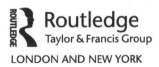
Routledge
Taylor & Francis Group

LONDON AND NEW YORK

First published 2020
by Routledge
4 Park Square, Milton Park, Abingdon, Oxon OX14 4RN
605 Third Avenue, New York, NY 10017

First issued in paperback 2023

Routledge is an imprint of the Taylor & Francis Group, an informa business

British Library Cataloguing-in-Publication Data
A catalogue record for this book is available from the British Library

Library of Congress Cataloging-in-Publication Data
Names: MacGregor, Susanne, editor. | Thom, Betsy, editor.
Title: Risk and substance use : framing dangerous people and dangerous places / edited by Susanne MacGregor and Betsy Thom.
Description: Abingdon, Oxon ; New York, NY : Routledge, 2020. | Series: Routledge studies in the sociology of health and illness | Includes bibliographical references and index.
Identifiers: LCCN 2019048425 (print) | LCCN 2019048426 (ebook) | ISBN 9781138491243 (hardback) | ISBN 9781351033503 (ebook)
Subjects: LCSH: Substance abuse—Social aspects. | Danger perception. | Threats. | Social groups. | Risk—Sociological aspects.
Classification: LCC HV4998 .R57 2020 (print) | LCC HV4998 (ebook) | DDC 362.29/12—dc23
LC record available at https://lccn.loc.gov/2019048425
LC ebook record available at https://lccn.loc.gov/2019048426

ISBN: 978-1-03-257028-0 (pbk)
ISBN: 978-1-138-49124-3 (hbk)
ISBN: 978-1-351-03350-3 (ebk)

DOI: 10.4324/9781351033503

Typeset in Times New Roman
by Apex CoVantage, LLC

Publisher's Note
The publisher has gone to great lengths to ensure the quality of this reprint but points out that some imperfections in the original copies may be apparent.

Contents

Tables

Figures

Acknowledgements

The editors thank all the contributors to this volume for their cooperation.

We would also like to thank members of CAATOD (Critical Approaches towards Alcohol, Tobacco and Other Drugs), an international group of addiction researchers meeting in Vienna under the umbrella of the Sigmund Freud Private University, for discussion of ideas and comments on early drafts of some papers.

A number of people acted as peer reviewers of chapters. We are very grateful to Shane Butler, Betsy Ettorre, Matilda Hellman, Zsuzsa Kalő, John Marsden, Alex Mold, Geoff Monaghan, Andrew Ryder, Franziska Schneider and Carla Treloar.

Contributors

Tamar M.J. Antin is Director of the Center for Critical Public Health and a senior research scientist at both the Prevention Research Center in Berkeley, California, and the Institute of Scientific Analysis in the San Francisco Bay Area, USA. Dr Antin received a master's degree in applied anthropology from the University of Maryland, College Park and a doctoral degree in public health from the University of California, Berkeley. Over the past 15 years, Dr Antin has conducted research on the social and cultural meanings of nicotine and tobacco as well as alcohol for youth and young adults. She is particularly interested in examining how the intersections of stigma – both the stigmas of social identities and the stigmas associated with substance use – combine to shape meanings related to the consumption of drugs. Dr Antin has received funding in the United States from the National Cancer Institute, the National Institute on Alcohol Abuse and Alcoholism and the Tobacco-Related Disease Research Program.

Virginia Berridge is Professor of History and Health Policy at the London School of Hygiene and Tropical Medicine, University of London, UK. Her research focuses on the contemporary history of public health, especially illicit drugs, alcohol, smoking, HIV/AIDS and the relationship between evidence (including history) and policy. Her most recent books are *Demons: Our Changing Attitudes towards Alcohol, Drugs and Tobacco* (Oxford University Press, 2013) and *Public Health: A Very Short Introduction* (Oxford University Press, 2016). She has had research funding from the Wellcome Trust, Economic and Social Research Council and other funders. She led the work package on addiction through the ages, part of the EU-funded ALICE RAP programme on drugs. She is currently principal investigator for a Wellcome Trust–funded cross-national study comparing the UK, the United States and Australia in terms of their divergent policy responses towards e-cigarettes. She edits the 'Addiction Lives' oral history interview series for *Addiction* and the Society for the Study of Addiction. Prof. Berridge is former president of the Alcohol and Drug History Society, former president of the European Association for the History of Medicine and Health and former chair of the Society for the Social History of Medicine. She is a Fellow of the Academy of Social Sciences.

Charlotte De Kock is a researcher at the Institute for Social Drug Research (Ghent University, BE), directed by Prof. Dr Tom Decorte, since 2015. She conducted several policy-oriented research projects for the Belgian Science Policy Office, including 'Patterns of substance use among migrants and ethnic minorities' (PADUMI, Belspo, 2015–2017) and 'Social prevention of drug related crime' (SOCPREV, Belspo, 2018, coordinated by Prof. Dr Lieven Pauwels). She is currently working on 'Mapping and enhancing substance use treatment for migrants and ethnic minorities' (MATREMI, Belspo, 2019, together with Prof. Decorte). Besides this policy-oriented research work and support in education, Charlotte is working on a PhD (funded by Ghent University) studying the accessibility and relevance of substance use treatment for migrants and ethnic minorities from a rights-based and eco-social perspective (ACCESS, Ghent University Fund, 2019–2022). She is part of a Ghent University network on migration and recovery (including Prof. Vanderplasschen and Prof. Vander Laenen). Charlotte is involved in the XChange prevention registry of the European Monitoring Centre for Drugs and Drug Addiction (EMCCDA) as an early career board member.

Karen Duke is Professor of Criminology and Co-Director of the Drug and Alcohol Research Centre at Middlesex University, UK. She is a criminologist and policy analyst, specialising in research on the development of drugs policy and the interfaces with the criminal justice system. She is one of the Editors in Chief of the journal *Drugs: Education, Prevention and Policy* and leads the MA programme in Comparative Drug and Alcohol Studies at Middlesex University, which is run jointly with universities in Italy, Denmark and Spain. She has conducted drugs-related research and consultancy for the European Commission, UNODC, Home Office, Department of Health, the former Central Drugs Co-ordination Unit (Cabinet Office) and the Royal Society for the Arts. Current research includes coordinating an EU-funded research project with Prof. Betsy Thom (EPPIC: Exchanging prevention practices on polydrug use among youth in criminal justice systems).

Christopher Hallam is a research associate at the Global Drug Policy Observatory at Swansea University, Wales, UK. He writes and conducts research on international drug policy and on the history and regulation of psychoactive drug consumption. Christopher obtained his PhD from the London School of Hygiene and Tropical Medicine, where he was supervised by Prof. Virginia Berridge. His first book was published in 2018; entitled *White Drug Cultures and Regulation in London, 1916–1960*, the book explores the formative heroin and cocaine cultures in Britain and the attempts by juridical and medical authorities to suppress them. He lives in Hampshire, where he is presently researching a biography of 'society drug addict' Brenda Dean Paul.

Rachel Herring is Senior Research Fellow and Co-Director of the Drug and Alcohol Research Centre at Middlesex University, UK. She is a former nurse turned social scientist with a particular interest in social and policy aspects of alcohol and drug use. Using primarily qualitative methods, she has undertaken a range of research, including studies on young people's drinking, young adults who drink little or no alcohol, innovative approaches and multi-component approaches to reducing alcohol-related harm at local level. Recent research includes a qualitative study of Polish drinkers accessing community-based treatment in London. She has worked with European partners on EU-funded research projects, including a current project on drug prevention interventions for young drug users in the criminal justice systems in six EU countries. She is also Co-Editor-in-Chief of the journal *Drugs: Education Prevention and Policy*.

Geoffrey Hunt is a social and cultural anthropologist. Currently, he is Professor at the Centre for Alcohol and Drugs Research at Aarhus University, Denmark and Senior Research Scientist at the Institute for Scientific Analysis in San Francisco, USA. Dr Hunt is the Principal Investigator (PI) on an NIH-funded project on Gender and Intoxication and also PI on a Danish Research Council project on Immigrant Youth Perceptions of the Police. His book publications include *Youth Drugs and Nightlife* (Routledge, 2010), *Drugs and Culture* (Ashgate, 2011) and *The Sage Handbook of Drug and Alcohol Studies* (2017).

Axel Klein is a social anthropologist with an interest in the culture of consumption of mind-altering substances. He has been fascinated by the changing status of cannabis, from menace to medicine. The spread of small-scale cannabis cultivation has been a fascinating process to be part of, with the changes in political rhetoric and the redefinition of growers and sellers as shamans and guerrilla medicine men. After heading the international unit at DrugScope and lecturing at the University of Kent, he worked on European Commission drug control projects and is currently with the Global Drug Policy Observatory at the University of Swansea, UK. His publications include *Collapse of the Global Order on Drugs: From UNGASS 2016 to Review 2019* (with Blaine Stothard, 2018), 'Poly and Tricky Dick: the drug war origins of the term "polydrug use"', *Nordic Studies on Alcohol and Drugs* (2018) and 'The three betrayals of the medical cannabis growing activist', *International Journal of Drug Policy* (with Gary Potter, 2018).

Torsten Kolind is Professor and Director of the Centre for Alcohol and Drug Research, Aarhus University, Denmark. He has published widely in the fields of criminal justice, prisons, ethnicity, young people, drug treatment, alcohol and drugs. He is Co-Editor-in-Chief of *Drugs: Education, Prevention and Policy*. He is Co-Editor of *The SAGE Handbook of Drug and Alcohol Studies* from 2017.

Susanne MacGregor is Emeritus Professor at Middlesex University London and Honorary Professor at the London School of Hygiene and Tropical Medicine, UK. Her first degree was in social anthropology and her PhD in politics. Since then she has worked in departments of social anthropology, social psychiatry, politics and sociology, social policy and politics, sociology, criminology and social policy, history and public health. She has concentrated on interdisciplinary and applied research on various social issues, especially drugs and alcohol, along with homelessness, unemployment, social security and urban development and policy. Her most recent book was *The Politics of Drugs: Perceptions, Power and Policies* (Palgrave Macmillan, 2017). She has been a scientific advisor to the UK Department of Health and was recently a member of an ACMD Working Group on the *Ageing Cohort of Drug Users* in the UK.

Emma Milne is Lecturer in Criminology at the University of Plymouth, UK. After completing her PhD in sociology at the University of Essex, Emma moved to Middlesex University, where she worked as a lecturer. Emma's research interests are in feminist criminology and social and legal responses to women who offend. The wider context of Emma's work considers social controls and criminal justice regulations on all women, notably in relation to pregnancy, sex and reproduction.

James Nicholls is Chief Executive Officer of Transform Drug Policy Foundation and Honorary Associate Professor at the Centre for History in Public Health, London School of Hygiene and Tropical Medicine, UK. He was previously Director of Research and Policy at Alcohol Research UK, during which time he sat on the Public Health England Alcohol Leadership Board and chaired the PHE National Licensing and Public Health Network. He is author of *The Politics of Alcohol: A History of the Drink Question in England* (Manchester University Press, 2009) and co-author of *Alcohol, Power and Public Health* (Routledge, 2017). His research interests include the history of drinking cultures, alcohol policy and changing ideas around addiction over time. James sits on the Executive Committee of the Alcohol and Drugs History Society, the International Editorial Board for *Drugs: Education, Prevention and Policy* and the Board of Trustees at Adfam.

Aileen O'Gorman is a sociologist whose research explores the living experience and problematisation of social issues such as poverty, health inequalities, drug and alcohol use and risk environments. She focuses on research that is participative, engages with the people and communities affected and that which has an impact on policy and practice. Aileen has worked as a researcher in academia, government and with marginalised communities in Ireland and the UK. Currently, she is a senior lecturer and programme leader for the postgraduate Contemporary Drug and Alcohol Studies programme at the University of the West of Scotland, UK. Recent research and publications include discussions of conceptualising polydrug use, the meaning of recovery, community approaches to drug problems and risk environments for drug-related deaths. She is a member of the Board of the European Society for Social Drugs (ESSD) research, on the International Editorial Board of the journal *Drugs: Education, Prevention and Policy* and on the steering group of the Drugs Research Network Scotland (DRNS).

Gary R. Potter is Reader in Criminology at Lancaster University Law School, UK. His research interests include drug policy and drug markets with a particular focus on cannabis cultivation. He is a founder member of the Global Cannabis

Cultivation Research Consortium (see worldwideweed.nl), a board member of the European Society for Social Drug Research and on the editorial boards of *Drugs and Alcohol Today* and *The International Journal of Drug Policy*. He also has an interest in researching the illegal wildlife trade and in green criminology more generally.

Emile Sanders is a research associate with the Center for Critical Public Health at the Institute for Scientific Analysis in Alameda, California, USA. During the study on which his contribution to this book is based, he was a research assistant at Prevention Research Center in Oakland, CA. Emile received a bachelor's degree in sociocultural anthropology from the University of California, Berkeley in 2017, where he focused also on LGBT and queer studies. He previously earned an associate degree in interdisciplinary studies with an emphasis on social and behavioural sciences. He is now interviewing study participants, conducting analyses and managing projects centred around the experiences of sexual and gender minority young adults in the San Francisco Bay Area. These current studies focus variously on alcohol intoxication, police interactions and tobacco harm reduction as a social practice.

Akihiko Sato (PhD, Kyoto University) is Professor of Sociology, Kwansei Gakuin University, Japan. His research interests concern the relationship between modernisation and social order. His work draws on historical, sociological and discursive analyses of both legal and illegal drug problems. On illegal drugs, he has been researching drug use and drug policy for 27 years both within and outside Japan. He has also conducted research on harm reduction in European countries over a decade. On legal drugs, he researches on drug-induced problems like the thalidomide incident and the issue of blood products contaminated with HIV. He is the author of *Drug and Discourse: Methamphetamine in Japan* (*Kakuseizai no Shakaishi, Toshindo, Tokyo, Japan*, published in Japanese, Japanese Association of Social Problems Academic Promotion Award [2007] and 7th Japanese Association of Sociological Criminology Promotion Award [2008]) and *Sociology of Drugs: Psychoactive Materials and Social Order* (*Drug no Shakaigaku, Sekaishisosha, Kyoto, Japan*, published in Japanese). He has published many articles and book chapters, including 'Methamphetamine use in Japan after the Second World War: transformation of narratives', *Contemporary Drug Problems*, 35/Winter 2008, 717–46, 2009.

Camille May Stengel is an early career researcher and Lecturer in Criminology at the University of Greenwich, UK. She is interested in drug policy, harm reduction, prison education and feminist and creative methodologies. She completed her EU-funded dual PhD in cultural and global criminology from the University of Kent in the UK and ELTE University in Hungary in 2016. Camille has previously worked as a research fellow and technical advisor at London School of Hygiene and Tropical Medicine, a media officer at Harm Reduction International and a research associate at the Canadian Institute for Substance Use Research. Camille is a trained Inside-Out Prison Exchange facilitator and has led undergraduate university courses in two English prisons. Outside of work, Camille can likely be found ambling along the streets of London on her bicycle.

Betsy Thom is Professor of Health Policy and Co-Director of the Drug and Alcohol Research Centre at Middlesex University, UK. She is a social scientist using largely qualitative research approaches. Her research interests include alcohol and drug policy, gender and substance use and community-based approaches to prevention and intervention. She is currently the prevention theme lead for the Drug Research Network Scotland (DRNS). She has been involved in several EU-funded projects and has worked as a consultant for UNODC and other national and European organisations. She was Editor-in-Chief of *Drugs: Education Prevention and Policy* for 20 years and a member of the board of the International Society for Addiction Journal Editors (ISAJE). Her work includes developing and running distance learning programmes in drug and alcohol studies including a collaborative programme with Denmark and Italy. Current research is looking at drug prevention interventions for young drug users in the criminal justice systems in six EU countries.

Alfred Uhl is Vice-Head of the English PhD Programme of the Sigmund Freud Private University (SFU) and Vice-Head of the Addiction Competence Centre of the Austrian Public Health Institute (GOEG), both in Vienna, Austria. He is a health psychologist and involved in empirical and theoretical research as well as teaching research methodology, statistics and substance abuse prevention at university level. He is a board member of several scientific journals and a member of the German Society for Addiction Psychology. He has been involved in several EU-funded projects and served as expert concerning prevention, evaluation and addiction policy for several Austrian, European and International governmental bodies and organisations, including the Federal Ministry of Health, the World Health Organization (WHO, Copenhagen), the German Society for Evaluation (DeGEval), the Pompidou Group of the Council of Europe (Strasbourg) and the European Monitoring Centre for Drugs and Drug Addiction (EMCDDA). His current research focus is on epidemiology, prevention, addiction policy, evaluation and research methodology.

Marie Claire Van Hout is Professor of Public Health Policy and Practice at the Public Health Institute, Liverpool John Moores University, UK. She has over 17 years research, education and clinical practice experience in various fields of public health and drug policy, with a particular interest in prescribed and illicit substance use, HIV/hepatitis C prevention, treatment, care and support, prison health, health and human rights and ethnic minorities and health. She has consulted for the Research Executive Agency, European Commission, the EMCDDA and United Nations Office on Drugs and Crime in Sub Saharan Africa, North Africa and the Middle East. She currently holds several honorary appointments at the South African Medical Research Council in Cape Town, the Centre for Research and Studies in Sociology, University Institute of Lisbon and University College Dublin.

1 Introduction

Risk and substance use

Betsy Thom and Susanne MacGregor

The aim of this collection of essays is to cast light on controversial issues by comparing across substances and across time, countries and cultures.

The book is concerned with the role of substance use (alcohol, illicit drugs and tobacco) as a key element in the framing of groups and spaces as 'dangerous', influencing the nature of responses to perceived threats. Case studies, drawn from different, mainly high-income countries, illustrate the processes through which a group or space is identified, defined and framed and the impact of such framing on informal responses as well as legal and regulatory responses, policies and practice. We consider framing processes against the wider context of economic, political, cultural and social environments and discuss how these processes change over time.

The chapters illustrate how, in the contemporary period, developments in social research methods, especially the rise of epidemiology, and their accompanying measurement techniques, by operationalising the concept of risk, have facilitated identification and characterisation of dangerous classes and dangerous spaces and have influenced policy and practice responses. They examine the roles of the media, advocacy and research, which have all played a part in building perceptions of dangerousness and risk regarding specific population groups and spaces. At the same time, there is resistance to, and avoidance of, negative stereotyping among affected social groups: several chapters look at how individuals and groups have developed alternative frames of understanding, devised strategies to deflect attention from their behaviours and create 'safe' spaces in which to live their lives as they choose. Issues of marginalisation, stigmatisation, human rights and social expectations are discussed and illustrated in the chapters.

Each chapter is based on theoretical perspectives and methodological approaches appropriate to the topic and the research data presented in the argument. However, 'framing' provides the main theoretical approach adopted throughout the book, and the concepts of 'frame', 'framing', 'risk' and 'danger' underpin each chapter. There is a vast literature around each of these concepts and, in the following sections, we can only touch on some of the main perspectives, arguments and critiques as they relate to the chapters in this book.

What do we mean by 'frame' and 'framing'?

To frame is to select some aspects of perceived reality and make them more salient in such a way as to promote a particular problem definition, causal interpretation, moral evaluation and/or treatment recommendation for the item described (Entman, 1993).

It is important to distinguish between 'frame' – a static state of knowing and understanding – and 'framing' – a process whereby a particular way of knowing or understanding comes to emerge, develop, fade away or re-emerge in an altered way of knowing.

Rein and Schön (1991) describe frames as providing guideposts for knowing, analysing, persuading and acting and for making sense of an amorphous, ill-defined, problematic situation. Frames are a central part of culture: they represent the 'taken-for-granted' and the beliefs and assumptions that guide everyday behaviour; they help us to define problems, diagnose causes, make moral judgements and suggest remedies. Frames are often – but not always – shared within a social group or culture: they can be widespread within a society or culture and can persist over long periods of time; and they serve to draw boundaries around the acceptable and the unacceptable, the included and the excluded. De Kock (Chapter 7), for instance, notes how the creation of ethnic boundaries can induce processes of 'othering' that frame seemingly static characteristics of populations as 'risk factors', with moralising consequences. This impacts on service providers, services and health systems and members of the same ethnic community, thereby influencing problem use, access to services and quality of care among (potential) clients.

Individuals may be framed in more than one way and the groups of interest in this book frequently suffer from intersecting negative labels. As Stengel describes (Chapter 6), Roma women, labelled as 'junkie Gypsy prostitutes', were seen as a triple threat to mainstream Hungarian social and moral values. Sanders, Antin and Hunt (Chapter 11) draw attention to the role of tobacco de-normalisation in creating a stigmatising smoker frame: 'The smoking body has come to be viewed, treated, and governed as a dangerous body, marked as a bearer of death and disease, of health risks, and of poor health'. In the case of lesbian, gay, bisexual, transgender and queer (LGBTQ) people, this negative smoker frame intersects with and compounds other stigmatising frames applied to those groups. Nicholls and Berridge (Chapter 2) discuss how race, space and class coalesced in anti-immigrant legislation in the UK in the early twentieth century.

While negative frames are more often attached to poor, immigrant or otherwise marginalised people and the spaces they inhabit, Hallam (Chapter 4) provides an example of negative framing applied to upper-class women in the interwar years in London; drug use and 'deviant' sexuality drew police surveillance and framed the women as a 'dangerous class', sometimes associated with 'the oriental' and the promiscuous mixing of races.

Once a characterisation of an issue, value, place or group of people is accepted, the frame can become institutionalised (Björnehed and Erikson, 2018); that is, it undergoes a process over time – often including a struggle between different frames of understanding and different groups of stakeholders – that results in a particular frame gaining influence and regulative function. We see this happening currently in the institutionalisation of the 'precautionary principle' as the dominant frame concerning alcohol consumption in pregnancy (Thom, Herring and Milne, Chapter 5).

Frames can gain or lose influence depending on their degree and level of institutionalisation. Medical cannabis, for instance, may be undergoing a frame shift as perceptions and regulatory systems change from seeing cannabis use, even for medical purposes, as illegal and harmful to accepting that its prescribed use for certain conditions may be beneficial (EMCDDA, 2018).

Any field of activity can have more than one frame (alternative frames) and some frames may be competing or in open conflict. For example, frames depicting alcohol consumption derived from the alcohol industry may be at odds with frames derived from public health advocates. People who smoke may frame their activity as coping with adverse circumstances or as an enjoyable (legal) way to relax, whereas those who object to smoking may see the behaviour as unhealthy and harmful to others. For many years, illicit drugs have been framed negatively, rejecting any alternative frame that focuses on the benefits or pleasures of drug use. Communities framed by the police, media and outsiders as 'no go' areas may be viewed in a very different – and more positive – light by residents (MacGregor and O'Gorman, Chapter 9). Counter-frames are common and may be intentionally developed as a form of resistance or challenge to existing frames. Potter and Klein (Chapter 12) report how home cultivation of cannabis is cast in positive terms as an activity undertaken for therapeutic purposes, often with altruistic intent, and how cannabis growers are at pains to distance themselves from being framed as part of the 'real' criminal world. Resistance can come from organisations as well as from individuals; MacGregor and O'Gorman (Chapter 9) note how local authority services resisted some of the shaming aspects of the 'Troubled Families' programme: 'almost all local authorities called their local troubled families work by another name'.

'Framing', on the other hand, as Vliegenthart and Van Zoonen (2011) argue, is a process. They draw attention to the importance of frame-building, how a frame comes about and frame effects, the consequences of the frame. Framing offers a way of understanding how a social phenomenon – such as the definition of a particular group or space as 'risky' or 'dangerous' – is constructed by stakeholders – the media, advocacy groups, political or social movements, researchers, practitioners or other actors. By considering framing as a dynamic process, we can also examine how frames alter and shift and the factors that prompt or hinder such changes. Several of the chapters in this book provide narratives that illustrate framing processes. Sato (Chapter 3) gives an account of how social and political forces, especially condemnation of specific groups of people (at various times – novelists, performers, students, Korean people), played important roles in how methamphetamine use was framed and how, over time, this led to the establishment of the *Stimulant Control Law* in Japan.

Framing occurs at individual and societal levels. While psychologically based research approaches framing from the individual (micro) level, studies coming from social movement research and from general sociology consider framing in a broader way as a macro-level or meso-level rather than an individual-level phenomenon (Scheufele and Iyengar, 2017). Clearly, these processes are not separate; there is a complex interactive relationship between frames and framing processes happening at the cultural, social group or institutional level and at the level of the individual actor and recipient. Different levels of coexisting frames and framing processes are explored by Duke and Kolind (Chapter 10); they note how international and national frames (macro-level) around drug problems in prison are interpreted and re-framed in institutional settings (meso-level) and how prisoners adapt and respond to the frames, sometimes reframing their involvement in drug use and drug supply in prison (micro-level). Equally, De Kock (Chapter 7) argues strongly for the adoption of an eco-social perspective on problem substance use, especially as it pertains to health inequalities (Solar and Irwin, 2010). This perspective draws attention to how factors at three levels – micro (client and treatment provider), meso (services) and macro (broader health and welfare systems) – intertwine to frame, in this case, Turkish migrants as 'at risk' and 'a risk', both within their own communities and in the wider society. It highlights the role of multi-level framing in influencing responses and in perpetuating marginal status and health inequalities.

Thus, framing is a critical activity in the construction of social reality because it helps shape the perspectives through which people see the world and which, if powerful, become embedded in policies and institutions. It operates interactively at different levels and it influences action; and it should be viewed as a dynamic process. A basic assumption underpinning the chapters in this book is that substance use is frequently a major part of the frames and framing processes that define certain social groups and the spaces they inhabit as 'dangerous' and, in some way, a threat, or an economic cost, to the wider society. Such framing is sometimes unintentional or an unwanted outcome from well-intentioned policy or advocacy; but it can also arise from struggles between political or group interests and from media sensationalism.

The concepts of 'risk' and 'danger' are prominent aspects of the frames and framing processes linked to substance use and a key element in the frames applied to the people and spaces discussed in this book.

The concept of risk

The term 'risk' has been applied to an enormous range of phenomena and, as Gabe (1995) noted, has led to the growth of a 'risk industry', incorporating research from many different disciplines. Furedi (2005) links the increasing emphasis on risk, risk averse policy and 'at risk' social groups to the politics of fear, commenting that it has fed into the paradigm of 'vulnerability', a cultural metaphor implying an intrinsic state of being which deprives individuals of a sense of agency and limits their choices. A similar view is taken by Brown and Wincup (2019) who argue that 'the current problematisation of vulnerability in English drug policy supports the operation of subtle disciplinary mechanisms to regulate the behaviour of those deemed vulnerable'. Being 'at risk' places an individual in a passive, dependent role requiring management and control while the risks themselves assume an active role that drives action. Very often, the social groups discussed in this book are seen as 'vulnerable' and 'at risk' but, at the same time, they – or their behaviours – are seen as posing a risk, again raising issues of the need for management and control. Risk, in contemporary discourses around substance use and users, implies negative outcomes predominantly due to individual behaviour (rather than external causes) and reflects implicit moral frameworks and judgements with the potential to arouse fear and anxiety and a sense of helplessness (Lupton, 1993).

As already noted, individuals can be both 'at risk' and pose a risk; for instance, young people involved in drug dealing in what has become known as 'county lines' (spreading drug dealing from major urban locations out to smaller towns and rural settings) are seen as both vulnerable victims of drug dealers and also as a risk to other young people and communities (Coomber and Moyle, 2017). Sato (Chapter 3) paints a similar picture of street kids and vagrant youth in post-war Japan who were seen as both victims of adult hoodlums and as adding to the problem of amphetamine and methamphetamine use that caused them to become involved in delinquent activity. However, as the chapters in this book make abundantly clear, individuals and groups occupy different structural positions in society, with varying access to resources such as power or information and varying experiences of environmental and situational hazards. Position within structural and organisational structures influences definitions and interpretations of reality, perceptions of risk and responses to risk.

In recent times, the concept of 'risk' has become an important element in contemporary thinking around health and in policy responses to perceived risks. A 2002 World Health report defined risk as 'a probability of an adverse outcome, or a factor that raises this probability' (WHO, 2002, p. xiii). The same report identified ten global risk factors responsible for a large proportion of the burden of disease, disability and death: underweight, unsafe sex, high blood pressure, tobacco consumption, alcohol consumption, unsafe water, sanitation and hygiene, iron deficiency, indoor smoke from solid fuels, high cholesterol and obesity. Within this wider health context, the substance use field has adopted the 'burden of disease' perspective (e.g. Rhem et al., 2009) and the emphasis on risk behaviour, risk perception and risk environments has grown exponentially. Enormous effort has gone into attempts to calculate and predict 'risk', various social groups have been labelled as 'at risk' and others as posing a risk to themselves, their communities or society at large because of their substance use.

In its original usage, 'risk' is neutral, referring to probability or the mathematical likelihood of an event occurring (Lupton, 1993). Risk can be understood as a statistical concept based on measures derived from screening instruments or underpinning lists of indicators and identification systems, all of which have proliferated in recent decades. These are viewed as allowing us to construct neutral, scientifically designed frames, but they also contain implicit value judgements: as Nutt et al. argued, the methodology and processes underpinning how risk is assessed and how conclusions are reached on the relative risk of one substance versus another lacks transparency and is contested (Nutt et al., 2007). More fundamental critiques of the 'risk factor' epidemiology that underpins much policy and intervention draw attention to the problems and deficiencies of epidemiological methods and make a plea for the incorporation of analyses of macro-level socio-economic, political and cultural forces and closer dialogue between epidemiology and social theory (Wemrell et al., 2016). Uhl (Chapter 13) addresses these issues in relation to research that informs alcohol policy. He argues that framing policy as 'evidence-based' suggests that policy can be derived from empirical facts alone and this camouflages the role value decisions actually play. He illustrates his argument by providing a critique of interpretations of research findings that frame international discourse on risks relating to 'harm to others due to alcohol' and 'drinking alcohol while lactating'.

The communication of risk and research findings on risk into the public domain is subject to many processes of ordering, selecting, deciding on the emphasis placed on one 'fact' compared to another and on balancing different priorities and stakeholder interests. Within these processes, the media has considerable power, frequently playing a prominent role in the translation of risk into the public arena, influencing how risks are portrayed and how the evidence of risk is communicated. Risk assessments are often inflated or distorted by media coverage, as illustrated in several chapters in this book. Hallam (Chapter 4), for instance, notes how the lives of a small number of celebrity 'bohemian' women were endlessly covered by the media, feeding into contemporary fears around gender and sexuality and perceived deviant behaviour among young women. The power of television, visible in programmes which portray welfare recipients – and their lifestyles – as responsible for their own poverty and wider social problems, is explored by MacGregor and O'Gorman (Chapter 9). The Internet has provided an unprecedented medium for the communication of risk across different forums. Advocacy groups, government departments, commercial enterprises and lay networks now promote and contest 'risk' claims in all spheres of life, including the use of alcohol, tobacco and drugs. Increasingly, social media are playing a role in risk communication across all fields of activity, bringing lay perspectives and alternative media coverage into the dynamics of risk communication and, if anything, expanding the range of available frames around substance use and problem use. Potter and Klein (Chapter 12), for example, give a hint of how alternative frames are shared and sustained through social media when they mention 'cannabis social clubs' and campaign groups. How this electronic explosion of risk communication will affect policy, practice and public attitudes and behaviours is beyond the scope of this book; but it is an important development and must remain an area for future examination.

The concept of danger

It is a key argument of this collection that the concept of risk has not escaped from more basic notions of danger. Scientific language is not clearly separated from wider public understandings of terms and ideas. People and places are still portrayed in the media, in public parlance and in policy as 'dangerous'. Indeed, it has been suggested that the use of 'risk' has come to mean danger and is the preferred term in professional discourse because the term 'danger' lacks the aura of science and the promise of precise calculation (Douglas, 1986, cited in Lupton, 1993). The chapters in this book are concerned with how risk and danger are linked to substances and patterns of substance use, to people and social groups deemed to be dangerous and a threat to society and to spaces – locations – seen as dangerous places to live or visit.

Certain substances have been defined as uniquely dangerous and subject to international prohibitions. They have been distinguished from other poisons and from foods and medicines and subject to different methods of regulation. They are seen as not only endangering the health of an individual but also as threatening the fabric of families, communities and societies. Perceptions of some substances as more dangerous than others are not new. For example, Hailwood (2015) notes, in eighteenth-century England, gin and whiskey were regulated differently, with much higher taxes applied to gin. The official reason for this was that gin was more dangerous than whiskey, but, Hailwood argues, the real reason was that gin was mainly consumed by the working class. Alcohol laws were used by the dominant class to control marginalised or potentially dangerous social groups. Then, as now, how substances and substance use are perceived and responded to is a window into social and political discourses and tensions. Views on the relative dangerousness of different substances are increasingly being challenged (e.g. Nutt et al., 2007) and international agreements are being modified in many countries (Csete et al., 2016). It is, however, difficult to shift public perceptions, professional structures built around the legal status of a drug and policy constrained by international agreements and stakeholder interests. Klein (2008) has argued that 'the prohibitionist stance in policy, while counterproductive in its effects, has maintained its predominance because it serves the interests of an international drug control bureaucracy, as well as, at national level, certain interests of state control and professional advancement' (reviewed in MacGregor, 2010). The chapters in this book draw attention to how the legal status of a substance is linked to interests and influences that have nothing to do with the property of the substance itself or to its effects and how, once framed in a particular way, substances take on significance beyond biological effects and health concerns.

The 'dangerous classes' was a term commonly used in the nineteenth century to describe sections of the population considered to be a threat to the political, economic or social status quo. As with other terms – the underclasses, the masses, the (lumpen) proletariat, the labouring classes – these labels are applied to a category of citizens who are seen as threatening social stability but who, through the use of pejorative frames, are located outside of respectable society (Morris, 1994). Lea (1999) argues that there has been an increase in the general criminalisation of the poor as a 'dangerous class' since the 1990s – a view taken up and examined in Chapter 9 (MacGregor and O'Gorman). But who is depicted as belonging to the 'dangerous classes', and even the concept itself, shifts over time and place (De Kock, Chapter 7).

The term 'dangerous classes' may now have fallen out of favour – and there have been changes in the groups subject to such 'othering' processes (see Jensen, 2011 for a discussion of 'othering') – but many of the assumptions it conveyed continue to influence contemporary debates and reappear in the discussions around 'risk', 'risk factors' and 'at risk'. Then, as now, the emphasis in policy and public concern is on moral failure, poor socialisation, lack of self-control, deviant personality types and indulgence in unhealthy behaviours. Drink, drugs and tobacco play a role here as signifiers of outsider status and as a rationale for a division between the worthy and unworthy citizens. Thus, the 'dangerous classes' or the 'underclass' have been variously defined. But what they have in common is that they are 'framed' through social processes which include media, political and research action. They are, or risk becoming, socially marginalised through their failure to live up to the social 'ideal' or conform to the notion of 'good citizens'. As such, behaviours, common across non-marginalised as well as marginalised groups and across social classes, are more heavily sanctioned (informally and formally) when they are part of the lifestyles of disliked classes. In this way, 'scapegoating', where outsider groups are portrayed as enemies who can be blamed for our national social and economic ills, can pave the way for special control and management measures from extremes, such as birth control and eugenic measures, separation and imprisonment, to surveillance through policing or professional intervention in private life. As the chapters in this book illustrate, social responses and policy measures tend to impact unequally on those defined as 'dangerous classes'.

Throughout the centuries, certain spaces have become defined as dangerous both by virtue of the types of people who gather there and because the space itself is seen as inherently hazardous. However, as Nicholls and Berridge (Chapter 2) illustrate:

> Judgements made about the location of substance use – whether that be the pub, the home, the street, the 'drug consumption room', the workplace, or internally in the female womb – both reflect and construct social ideas about what is normal, pleasurable, acceptable, morally approved or beyond the pale.

Again, gender, race and class are potent elements contributing to how spaces are framed. In some eras, public houses were deemed dangerous for (respectable) women; at various times, locations such as coffee houses or 'opium dens' and areas populated by particular sections of the population – often immigrant communities – have been labelled as 'dangerous' spaces. Van Hout (Chapter 8) writes of Irish Travellers whose 'situation in societal spaces in halting sites, group housing schemes, and social housing areas' is seen as creating dangerous spaces and responded to with harassment from local communities. Some urban districts – inner cities, outer estates, ghettoes, 'city centres' – have been considered as 'no go' areas. In those spaces, norms may be challenged, authority relations may be contested and alternative forms of social control, such as street gangs, may fill a vacuum. These are the kinds of spaces where substances and substance users are seen to flourish. A striking research finding is of the displacement of danger – how the perception of danger or safety rests with the viewer. In other words, 'risk' is not a mere 'fact'; it is a social phenomenon and we need to ask why and how something, someone, some spaces are considered to be a risk (Boholm and Corvellec, 2011). Specific spaces may be designated as dangerous or safe, but this varies between insiders and outsiders – what is safe to an insider may be perceived as dangerous to an outsider and vice versa. For some groups, like the Roma women drug users discussed by Stengel (Chapter 6) and the 'queer adults' described by Sanders, Antin and Hunt (Chapter 11), the everyday world is a dangerous place and evokes the need to create safe spaces. As noted already, we see resistance emerging from those who have been marginalised, often with little visibility, as in the case of cannabis cultivation in the relative safety of the home (Potter and Klein, Chapter 12), sometimes in the intentional creation of 'safe spaces' by concerned professionals (Stengel, Chapter 6) or by groups themselves when they can muster a united front or have the resources to set up alternative spaces (Sanders, Antin and Hunt, Chapter 11).

The literature on framing, risk and danger is vast and the preceding sections merely touch on some of the theories, critiques and ideas most relevant to the chapters in this book. Hopefully, it is sufficient to stimulate further discussion.

The chapters

Historical accounts of how views on substance use and substance users have emerged and changed over time are provided in the following three chapters (Nicholls and Berridge, Chapter 2; Sato, Chapter 3; Hallam, Chapter 4). Drawing on examples from the UK and Japan, and from alcohol, drugs and tobacco, these chapters illustrate how concerns about substance use convey judgements about the substance itself – modified by perceptions of the gender, class, race or sexuality of the user – and also act as the vehicle for concern about broader social norms, values and behaviours. Taking examples from British history, Nicholls and Berridge analyse how the construction of alcohol, opiates and tobacco as social and public health 'problems' relates to the framing of *who* uses the substances and *where*. They argue that this framing then shapes the control mechanisms that come to be established in response. Therefore, if we wish to understand how the control of substances operates, and why it takes the forms it does, we need to think about the historical contexts that these mechanisms reflect. Sato examines the framing processes around the establishment and subsequent amendments from 1951 of Japan's *Stimulant Control Law*. His case study illustrates how some specific groups (at various times, celebrity performers, youth gangs and foreigners) were blamed for the perceived prevalence of methamphetamine and the perceived problems associated with its use. Hallam's chapter considers how drug using young celebrity women in London in the interwar period became the object of police surveillance and media hounding that brought them to the attention of the courts. Their drug use and lesbianism were seen to typify the problems of 'modernism' and the threat posed by a new and surprising 'dangerous class', inhabiting the dangerous spaces of nightclubs and doctor's surgeries.

The next two chapters (Thom, Herring and Milne, Chapter 5; Stengel, Chapter 6) pick up the gender theme. Thom, Herring and Milne consider risk communication concerning alcohol consumption by pregnant women. In particular, they look at how the evidence on risk is interpreted and communicated through advocacy and policy mediums and how the 'precautionary principle' has become dominant in public health messages to women. They note that moral frameworks and value judgements still underpin attitudes and approaches towards alcohol consumption in pregnancy and raise questions regarding female autonomy in relation to the rights of the foetus and the responsibility of the mother. Stengel gives an account of how practitioners in Hungary attempted to provide a safe space for Roma women who injected drugs and who also experienced danger through their precarious physical, emotional, financial and sociocultural conditions. The intersecting labels as 'the junkie Gypsy prostitute' meant that clients were constructed as a triple threat to mainstream Hungarian social and moral values. Located in a deprived area of Budapest, 'Chicks Day' provided weekly harm reduction services for these women until it was closed.

Ethnicity and race have also been a key element in linking substance use with perceptions of risk and danger; this is addressed in Chapter 7 (De Kock) and Chapter 8 (Van Hout). De Kock explores the complex ways in which Turkish drug users in Ghent experience their identities as 'Turkish' and 'Muslim' and the consequences of perceived negative framing in the Turkish community (because of drug use) and in society (i.e. as 'Turkish' or 'Muslim') on help seeking and drug treatment. The findings from her study indicate the importance of clients' own feelings of exclusion in their perceived ethnic community and in general society, the need to build trust to help clients disentangle what ethnic boundaries mean to them, what determines the construction of these boundaries and which other issues, in other life domains, are hindering their personal recovery. At the same time, it is important not to downscale the socio-economic causes that contribute to problem use in these populations. De Kock suggests that 'cultural traits' are often used to constitute a specific group of 'others'; this may prevent service providers challenging dominant treatment paradigms and locate the 'problem' in the culture of the client as risk factors. The second ethnic group is the Irish Traveller community. As Van Hout argues, historically they have been viewed as a 'dangerous class' within Irish society. Their limited interaction with settled people and inner community boundaries contributed to public prejudice of the *'itinerant way of life'* and the labelling of Travellers as criminals. However, while their traditional way of life offered some protection from the problems of illicit drug use and addiction, since the 1950s, strict assimilation policies by the Irish government have contributed to the erosion of Traveller cultural identity, values, norms and traditions with a resultant rise in harmful substance use. Drug exposure and activity, whether consumption or dealing, contribute to the renewed framing of the Traveller community as a *'dangerous class'* operating within contemporary criminal environments.

Chapters 9–12 focus on different marginal and negatively framed groups: the 'pathological poor'; prisoners; lesbian, gay, bisexual and transgender people; cultivators of cannabis.

MacGregor and O'Gorman (Chapter 9) discuss ways in which drug and alcohol use has been presented to construct an image of the 'pathological poor' and how these problematisations have influenced policy. It is argued that it is social status which determines how much people are demonised rather than their pattern of drug or alcohol use. In turn, such ideas, framing perceptions of and policies towards social groups, are set within overarching paradigms of social, economic and political arrangements. These have varied from welfare state, to malign or benign neoliberalism, to the currently rising populism. The chapter examines the role of the media and reviews: proposals for compulsory drug testing of recipients of social assistance in the UK, the United States and Australia; the category 'troubled families' and its place in policy shifts in the UK; the reframing of drug use from 'welfare queens' to the 'diseases of despair' in the United States.

In Chapter 10, Duke and Kolind look at prison contexts where drug problems are simultaneously framed as both problems of crime and control and problems of well-being and health, and prison populations involved in drugs are framed as both criminal and in need of treatment. These frames often compete, conflict and converge with each other, but in the prison space, conflicts and convergences within the drugs debate are intensified. The authors look at ways in which those imprisoned adapt and respond to these frames and how they frame and re-frame their involvement with drug use and supply in prisons.

The focus in Chapter 11 is on 'queer adults' (lesbian, gay, bisexual, transgender) and the ways that smoker-related stigma intersects with other forms of health-based stigma affecting bodies that, on the basis of non-heteronormative sexual and/or gender variance, have been historically constructed as pathological, risky and deviant within the dominant health establishment. Sanders, Antin and Hunt provide an account of how such negative framing has affected these groups and explore the implications and unintended consequences of a tobacco control policy environment that mobilises stigma to make smoking socially unacceptable. The chapter brings to the fore (as do other chapters) issues of control and the management of behaviour and highlights how control measures impact unequally on different social groups.

Potter and Klein (Chapter 12) discuss the proliferation of small-scale cannabis grow operations that now provide the bulk of the cannabis consumed in the UK. These home growers have to hide their growing and dealing operations and have developed various strategies to conceal their production from the police, neighbours, family and friends, competitor growers and criminal groups. The authors describe the discrepancy between the image conjured up by the idea of large-scale criminal supply and the banal reality of home-based, small-scale production. They record the justification growers give for their lifestyle choices, their suggestions for changes in the legislative framework for cannabis and the ways in which they reject the criminal framing of their activities.

In Chapter 13 (Uhl), we return to an issue that has relevance across the chapters and has important implications for policy responses to substance use. Drawing on examples from the alcohol field, Uhl considers how research approaches, methods and interpretation frame the evidence base that informs policy, noting, at the same time, that political interests and policy needs may determine what is researched and how it is researched. He argues that basic convictions related to specific worldviews shape the way facts are selected or omitted to frame lines of argumentation. Examination of the production and use of evidence around 'harm to others' from drinking and 'alcohol consumption while lactating' provides the basis for the critique of current research and for the contention that we need to strive for more meaningful research approaches and methods that allow problem areas to be described more precisely and a more detailed understanding of the mechanisms of problem genesis to be generated.

Finally, in the conclusion (Chapter 14), we discuss implications for policy and practice. The chapters in the collection demonstrate that policies change – none more striking than attitudes towards tobacco and more recent changes in policies on cannabis. The design and implementation of policies has been largely determined by the desire to control specific groups and behaviours in specific places, and in practice, sanctions have varied for different social groups. Policies involve the use of state power and questions thus arise about the legitimacy of the use of state power, especially when and where can and should the state intervene? Generally, this is justified in terms of concern for social order or public health. The conclusion pays particular attention to the development of public health approaches and most recently the use of the precautionary principle. This chapter develops the critique presented by Sunstein (2005) with its distinction between weak and strong versions and considers the implications for policies regarding substance use, continuing the discussion raised by Uhl (Chapter 13) of the balance between freedom and paternalism, especially with reference to the responsibilities of researchers.

References

Björneheda, E., and Erikson, J. 2018. Making the most of the frame: Developing the analytical potential of frame analysis. *Policy Studies* 39 (2), pp. 109–26.

Boholm, Å., and Corvellec, H. 2011. A relational theory of risk. *Journal of Risk Research* 14 (2), pp. 175–90.

Brown, C.E., and Wincup, E. 2019. Producing the vulnerable subject in English drug policy. *International Journal of Drug Policy* 13 (3), pp. 1–17.

Coomber, R., and Moyle, L. 2017. The changing shape of street-level heroin and crack supply in England: Commuting, holidaying and cuckooing drug dealers across 'County Lines'. *The British Journal of Criminology* 58 (6), pp. 1323–42.

Csete, J., Kamarulzaman, A., Kazatchkine, M., et al. 2016. Public health and international drug policy. *Lancet* 387 (10026), pp. 1427–80.

EMCDDA. 2018. *Medical Use of Cannabis and Cannabinoids. Questions and Answers for Policy Making.* Lisbon: European Monitoring Centre for Drugs and Drug Addiction.

Entman, R.M. 1993. Framing: Towards clarification of a fractured paradigm. *Journal of Communication* 43 (4), pp. 51–8.

Furedi, F. 2005. *Politics of Fear. Beyond Left and Right*. London: Continuum.

Gabe, J. (Ed.) 1995. *Medicine, Health and Risk*. Oxford: Blackwell, pp. 1–14.

Hailwood, M. 2015. *Alehouses and Good Fellowship in Early Modern England*. Woodbridge: Boydell and Brewer.

Jensen, S.Q. 2011. Othering, identity formation and agency. *Qualitative Studies* 2 (2), pp. 63–78.

Klein, A. 2008. *Drugs and the World*. London: Reaktion Books.

Lea, J. 1999. Social crime revisited. *Theoretical Criminology* 3 (3), pp. 307–25.

Lupton, D. 1993. Risk as moral danger: The social and political functions of risk discourse in public health. *International Journal of Health Services* 23 (3), pp. 425–35.

MacGregor, S. 2010. Alex Klein. Drugs and the world. Book review. *Social History of Alcohol and Drugs* 24 (1), pp. 62–3.

Morris, L. 1994. *Dangerous Classes. The Underclass and Social Citizenship*. London: Routledge.

Nutt, D., King, L.A., Saulsbury, W., et al. 2007. Development of a rational scale to assess the harm of drugs of potential misuse. *Lancet* 369, pp. 1047–53.

Rein, M., and Schön, D. 1991. Frame-reflective policy discourses. In: Wagner, P., Hirschon Weiss, C., Wittrock, B., and Wollman, H. (Eds.), *Social Sciences and Modern States*. Cambridge, NY: Cambridge University Press, ch. 12, pp. 262–89.

Rhem, J., Taylor, B., and Room, R. 2009. Global burden of disease from alcohol, drugs and tobacco *Drug and Alcohol Review* 25 (6), pp. 503–13.

Scheufele, D.A., and Iyengar, S. 2017. The state of framing research: A call for new directions. In: Kenski, K., and Hall Jamieson, K. (Eds.), *The Oxford Handbook of Political Communication*. Oxford: Oxford University Press, ch 43, pp. 619–32.

Solar, O., and Irwin, A. 2010. A conceptual framework for action on the social determinants of health. *Social Determinants of Health Discussion Paper 2 (Policy and Practice)*. Geneva: World Health Organisation.

Sunstein, C.R. 2005. *Laws of Fear: Beyond the Precautionary Principle*. Cambridge: Cambridge University Press.

Vliegenthart, R., and Van Zoonen, L. 2011. Power to the frame: Bringing sociology back to frame analysis. *European Journal of Communication* 26 (2), pp 101–15.

Wemrell, M., Merlo, J., Mulinari, S., and Hornborg, A.C. 2016. Contemporary epidemiology: A critical review of critical discussions within the discipline and a call for further dialogue with social theory. *Sociology Compass* 10 (2), pp. 153–71.

WHO. 2002. *The World Health Report. Reducing Risks, Promoting Healthy Life*. Geneva: World Health Organisation.

2 Substance use, dangerous classes and spaces

A historical perspective

James Nicholls and Virginia Berridge

Introduction

Public and political concerns about substance use are never simply about substances themselves or their specific intoxicating effects. They are always also about *who* takes (or is assumed to take) them, in what contexts and with what perceived impacts on social order, cohesion or control. They are also about *where* those substances are taken and what those spaces signify. Judgements made about the location of substance use – whether that be the pub, the home, the street, the 'drug consumption room', the workplace or internally in the female womb – both reflect and construct social ideas about what is normal, pleasurable, acceptable, morally approved or beyond the pale.

How such spaces are morally evaluated, and how this differs in regard to who is making the evaluation, are inevitably inflected by gender, race and class. As this chapter will demonstrate, for instance, the same spaces may be identified with very different risks and moral hazards depending on whether they are associated with, or utilised by, men or women. In many countries, for example, public drinking places have historically been, if not taboo to women, then certainly places that 'respectable' women avoided. Similarly, the health problems associated with, and the wider social implications of such issues, are often inextricable from gender – as will be shown in the following example of smoking in pregnancy.

What, and how, substances are consumed is also gendered. In Britain, for example, wine has been much more popular among (and heavily marketed to) female consumers since the expansion of the wine market in the 1960s (Purshouse et al., 2017). Meanwhile, beer (especially traditional cask ales) was conventionally viewed as a male drink – though this has changed markedly in recent years as the gender balance of beer-drinking has shifted and brewers have made sustained efforts to tap the female market (Thurnell-Read, 2015).

This chapter will look at how space, race, class and gender have intersected in the construction of 'danger' around substance use from a historical perspective and how, more recently, the concept of 'risk' has fulfilled similar functions. Focusing on the UK, it will show how public discourse on alcohol, tobacco or opium use often provides a mode for conversations about the boundaries of acceptable behaviour more broadly, and how that is articulated through the lens of *where* drinking, smoking or opium use took place: the public bar, the street, the home, the 'opium den' and so forth. Again, gender, race and class provide filters through which such spaces are understood. In other words, two processes are often in operation when substance use is the subject of public discourse: one is a series of judgements being made about the substance itself (and such judgements have tended to vary historically depending on the gender, race and class of the assumed 'user'); the other is a vicarious set of discussions about social norms, values, behaviours, etc. expressed via an ostensible debate on a particular substance. Intoxicants, then, can function as both the direct object of public concern and as the vehicle for the articulation of broader, underlying social values.

Alcohol and gender

It would be wrong to assume that drinking places have, until recently, been an exclusively male preserve. In early modern England, for example, women commonly frequented the alehouses that served the rural poor (Hailwood, 2014). Victorian court records reveal that women were often arrested for drunkenness in pubs (Jennings, 2012). Women also formed a large percentage of serving staff in nineteenth- and twentieth-century pubs (Beckingham, 2017). According to Langhamer (2003, p. 426), in the 1920s and 1930s, women made up 'anywhere between 12.5% and 41.5% of total pub attendance'. Nevertheless, women drinkers were always in the minority and subject to far more intense levels of moral judgement than men. Those judgements also applied differently depending on location. Hailwood (2014), for instance, notes a clear 'drinking double standard' in early modern England; one by which women's drunkenness was subject to far more severe moral, and legal, censure than men's. Describing the situation 400 years later, Wright and Chorniawry observed that women drinkers in Edwardian England faced a double jeopardy: 'If a woman went to a public house to drink, her respectability could be questioned. If she drank at home, she could be accused of secret drinking' (Wright and Chorniawry, 1985, p. 128). This double judgement remains a characteristic of recent media discourse on alcohol, in which public drinking by women is associated with sexual impropriety while drinking in the home is construed as evidence of furtive dependence (Emslie et al., 2016).

The maintenance of conventional gender relations, as distinct from the matter of policing sexual behaviour, was one of the many reasons that drinking places, particularly those frequented by the poor, became the object of intensive legislative action from the mid-sixteenth century onwards. In addition to concerns about political sedition and idleness among the poor (Clark, 1978; Wrightson, 1981; Warner, 1995), alehouses functioned as spaces in which conventional social boundaries (including gender and sexual relations) were blurred and loosened. That is, places that facilitated a 'carnivalesque' transgression of social, political and gender norms: something that has long been associated with drinking (see Roth, 1997; Hackley et al., 2013; Haydock, 2015, 2016). The development of licensing legislation in the early modern period can be understood as, in one aspect at least, the establishment of the boundaries within which 'carnival' would be tolerated and, perhaps, neutralised.

While alehouses provided the primary lens for regulatory action in the seventeenth century, increasing urbanisation and the sudden expansion of distillation as a production method dramatically shifted the focus of concern in the eighteenth century towards women and towards the street. The period in England from around 1720 to 1750 would later become popularly known as the 'Gin Craze' (Dillon, 2002; Warner, 2003). During this period, the consumption of distilled spirits boomed, especially in London, creating a wave of political anxiety over public drunkenness, morality and the long-term consequences for the economy. In just over 20 years, eight Acts of Parliament were passed, either introducing new controls or repealing ones that had failed – spectacularly, in some cases.

The period also saw the development of the first organised anti-alcohol campaigns in the modern West. Under the leadership of prominent clerics, medics, writers and politicians, successive efforts were made to lobby Government to introduce controls on spirits consumption, ranging from stricter licensing to outright prohibition (Nicholls, 2009). Anti-gin campaigners were largely members of the social and political elite, but they were concerned almost exclusively with alcohol consumption among the urban poor – and, in particular, poor women (Warner and Ivis, 2000; White, 2003).

In the newly emerging popular press, stories describing instances of drunken child neglect energised the developing anti-spirits campaigners, as did an apparent rise in child mortality (Dillon, 2002, pp. 95–7). Many of the leading anti-gin campaigners expressed particular anxiety about the impact of spirits on women. Henry Fielding, for example, echoed a common trope in asking how children 'conceived in gin' could become 'our future sailors and our future grenadiers' (Fielding, 1988, p. 90). That is to say, poor women's drinking was not simply a threat to the women involved but also to the economic prospects of the entire country insofar as it relied on their male children to provide both its workforce and military rank and file. The most famous image of this period, William Hogarth's 1751 engraving 'Gin Lane', captures the manner in which the problem was commonly framed. In depicting a drunken prostitute carelessly dropping a naked baby down a flight of steps, it illustrates the extent to which women's drinking was construed not only as poisoning maternal instincts but also as embodying wider social chaos.

Georgian anti-spirits campaigners were not, of course, exclusively concerned with women's drinking. Male drinkers were condemned as unproductive at work, violent or criminal in public, and financially irresponsible in the home. Women's drinking, by contrast, posed a series of narrower but potentially more catastrophic risks. In the private domain, so campaigners argued, it destroyed natural maternal instincts, leading to both child neglect and domestic conflict; in the public domain, not only was there a broad challenge to sexual morality, but also the risk to unborn (male) children was construed as a direct economic and political threat. Women, in this framing, were less the model for moral purity against which men were expected to measure themselves (as was more common in the nineteenth-century temperance literature), they were rather the producers of the male bodies that would ensure the productivity and military competence of the nation in the future.

The anti-spirits campaigns of eighteenth-century England prefigured the later temperance campaigns: they responded to shifts in the availability and afford-ability of alcohol; they dwelt especially on the behaviour of the poor and they constructed alcohol harms as varying by gender. However, where the Georgian anti-spirits movement was essentially an elite campaign, Victorian temperance quickly became a mass social movement. Where anti-spirits campaigners saw little harm in wine or beer, abstinence from *all* alcohol would come to dominate Victorian century temperance; and where poor women were the primary object of anti-gin campaigners' anxieties, in Victorian temperance, women were more often construed as the primary agents of change – whether as mothers, wives or daughters.

The Victorian temperance movement emerged independently of the Georgian anti-spirits campaigns, though there are some channels of influence such as the work of Benjamin Rush in America and Basil Montagu in Britain (Nicholls, 2011a). Temperance certainly began as a relatively elite anti-spirits campaign (Harrison, 1971). However, the adoption of temperance principles by working-class men, the radicalisation of those principles in the notion of total abstention from all alcohol and the leadership of idealistic campaigners such as Joseph Live-sey transformed temperance from a loosely organised attempt at the improvement of civility to a mass movement founded on a utopian notion of social reform (Gusfield, 1986; Nicholls, 2009; McAllister, 2014).

The front line of that battle, however, was not only occupied by the firebrand speakers and reformed drinkers who led the marches and published the volumi-nous newspapers and magazines dedicated to the cause. It was also, in the tem-perance imagination at least, held by the wives and daughters of those drinkers. Wives and daughters were often depicted as the primary victims of male drunken-ness, experiencing both violence and financial ruin as a consequence. However, they were also depicted as the most powerful catalyst for change – albeit often necessitating that transformation through their own suffering (Shiman, 1988; Berridge, 2005).

The trope of the neglected daughter, for example, was widespread in temper-ance literature (Reynolds and Rosenthal, 1997). Temperance narratives would commonly recount the catastrophic impact of a father's drinking on his daughter, often concluding in a tragedy which, too late for the child, would shock the father into reform. Wives often played a similar role. In William Cruikshank's famous series of temperance cartoons 'The Bottle' (1847), a father's drinking progres-sively drags his family from prosperity to poverty until, in an act of drunken violence, he kills his wife in front of their children and is committed to an asylum. In a later series, 'The Drunkard's Children' (1848), Cruikshank depicts a simi-lar course of domestic moral collapse, this time concluding in the suicide of the drinker's daughter by throwing herself from a bridge.

In the temperance imagination, then, drinking spaces were clearly demarcated by gender. In the public house, masculinity was both cheapened and exploited.

By contrast, in the (female) domestic sphere, the wider Victorian values of character, thrift, hard work and future-facing sacrifice were nurtured and inculcated. By personifying the domestic ideal, mother and daughter came to personify the temperance ideal.

Of course, temperance did not simply construct women as the idealised guarantors of moral purity. Like earlier anti-alcohol movements, it saw women's drinking as especially pernicious. Precisely because the (male) pub and the (female) home were set at odds, women who drank presented a double transgression: they both amplified the moral hazard of the pub and undermined the moral stability of the home. One of the few occasions on which temperance campaigners and leading brewers united was when William Gladstone attempted to liberalise alcohol licences for shops in 1860. For brewers, this was a direct threat to their control of the trade through 'tied' pubs; to temperance campaigners it widened the availability of alcohol – something they saw as directly associated with increased consumption. For both, the figure of the furtive female drinker provided the moral threat with which they opposed a change in the law. Both insisted that the introduction of a 'grocer's licence' would allow women easier access to alcohol and encourage more drinking in the home (Nicholls, 2011b).

A different, but striking, illustration of how gender shaped the Victorian moral policing of alcohol is found in the story of the 'inebriate asylums', which appeared in the late nineteenth century as a novel means to address 'habitual drunkenness' through an early form of mandated treatment (Brown, 1985). Inebriate asylums were first promoted by progressive medics seeking to redefine habitual drunkenness as a disease rather than a moral failing. As one leading proponent put it, the imprisonment of habitual drinkers was 'a deliberate injustice and inhumanity in . . . permitting a man to expose himself to the penalties of the law, when it has long been apparent that he has not the powers to govern his own will and reason' (Peddie, 1858, p. 15).

In Britain, inebriate asylums began as private institutions where inmates would voluntarily commit to treatment. However, new legislation in 1898 allowed for the development of state-run asylums and the commitment of offenders to treatment by the courts. Under this law, anyone whom the court deemed to be a 'habitual drunkard', or who was arrested four times for a drink-related offence, could be referred to an asylum for up to three years, whether willing or otherwise (Nicholls, 2009, pp. 164–6). However, while men were far more likely to drink, and get drunk, women were far more likely to be committed to reformatories than men – mostly either charged with child neglect or prostitution (Kelynack, 1904, pp. 123–7; Valverde, 1998, p. 77; Johnstone, 1996, p. 44). Not only, then, was women's drinking subject to more intense policing and moral condemnation but the policing of drunkenness also acted as a means to regulate women's behaviour more broadly.

Inebriate asylums began to fall into abeyance after World War I, at the same time as the influence of Victorian temperance began to wane in the political sphere. A dramatic fall in alcohol consumption across the population, economic hardship associated with the Great Depression and the gradual emergence of alternative leisure options, such as cinema, spectator sports and radio, eroded the intensity of public concern over drinking. At the same time, the necessary relaxation of social taboos on women's work and leisure that occurred during World War I increased the acceptability of women's drinking to some degree (Langhamer, 2003; Gutzke, 2013). By the 1940s, anthropological studies of pub culture were finding that up to a third of customers were women (Mass Observation, 1943).

Indeed, as pubs sought to attain greater 'respectability' in the early twentieth century, gender diversity became something of a feature of their marketing (Gutzke, 2006; Jennings, 2007). The 'traditional' pub (itself a Victorian invention) was characterised by snugs and booths – relatively isolated spaces which encouraged intimacy and by extension could facilitate otherwise illicit encounters between men and 'unrespectable' women. In the 1920s, as brewers sought to make pubs more attractive to affluent drinkers, 'improved pubs' began to appear, which featured much brighter, open spaces, table service and food. This was a deliberate attempt to make the pub a destination for respectable couples, even whole families, who would otherwise avoid the dark, smoky atmosphere of the more traditional 'local'.

Much later in the twentieth century, as both changing gender politics and opportunistic developments in the marketing of alcohol further normalised drinking across genders, interior design would again become a key feature in opening up public drinking to women. The 1980s fad for wine bars provided a successful 'proof of concept' for drinking spaces designed to contrast with the traditional pub, and in doing so demonstrated a large market for mixed-gender (and women-only) drinking (Barr, 1998). Subsequently, as themed bars became an increasingly common feature of the high street from the 1990s, pub companies used interior designs that consciously used light, space and open-plan seating to both attract more mixed clientele and to reduce levels of violence through both increasing the capacity for surveillance and reducing the number of 'pinch points' that research had demonstrated often triggered conflict (Hadfield, 2006, pp. 81–121).

The second half of the twentieth century witnessed a transformation, across British society, in how alcohol was consumed, where, by whom and in what quantities. In 1964, for example, wine consumption stood at around 3 L per person annually; by 2004, it was 22 L (British Beer and Pub Association, 2013). The enormous inflation in per capita consumption was to some extent driven by higher levels of consumption per person but also by an absolute increase in the amount of alcohol women drank, which drove a dramatic rise in wine sales especially (Purshouse et al., 2017).

As alcohol consumption reached a historical peak in the 1990s and early 2000s, women's drinking could be viewed as both a reflection of improved gender equality and very good for the alcohol industry – especially the wine sector. However, this shift also led to increased public and political concern over the impact of alcohol on society. Throughout the 2000s, led by a coalition of public health advocates and fuelled by a news media increasingly fascinated by images of drunken excess, alcohol rose up the political agenda (Plant and Plant, 2006; Nicholls, 2012). In doing so, old concerns about women's drinking began to re-emerge.

Content analysis of the UK media coverage showed not only that women appeared in the majority of images used for alcohol-related news stories, but also that those women were usually young, often in a state of apparent collapse in a public street, and either partially dressed or scantily clad (Mellows, 2012; Patterson et al., 2016). By contrast, images of men tended to involve public violence (Patterson et al., 2016). Analysis of court records also found that women were treated as 'doubly deviant' in cases of alcohol-related public disorder, routinely receiving harsher sentences than men for similar crimes (Lightowlers, 2018). Media concern over women's drinking in the home has also increased – often represented through the trope of 'wine o'clock' (e.g. Brennan, 2018). Hence, the growth of home drinking has become particularly associated with concerns about women's health and moral responsibility. Thus, in mainstream media reporting at least, the risks of drinking are routinely tied to underlying, and often unarticulated, positions on motherhood, sexual propriety and the 'dark side' of gender equality (e.g. Woods, 2018; Sperkova, 2018), despite the fact that women remain far less likely to either drink or get drunk than men, and that alcohol performs a complex array of social and psychological functions for both (Hutton et al., 2013; Lyons et al., 2014; Emslie et al., 2015, 2016; Scottish Health Action on Alcohol Problems, 2018)

The threat of women's drinking for unborn children also re-emerged in debates over the impact and prevalence of foetal alcohol spectrum disorder, shading in some cases towards calls for all women of child-bearing age to avoid alcohol in order to minimise risk (Brown and Trickey, 2017; British Pregnancy Advisory Service, 2017). In revising the official guidelines on risky drinking, the UK Chief Medical Officers opted to adopt the 'precautionary' recommendation that pregnant women should avoid alcohol altogether – despite evidence on the relationship between low levels of consumption and harm being far from conclusive (Department of Health, 2016). Hence, tabloid journalists and public health activists were often united in expressing concern that the increasing social acceptability of alcohol consumption by women pointed to a problem at the heart of improved gender equality.

Despite dramatic changes in gender relations, then, the broad structure of public debates on problematic alcohol consumption has remained remarkably consistent, with men's drinking primarily associated with public spaces and public disorder, while women face a 'double deviancy': association with sexual risk and promiscuity when drinking in public, furtive loss of control when drinking at home and irresponsibility towards future generations when drinking in either context.

Opiates: the role of race and the 'opium den'

Gender, class and race also underpinned early responses to the use of opiates. In particular, there were concerns about the impact of opium use by working-class mothers – whether their own use or their use of opium as a way of calming children while they were at work. The latter was seen as a concern especially where working mothers were absent, leaving their child to suffer 'ignorant nursing' in so-called baby farms. In a series of public lectures in the 1850s and 1860s, for example, the Manchester and Salford Sanitary Association pointed to the 'injurious influence of certain narcotics upon human life, both infant and adult'. Such concerns led to calls for regulation, which generally focused less on *where* opium might be consumed than on establishing professional regulation of the opiates and patent medicines that were much used by the poor. Some of this was eventually achieved in the *1868 Pharmacy Act*, although patent medicines were not regulated until the early twentieth century.

Race was also a key concern in the nineteenth-century process of gradual marginalisation of the opiates. The perceived association between opium use and supply and the Chinese community in the dockland areas of East London was a central image in anti-opium literature. The increasingly notorious 'opium den' in its literary presentation and in social commentary opened up powerful imagery, which later helped to drive regulation at the international level. Here is a depiction in the Sherlock Holmes adventure, *The Man with the Twisted Lip*, published in 1891:

> Through the gloom one could dimly catch a glimpse of bodies lying in strange fantastic poses, bowed shoulders, bent knees, heads thrown back and chins pointing upwards, with here and there a dark lack lustre eye turned upon the newcomer. Out of the black shadows there glimmered little red circles of light, now bright, now faint, as the burning poison waxed or waned in the bowls of the metal pipes. The most lay silent, but some muttered to themselves, and others talked together in a strange, low monotonous voice, their conversation coming in gushes, and then suddenly tailing off into silence, each mumbling out his own thoughts and paying little heed to the words of his neighbour.
>
> (Conan Doyle, 1892)

Such imagery was constantly repeated in the social investigations of the late nineteenth and early twentieth century. It was often accompanied by concern about the relationships between Chinese men and white women. This was in some respects part of a more general fashion, from the 1870s onwards, for investigating the lower depths of society – with the Chinese character of the opium den providing an orientalist twist. However, it was also tied to very real race politics, which came to a peak at the turn of the century. Race and drugs became a focus of unease within 'respectable' society at the threat of 'outcast London' and at how the housing crisis and overcrowding were bringing the poorer classes and the criminal classes together. The existence of a 'residuum' of chronically poor and unemployed people was seen by many social commentators as substantial and growing, poised to engulf civilised London (Stedman Jones, 1971). The fog-shrouded East End of London symbolised this fear, and opium smoking was part of it. Fear over opium became tied also to wider concerns about immigration in the late nineteenth century, primarily directed at Jewish immigration into East London but also encompassing the Chinese and their 'alien practices' (Berridge, 2013, pp. 77–95).

Race, space and class coalesced in anti-immigrant legislation in the early twentieth century, and the Chinese were subject to control via the regulation of spaces with which they were associated. In London, the political response saw the establishment of a licensing system for seamen's 'lodging houses'; and evidence of opium smoking could lead to withdrawal of such a licence. Oral history investigations have shown that the reality of the 'opium den' was far from the mythology. One old man living in Limehouse in East London had run errands for the Chinese seamen in the early 1900s and took a pragmatic view:

> In every house I have been in, there's been a bed or two. It was quite natural for the people that come in here and have their pipe, because they're laid off from the shipping and they have their pleasure time in the Causeway as long as their money lasts.
>
> (Cecil, quoted in Berridge, 1978)

Opium-smoking was, therefore, a real social phenomenon and, in parts of London at least, was particularly prevalent among some migrant communities. However, the amplification of anxieties about the link between drugs and immigration, especially when achieved through raising the fear of the sexual exploitation of white women by non-white men, served a wider political purpose: both to demonise immigrant communities and to raise pressure for the prohibition of the substances with which they were associated. Similar dynamics underpinned hostile responses to the 'opium den' in the United States (Ahmad, 2007). Although opium smoking was never a mainstream activity in these societies, the stoking of racially oriented anxieties became a critical component of legislative responses to drug use, particularly in the United States. The widespread imagery of degenerate Chinese infecting respectable, white society by encouraging the adoption of opium use by upper- and middle-class visitors, or through sexual relationships with white women, helped to raise concern about the role of the Chinese and opium smoking, which ultimately fed into the moves towards international control of drugs prior to and after World War I.

The racial politics of drugs remained an important dynamic in the US prohibitionist response down the years, although less so in the UK. Indeed, the long-standing liberal response to drugs of the British medical profession established both before and after the Rolleston Report in the 1920s owed much to the fact that their clientele was primarily middle class. The so-called British System was not merely a reflection of different clinical assessments of potential drug harms but a very different construction of the role of race and class in both use and social consequences. Working-class consumption, for example, the use of the patent medicine chlorodyne, mostly fell under the radar by the 1920s and was excluded from consideration by the Rolleston Committee. The belief in continued maintenance on opiate drugs was largely founded on the unthreatening nature of the consumers and their adherence to dominant respectable social norms (Berridge, 1999).

Smoking and the rise of 'risk groups'

Smoking and tobacco emerged as a political concern later than drugs and alcohol, and not substantially until after the groundbreaking epidemiological work of Hill and Doll in the UK and Wynder and Graham in the United States demonstrated the links between smoking and lung cancer. Anti-smoking campaigns epitomised a new style of public health: away from the environmentalism, the focus on drains, sewage and housing of the nineteenth century, towards a focus on the modification of individual behaviour and what became known as 'lifestyle' diseases. Central to this new version of public health was the science of risk factor epidemiology and the notion of long-term risk and 'risk groups'. Nevertheless, although the language of public health was different, some familiar patterns of concern began to emerge which replicated and developed the nineteenth-century concerns around class and gender. In 1962, when the first Royal College of Physicians (RCP) report on smoking was published, smoking was ubiquitous in all classes of society; however, the main area of public and scientific concern was working-class smokers and their children. In 1962, Penguin published a special paperback called *Commonsense about Smoking* in tandem with the Royal College of Physicians' first report on smoking. Its cover image featured a group of wizened working-class child smokers, epitomising the enduring concerns of the time about transmission of the habit within the working class despite the fact that smoking was a widespread activity and the focus at that stage was still to stop and prevent its spread in the population as a whole.

But this focus changed as the new style of public health consolidated. The new model involved advocating for fiscal interventions at the population level (chiefly higher duties and taxation), campaigns for behaviour modification and both the regulation of advertising and its use as a tool for inculcating behavioural norms. Mass media advertising became a key site, and target, of the new public health advocacy. The strategy was a twin one: advertising was to be regulated so that tobacco was not visible – as with control of advertising on television in the 1960s – while, in contrast, it was to be used so that public health messages and persuasion would be visible through posters and national campaigns, often on television. In Britain, the Cohen Committee of 1964 carried through a new centralised and technocratic agenda for health education, which began to make greater use of the techniques of mass persuasion. A central health education agency, the Health Education Council (HEC), was set up and government began to use advertising agencies for key campaigns.

The new style of behavioural public health brought the role of women to the fore. But the framing of the issue owed much to the nineteenth-century public health trope of the culpability of women as mothers. This role was key to one of those early mass campaigns, created in 1973 by the HEC. A powerful image of a naked pregnant woman smoking was the main image in a campaign which took up nearly two-thirds of the HEC's anti-smoking budget for the year. The Council's main preparatory work for the campaign had been based on a clothed model, but the director of the Council later explained that the nude version emerged out of a conversation he had had with his chief medical officer: 'I can remember thinking in a crude way what a tremendous topic this was for public relations work'. Nevertheless, the at-risk foetus was definitely male. The text of the advertisement referred to a male baby-to-be and the press release for the campaign also made it clear that the concern was for a male baby. Echoing the concerns of anti-gin campaigners two centuries earlier, the campaign framed women in their reproductive role as a classic 'vector of infection' (Berridge, 2007). In the 1970s, the mothers whose role was criticised fought back. A research project led by the sociologist Hilary Graham captured the hostility of working-class mothers who felt they were stigmatised by the campaign. Their opposition was based on a different view of 'the evidence', and it was a view which based decision-making on family needs (Graham, 1987). Noticeably, public space did not figure in this campaign. Women were using cigarettes in a way which affected the unborn foetus, so the affected space was the interior of their own bodies, made visible also through the advent of foetal monitoring technology at that time.

Public health at this stage had dropped the environmentalism of the nineteenth century, but that was to change by the 1980s. Public and domestic space came more centrally onto the agenda, driven by a newer style of epidemiology but also by concerns that the public health agenda of the 1970s had stalled and new directions were needed for anti-smoking campaigns. Environmentalism revived in the 1970s through issues such as car transport and lead in petrol but smoking itself had only a weak environmental dimension. Although the RCP reports had always mentioned the pollution of the environment by smoking, little had been done about it. The pressure group, the National Society of Non-Smokers (NSNS), were concerned about the environmental impact of smoking but argued on moral grounds that this was a selfish habit. Initiatives such as the Order of Fridayites whose members took a pledge to abstain from smoking on one day a week gave the environmentalist case against smoking a fusty temperance tinge.

What changed the situation? Firstly, the public health case against smoking began to harden in the 1970s. Secondly, smoking became increasingly stratified by class: middle-class smokers were giving up in larger numbers while working-class smokers were more likely to continue. For anti-tobacco campaigners, smokers were in the process of becoming 'the other' rather than a mainstream cultural phenomenon. Smoking as a 'waste of working-class life' was widespread terminology among the emergent public health discipline of health economics. The claim that smoking led to a pollution of public space was more actively pursued. Initially, the 'selfish' moral argument of the NSNS was redefined as a rights-based stance, in which the rights of the non-smoker were put at risk by public smoking. However, the argument that smoke was a public inconvenience only carried limited weight in a culture where public smoking remained firmly embedded as a social norm.

Scientific research, however, was starting to focus on the impact of 'passive smoking' on health and, by the early 1980s, began to provide an altogether more compelling environmental justification for restrictions on the rights of smokers.

In 1981, papers by the Japanese epidemiologist Hirayama and others, published in the *British Medical Journal*, showed that the non-smoking wives of heavy smokers had a much higher risk of lung cancer. This scientific fact quickly acquired considerable policy salience, and the reality of passive smoking soon became accepted in policy documents in the United States and in Britain. The risk to the unborn child, which had featured in the advertising campaigns of the 1970s, also re-emerged through the prism of science. The previously invisible 'passive smoker' came into view and the 'innocent victim' of smoking became the driver of policy – facilitating arguments for the restriction of liberties among a section of the population (smokers) in pursuit of the greater social good. As this shift occurred, women, who had been 'victims' in the early passive smoking research, were once again framed as the vectors of infection within the family through their own smoking. The science of passive smoking, although controversial and not seen as central by some leading epidemiologists, nevertheless had policy significance in justifying the stringent regulation of public spaces – as far as smoking was concerned – which came into law in England (following Ireland and Scotland) in the early twenty-first century.

Concluding remarks

The history of attitudes towards substance use, and the regulation of substances, is never just about the substances in themselves. Drugs, in all their forms, provide a focus for the panoply of social attitudes, anxieties and beliefs around which their use occurs. These concerns also tend to be articulated through an emphasis on *where* the substances are consumed, and what these spaces signify in terms of gender, class and race, as much as their specific psychoactive effects. It is striking how durable some of the emergent patterns of thought and representation are, although framed within different variants of public health, from the 'dangerous classes' of the nineteenth century to the 'risk groups' of post–World War II society. Substance use by women, for instance, is framed repeatedly as creating risks to wider society through the impact on unborn children; the consumption of substances in public spaces is associated with both sexual risk and a threat to sexual propriety; substance use in private, however, is similarly condemned as furtive, pointing towards dependence or moral weakness.

Similarly, moral and public health concerns over the effect of substance use invariably fall more heavily on the poor and the proposed solutions often impact most heavily on the poorest communities. One change in the post-war years has been the greater reference to science as justification for these long-standing concerns. Initially this was through risk factor epidemiology and the concept of the 'risk group'. But as time has passed, other variants of science have developed, most notably health economics. Recently, for example, 'minimum unit pricing' has become a flagship policy idea, gaining almost universal support among alcohol health advocates; however, it unavoidably impacts disproportionately on poorer drinkers. The justification often given is that this is ethical because, on average, less affluent communities experience higher rates of alcohol harm – despite drinking less in general (e.g. Holmes et al., 2014). This perspective, in which the poor are treated as a social block rather than a collection of individuals, and in which their best interests are defined on their behalf by moral and medical elites, is in keeping with the work of moral reformers going back centuries.

Although race has only been touched on briefly here, there is no doubt that the construction of drug consumption as a racial issue played a critical role in the establishment of drug prohibition in the early twentieth century, and its continuation as a global policy decades after alcohol prohibition was largely abandoned (Hari, 2015). Constructing psychoactive substances as inherently dangerous, and asserting that they make social groups who are already framed as a threat even more dangerous, achieves a reciprocal effect: it justifies state action to control both drug users and the 'dangerous classes' who have come to be associated with those drugs (whether fairly or not).

This chapter has only set out this case in the broadest sense. Its key purpose is less to provide a detailed investigation of the examples discussed than to establish the principle that any critical analysis of substance use control – whether smoking bans, alcohol licensing or drug prohibition – needs to start from the principle that such actions are only motivated in part by an understanding of, or concern for, the specific effects of the substance at hand. More generally, they will reflect how attitudes to that substance among powerful social groups (the media, the medical profession, the police, etc.) are inflected by, and express, wider attitudes about who needs to be controlled, how and where. That the subjects of such control are more often women, the poor and minority communities is not a surprise; but the extent to which this defines both the analysis of and the response to the 'problem' of substance use should not be underestimated.

References

Ahmad, D.L. 2007. *The Opium Debate and Chinese Exclusion Laws in the Nineteenth-century American West*. Reno and Las Vegas: University of Nevada Press.

Barr, A. 1998. *Drink: A Social History*. London: Pimlico.

Beckingham, D. 2017. Banning the barmaid: Time, space and alcohol licensing in 1900s Glasgow. *Social and Cultural Geography* 18 (2), pp. 117–36.

Berridge, V. 1978. East end opium dens and narcotic use in Britain. *London Journal* 4 (1), pp. 3–28 interview with Mr Cecil by author.

Berridge, V. 1999. *Opium and the People. Opiate Use and Drug Control Policy in Nineteenth and Early Twentieth Century*. England and London: Free Association Books Expanded Edition.

Berridge, V. 2005. *Temperance: Its History and Impact on Current and Future Alcohol Policy*. York: Joseph Rowntree Foundation.

Berridge, V. 2007. *Marketing Health. Smoking and the Discourse of Public Health in Britain, 1945–2000*. Oxford: Oxford University Press.

Berridge, V. 2013. *Demons. Our Changing Attitudes to Alcohol, Tobacco and Drugs*. Oxford: Oxford University Press.

Brennan, S. 2018. Mother who downed a bottle of red a night reveals how quitting has made her happier and boosted her libido and warns that the 'wine o'clock' is a hidden epidemic among mums. *Daily Mail*. Available at: www.dailymail.co.uk/femail/article-5783125/Mother-reveals-wine-o-clock-ruined-life.html (Accessed September 15, 2018).

British Beer and Pub Association. 2013. *Statistical Handbook, 2013*. London: BBPA.

British Pregnancy Advisory Service. 2017. *Alcohol in Pregnancy: What are the Issues?* Available at: www.bpas.org/get-involved/campaigns/briefings/alcohol-in-pregnancy/ (Accessed December 18, 2018).

Brown, C., and Trickey, H. 2017. Communicating public health alcohol guidance for expectant mothers: A scoping report. *Alcohol Change UK*. Available at: https://alcoholchange.org.uk/publication/communicating-public-health-alcohol-guidance-for-expectant-mothers-a-scoping-report-1 (Accessed December 18, 2018).

Brown, E.M. 1985. 'What shall we do with the inebriate?' Asylum treatment and the disease concept of alcoholism in the late nineteenth century. *The History of the Behavioural Sciences* 21 (1), pp. 48–59.

Clark, P. 1978. Alehouses and alternative society. In: Pennington, D., and Thomas, K. (Eds.), *Puritans and Revolutionaries: Essays in Seventeenth-Century History*. Oxford: Clarendon.

Conan Doyle, A. 1892. *The Man with the Twisted Lip in the Adventures of Sherlock Holmes*. London: George Newnes, originally published in the Strand Magazine, 1891.

Cruikshank, G. 1847. *The Bottle*. London: David Bogue.

Cruikshank, G. 1848. *Drunkard's Children*. London: David Bogue.

Department of Health. 2016. *How to Keep Health Risks from Drinking Alcohol to a Low Level: Government Response to the Public Consultation*. Available at: https://assets.publishing.service.gov.uk/government/uploads/system/uploads/attachment_data/file/545911/GovResponse2.pdf (Accessed December 12, 2018).

Dillon, P. 2002. *The Much-Lamented Death of Madam Geneva: The Eighteenth-Century Gin Craze*. London: Review.

Emslie, C., Hunt, K., and Lyons, A. 2015. Transformation and time-out: The role of alcohol in identity construction among Scottish women in early mid-life. *International Journal of Drug Policy* 26 (5), pp. 437–45.

Emslie, C., Patterson, C., and Hilton, S. 2016. When media use pictures of drunk girls in alcohol stories we are being misled. *The Conversation*. Available at: https://theconversation.com/when-media-use-pictures-of-drunk-girls-in-alcohol-stories-were-being-misled-70714 (Accessed September 15, 2018).

Fielding, H. 1988. *An Enquiry into the Causes of the Late Increase of Robbers and Related Writings*. Oxford: Clarendon Press.

Graham, H. 1987. Women's' smoking and family health. *Social Science and Medicine* (25), pp. 47–56.

Gusfield, J. 1986. *Symbolic Crusade: Status Politics and the American Temperance Movement*. Chicago: University of Illinois Press.

Gutzke, D. 2006. *Pubs and Progressives: Reinventing the Public House in England, 1896–1960*. Dekalb: Northern Illinois University Press.

Gutzke, D. 2013. *Women Drinking Out in Britain Since the Early Twentieth Century*. Manchester: Manchester University Press.

Hackley, C., Bengry-Howell, A., Griffin, C., et al. 2013. Young adults and 'binge drinking': A Bakhtinian analysis. *Journal of Marketing Management* 29, pp. 933–49.

Hadfield, P. 2006. *Bar Wars: Contesting the Night in Contemporary British Cities*. Oxford: Oxford University Press.

Hailwood, M. 2014. *Alehouses and Good Fellowship in Early Modern England*. Woodbridge: Boydell Press.

Hari, J. 2015. *Chasing the Scream: The First and Last Days of the Drug War*. London: Bloomsbury.

Harrison, B. 1971. *Drink and the Victorians: The Temperance Question in England 1815–1872*. London: Faber and Faber.

Haydock, W. 2015. Understanding English alcohol policy as a neoliberal condemnation of the carnivalesque. *Drugs: Education, Prevention and Policy* 22 (2), pp. 143–9.

Haydock, W. 2016. The consumption, production and regulation of alcohol in the UK: The relevance and ambivalence of the carnivalesque. *Sociology* 50 (6), pp. 1056–71.

Holmes, J., Meng, Y., and Meier, P.S., et al. 2014. Effects of minimum unit pricing for alcohol on different income and socioeconomic groups: A modelling study. *Lancet* 383 (9929), pp. 1655–64.

Hutton, F., Wright, S., and Saunders, E. 2013. Cultures of intoxication: Young women, alcohol and harm reduction. *Contemporary Drug Problems* 40, pp. 451–80.

Jennings, P. 2007. *The Local: A History of the English Pub*. Stroud: History Press.

Jennings, P. 2012. Policing drunkenness in England and Wales from the late eighteenth century to the First World War. *Social History of Alcohol and Drugs* 26 (1), pp. 69–92.

Johnstone, G. 1996. From vice to disease? The concepts of dipsomania and inebriety, 1860–1900. *Social and Legal Studies* 5 (1), pp. 37–56.

Kelynack, T.N. 1904. Medico-legal aspects of inebriet. *The British Journal for the Study of Inebriety* 2 (1), pp. 117–29.

Langhamer, C. 2003. 'A public house is for all classes, men and women alike': Women, leisure and drink in Second World War England. *Women's History Review* 12 (3), pp. 423–43.

Lightowlers, C. 2018. Drunk and doubly deviant? The role of gender and intoxication in sentencing assault offences. *British Journal of Criminology* 59 (3), pp. 693–717.

Lyons, A., Emslie, C., and Hunt, K. 2014. Staying 'in the zone' but not passing the 'point of no return': Embodiment, gender and drinking in mid-life. *Sociology of Health and Illness* 36 (2), pp. 264–77.

Mass-Observation. 1943. *The Pub and the People: A Worktown Study*. London: Victor Gollancz.

McAllister, A.M. 2014. *Demon Drink: Temperance and the Working Class*. London: Amazon e-book.

Mellows, P. 2012. Widdecombe, bench girl and fear of the hoyden. *Morning Advertiser*. Available at: www.morningadvertiser.co.uk/Article/2012/04/30/Widdecombe-Bench-Girl-and-the-fear-of-the-hoyden (Accessed November 18, 2018).

Nicholls, J. 2009. *The Politics of Alcohol: A History of the Drink Question in England*. Manchester: Manchester University Press.

Nicholls, J. 2011a. On the origins and progress of temperance: Basil Montagu's some inquiries into the effects of fermented liquors (1814) in context. *Social History of Alcohol and Drugs* 25, pp. 15–25.

Nicholls, J. 2011b. Wine, supermarkets and alcohol policy. *History and Policy*. Available at: www.historyandpolicy.org/policy-papers/papers/wine-supermarkets-and-alcohol-policy.

Nicholls, J. 2012. Time for reform? Alcohol policy and cultural change in England since 2000. *British Politics* 7 (3), pp. 250–71.

Patterson, C., Emslie, C., Mason, O., Fergie, G., and Hilton, S. 2016. A content analysis of UK newspaper and online news representations of women's and men's 'binge' drinking: A challenge for communicating evidence-based messages about single-episodic drinking? *BMJ Open* (6), p. e013124. doi:10.1136/bmjopen-2016-013124.

Peddie, A. 1858. *The Necessity for Some Legislative Arrangements for the Treatment of Dipsomania, or the Drinking Insanity*. Edinburgh: Sutherland and Knox.

Plant, M., and Plant, M. 2006. *Binge Britain: Alcohol and the National Response*. Oxford: Oxford University Press.

Purshouse, R.C., Brennan, A., Moyo, D., Nicholls, J., and Norman, P. 2017. Typology and dynamics of heavier drinking styles in Great Britain, 1978–2010. *Alcohol and Alcoholism* 52 (3), pp. 372–81.

Reynolds, D., and Rosenthal, D. 1997. *The Serpent in the Cup: Temperance in American Literature*. Amherst: University of Massachusetts Press.

Roth, M. 1997. Carnival, creativity and the sublimation of drunkenness. *Mosaic* 30 (2), pp. 1–18.

Scottish Health Action on Alcohol Problems. 2018. *Women and Alcohol: Key Issues*. Available at: www.ias.org.uk/uploads/pdf/IAS%20reports/rp29032018.pdf (Accessed December 10, 2018).

Shiman, L.L. 1988. *Crusade Against Drink in Victorian England*. Abingdon: Palgrave Macmillan.

Sperkova, K. 2018. Time's up for big alcohol exploiting feminism. *IOGT*. Available at: http://iogt.org/blog/2018/03/07/times-big-alcohol-exploiting-feminism/ (Accessed December 10, 2018).

Stedman Jones, G. 1971. *Outcast London. A Study in the Relationship Between Classes in Victorian Society*. Oxford: Oxford University Press.

Thurnell-Read, T. 2015. Beer and belonging, real ale consumption, place and identity. In: Thurnell-Read, T. (Ed.), *Drinking Dilemmas: Space, Culture and Identity*. Abingdon: Routledge, pp. 45–61.

Valverde, M. 1998. *Disease of the Will: Alcohol and the Dilemmas of Freedom*. Cambridge: Cambridge University Press.

Warner, J. 1995. Good help is hard to find: A few comments about alcohol and work in preindustrial England. *Addiction Research* 2 (3), pp. 259–69.

Warner, J. 2003. *Craze: Gin and Debauchery in the Age of Reason*. London: Profile.

Warner, J., and Ivis, F. 2000. Gin and gender in early eighteenth-century London. *Eighteenth-Century Life* 24 (2), pp. 85–105.

White, J. 2003. The 'slow but sure poison': The representation of gin and its drinkers, 1736–51. *Journal of British Studies* 42 (1), pp. 35–64.

Woods, J. 2018. Wine o-clock has damaged an entire generation of women. *Daily Telegraph*. Available at: www.telegraph.co.uk/women/life/wine-oclock-has-damaged-entire-generation-women/ (Accessed December 10, 2018).

Wright, D., and Chorniawry, C. 1985. Women and drink in Edwardian England. *Historical Papers* 117 (310), pp. 117–31.

Wrightson, K. 1981. Alehouses, order and reformation in rural England 1590–1660. In: Yeo, E., and Yeo, S. (Eds.), *Popular Culture and Class Conflict 1590–1914*. Sussex: Harvester.

3 Methamphetamine users and the process of condemnation in Japan

Framing and influence

Akihiko Sato

Introduction

Methamphetamine, known as 'ice' and 'crystal' on the streets of Western countries, was discovered in Japan in 1888 (Nagai, 1893). It is categorised as an amphetamine-type stimulant (ATS). Japan was one of a first few countries to establish a law to control ATS. The *Stimulant Control Law* in Japan was passed in 1951 and has been amended more than 20 times since then.

The dominant story on methamphetamine today

Official documents and researchers who discuss the establishment of the *Stimulant Control Law* still refer back to the story regarding the spread of stimulants which led to the passing of this law. Japan had a recognisable methamphetamine problem soon after World War II as post-war problems led many people to use stimulants as a way to relieve their mental stress. This increased the prevalence of stimulant addiction and psychosis leading to the establishment of the law. This story is often referred to in relation to some statistical data depicting the numbers of arrests for violating the law since 1951 (Figure 3.1).

However, as discussed previously by the author, the aforementioned story has been constructed from a retrospective point of view (Sato, 2006, 2009) and is often misunderstood. It can be called a 'post-1954 framing' and its effect will be discussed later. When the processes of the establishment and amendment of this law are traced systematically, it becomes apparent that some other stories did exist in post-war Japanese society. Those fragments of stories were searched for, identified and collected in this chapter to describe a different picture of drug scenes in Japan after the war.[1] The discourses that contributed to constructing such framing will come to light. Subsequently, it will be revealed that some social and even political factors, especially condemnation of specific groups of people, played important roles in the process of the establishment and amendment of the law in Japan in the 1950s.

Framing and framework

Before describing the processes, the concepts of framing and framework are discussed briefly. The idea of framing became more popular following Entman's

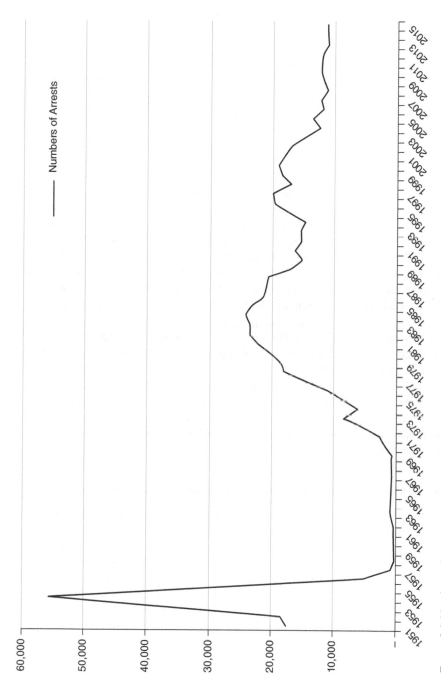

Figure 3.1 Numbers of arrests for violations

Source: Ministry of Justice 2016.

discussion of its importance in communication research. He defined framing as follows:

> To frame is to select some aspects of a perceived reality and make them more salient in a communicating text, in such a way as to promote a particular problem definition, causal interpretation, moral evaluation, and/or treatment recommendation for the item described.
>
> (Entman, 1993, p. 52)

His definition seemed to emphasise the aspect of salience.

In the field of sociology, frame and framework have been key concepts in the analysis of interaction. Goffman successfully introduced the concepts of frame and framework to help understand how the situated order is constructed through interactions. He used Bateson's term 'frame' and defined it, noting, 'I assume that definitions of a situation are build up in accordance with principles of organisation which govern events – at least social ones – and our subjective involvement in them' (Goffman, 1974, pp. 10–11). The key point is how the meaning of talk and behaviour arise. Meaning is not determined intrinsically but requires the process of social framing (Goffman, 1974, p. 22). Social frameworks provide the context of the situation within which people can define what goes on in that situation. However, social frameworks are not always single but sometimes multiple. He pointed out, 'during any moment of activity an individual is likely to apply several frameworks' (Goffman, 1974, p. 25). Viegenthart and van Zoonen (2011, p. 103) also pointed out that, 'this notion of multiple and intersecting frames' is crucial when analysing social phenomena. It means that several framing processes with suitable discursive resources might be ready for use in every situation. Such aspects of framing are worth noting when describing the process of stigmatisation of methamphetamine use.

Post-war drug use in Japan and the beginning of control

ATS, that is methamphetamine and amphetamine, have been available for commercial use in Japan since 1941 during the beginning of the Pacific War. The number of patented drugs containing ATS in the 1940s in Japan was 24. That included Hospitan (methamphetamine), Philopon (methamphetamine), Zedrin (amphetamine), etc. (Ikuta, 1951). Philopon was one of the most famous and popular ATS and its name was synonymous with ATS until the 1970s. The list of patented ATS in the 1940s showed that methamphetamine was more popular than amphetamine (Sato, 2009, p. 721). During wartime, ATS was used even by the Imperial Japanese Armed Forces.

Post-war ATS use and its control

After the war, the Armed Forces' stockpiles of those drugs were dispersed through multiple channels. These are impossible to trace today. However, elderly veterans once admitted to the author that they collected the drugs from the Armed Forces and took them back home after the war. Those drugs were used to stay awake for studying throughout the night (Sato, 2009, pp. 720–1). Some other contemporary documents also suggested that many people recognised that ATS was useful for their work and study in the period when provisions were scarce in the city. One such example can be found in the minutes of the National Diet as follows.

In March 1949, the Ministry of Health and Welfare revealed it had designated ATS as a powerful drug. This meant that ATS was strictly controlled with imposed sales restriction (Asahi Shinbun, 1949, March 29). A powerful drug could not be purchased by any person below 14 years of age and could not be bought without a prescription. In the autumn of 1949, the Ministry also issued administrative guidelines (i.e. order without legal basis) and regulations to every pharmaceutical company to refrain from the production of ATS. Both measures were enforced on the basis that some users, such as novelists, performers and students, were abusing ATS (Ikuta, 1951; National Diet, 1950, December 5).

However, one representative of the Diet called such administrative measures into question on November 24, 1949. He claimed,

> I have some questions about the Philopon problem. The Ministry of Health and Welfare, in the name of the permanent undersecretary asked every pharmaceutical company not to produce or reduce the amount of production of Philopon and other stimulants. However, the general working public and the industry have been suffering from such measures. According to medical and pharmaceutical points of view, the stimulants represented by Philopon are excellent drugs.
>
> (National Diet, 1949, November 24 p. 1116)

He added that the problems associated with Philopon were confined to small groups of users and that it would be better to enforce strict control over those abusers rather than controlling the entire population.

These comments indicated that people in the late 1940s still talked about the positive actions of ATS even after it was claimed to be dangerous or problematic. Additionally and importantly, the problems associated with ATS were attributed not to the drug and its effect but to the specific groups or persons who used it. It could be called the first stage of a framing process of stigmatisation of ATS use in Japan.

Drug use and some conspicuous deaths

Now the question arises why novelists, performers and even students were accused of abusing such a drug when the 'general working public' also used the same drug. This was the crucial point regarding the control of ATS at the first stage after the war.

One of the reasons behind adopting these measures by the Ministry could be found ahead of the designation of a powerful drug status and the establishment of guidelines for ATS production in 1949. Two conspicuous deaths of celebrities entered the limelight. On October 14, 1946, a famous comedienne, Miss Wakana, died of a heart attack on the platform of Nishinomiya Kitaguchi station near Osaka. Her death was attributed to Philopon as she was known to use it regularly. On December 4, 1947, a popular novelist, Sakunosuke Oda, was admitted into hospital with expectoration of blood. He died the following month on January 10, 1948. He was also well known for using Philopon and so many people thought that he died because of it.

After Miss Wakana's death, the very first medical paper that claimed there was a problem of ATS after the war in Japan was presented at a conference on internal medicine in 1947. It mentioned just one case related to acute intoxication from methamphetamine. Following that, the attendees of the conference insisted on the need for control of ATS by medical doctors, referring to Miss Wakana's death and ATS abuse by different performers (Nakazaki and Mori, 1947; Iwata, 1947; Horimi, 1947). These comments suggest that ATS abuse by specific users was thought to be problematic after these two conspicuous deaths.

Drug abuse and moral judgements

The remarks in the Diet suggested that many people other than novelists and performers used ATS even after those two deaths. These facts do not comprehensively cover the reason why novelists and performers drew people's attention to drug use.

One of the comments by Shigeo Iwata at the aforementioned conference suggested one such reason behind it. He pointed out that ATS was used by performers and added that junior high-school students frequently used the drug during examinations, but they were unable to concentrate on studying because they often needed to urinate. Using such a drug is suitable for workers who do not need to behave responsibly when working, but unsuitable for workers who need to work conscientiously (Iwata, 1947, p. 99). He suggested that many of the users like performers were working irresponsibly and their consciences were numbed.

Other discourses around this period help to understand the reason why such people, especially post-war novelists, were accused of abusing ATS. Those novelists who were known to use ATS in public were categorised as novelists of the 'après-guerre' (post-war) generation. Sakunosuke Oda, as mentioned, was one of the representatives of this generation. They were very famous and popular at that time when common means of amusement were scarce, except for novels and performances.

One example of such discourses can be found in an essay written in 1949 by a famous poet, Imao Hirano. He accused the novelists of the après-guerre generation as 'good-for-nothing and antisocial' and even described them as 'non-productive, unhealthy, being like petty bourgeois, passive, nihilistic, being like Kamikaze, regressive' (Hirano, 1949, p. 69). Interestingly, the word Kamikaze can be found in his writings. He also claimed that ATS was the drug that the Imperial Japanese Armed Forces used to make young people engage in Kamikaze attacks. It means that using ATS sometimes functioned as a symbol of the darkness of wartime at this time. Novelists and performers who used ATS were framed as immoral people who tend to re-enact such wartime darkness.

On the other hand, one representative medical review article on ATS in 1950 suggested that healthy office workers could use it without becoming addicted. This was because the reason for their drug use was not due to any internal craving but just because of a superficial reason, such as that they had to finish loads of work (Kasamatsu and Kurino, 1950). There were similar discourses around in the medical societies as well. One example can be traced in the editorial note of a medical journal:

> When I met many journalists in a meeting and asked them about its use, I was very surprised to find that almost all of them have been using it regularly. Of course they suggested that its use is not due to addiction but to the need to make work productivity rise.
>
> (Japan Medical Association, 1950, p. 141)

Moral judgement and medical (or scientific) evaluation worked together to delineate the boundary between ATS use by ordinary people and abuse by immoral people like performers and novelists. Immoral people were also often interpreted in medical journals as psychopaths, and such a diagnosis functioned as the reason for addiction (e.g. Kasamatsu and Kurino, 1950). These discourses indicate that ATS users in some particular categories were marginalised in society and were blamed for their actions. In other words, there were several different frames with moral judgements simulating scientific evaluation. In such framings, the risk of social unrest was attributed to some particular categories of people. It was a typical process of 'othering' which will be discussed again later.

Establishment of the *Stimulant Control Law* in 1951

Ordinary people still used to talk about the effects of ATS around 1950 in a positive note even after the two conspicuous deaths mentioned. It was because the problems related to ATS were often not attributed to the drug but to users. It means that ATS itself was not interpreted as being problematic enough to require strict control. This implies that other crucial factors were needed to establish strict control like total prohibition on ATS.

Problems with youth after the war

During the same period in 1949 and 1950, ATS was often associated with a different problem. This was related to juvenile vagrants or street kids, one-third of whose parents became victims of the war because of the frequent air raids in the cities or of the troubles encountered in coming home from overseas colonies. The population of orphans and street kids was huge. Even the official statistics in 1948 showed that the number of orphans was 123,511 and only 12,202 of them (9.8 per cent) were housed (the findings of the national research on orphans in

February 1948 by the Ministry of Health and Welfare). This was one of the largest problems in post-war Japanese society which was sometimes attributed to ATS use by the newspapers and news magazines.

However, street kids were not so much blamed for their ATS use but were rather seen as some kind of victims of adult hoodlums. For example, a newspaper article in 1949 pointed out that the street kids were often exploited by adults who offered them ATS in exchange for stealing things (Asahi Shinbun, 1949, November 22). This was because kids could not purchase ATS by themselves as it was designated a powerful drug, as mentioned. Some news magazines also reported that adult gangsters used to teach kids how to use ATS (Shukan Asahi, 1949, December 16).

As such, ATS abuse was often considered as one of the most important factors behind youth problems, especially the problem of delinquent kids in the cities, during that period. That is why the very first reference to ATS in the Diet was in a representative's remark that was about the connection between street kids and ATS use in 1949 (National Diet, 1949, October 24).

In December 1950, youth problems were intensively discussed in the National Council of Youth Problems (NCYP), which was constituted by representatives from all prefectures and the Ministries (NCYP, 1950). One particular division (No. 5) of the Council was organised to discuss the factors behind youth delinquency in which ATS-related problems were argued as one of the major factors along with smoking, drinking and other related behaviours.

However, the contents of the discussion about ATS-related problems showed that the problem was examined not just because of drug use but because it caused young people to become involved in delinquency, like stealing. The root of the problems was not the youths themselves but the smugglers who used to distribute ATS to the youths. The youths were perceived as objects for protection and education and so the victims of the misdeeds of adults.

The trouble with a company's production quota

The minutes of NCYP in 1950 did not indicate that young ATS users were to be blamed for its use. The problems were identified as resting in other activities like production, distribution and sale of ATS. This was a typical framing of the young ATS users of that period and one of the most important framings to influence the *Stimulant Control Law*.

For example, a representative of Fukuoka Prefecture insisted that they needed a law to prohibit the production of ATS because they were facing its unregulated distribution (NCYP, 1950, p. 97). This was because the *Pharmaceutical Affairs Law* that controlled the production of all approved drugs, including ATS, was enforced mainly to control fake drugs. As already pointed out, only administrative guidelines without legal basis could be issued by the Ministry to control production. It meant that the traditional method of control over ATS was not thought to function well enough to solve the problems. The attendees from other prefectures, Ministries and National Police Headquarters also insisted that legal measures to control production and distribution of ATS were needed.

One incident, which had already happened in Saitama Prefecture, was utilised by those who demanded the need to establish a new law to control ATS. The Saitama Mass Sexual Assault Incident came to light in October 1950, just before the Council, and over 100 men and women were arrested for it. A local newspaper, *Saitama Shinbun*, disclosed that the cause behind the incident was lack of education among young people and later that there was a shortage of policemen posted in the village to control such behaviours (Saitama Shinbun, 1950, October 1, 20, and 23). However, the National Police Headquarters subsequently insisted that the incident was caused by ATS. They also discovered that Toyama Chemical, a pharmaceutical company, produced over 10 million ampoules of ATS quarterly whereas its production quota by the Ministry was set at only 51,000. However, the quota limit had no legal basis and, as a result, Toyama Chemical was fined only 5,000 yen (about five GBP in the 1950s). This was called the Toyama Chemical Incident. Because of it, the National Police Headquarters strongly stressed the need to establish a new law to control ATS.

The reason for the prohibition of possession

Kondo (1955), Tamura (1982) and other researchers, based on their accounts of the establishment of ATS control, insisted that the Saitama Incident was the turning point for the establishment of the new law. They claimed that some psychopathological effect caused by ATS was the main reason behind the establishment. However, they might have misunderstood how the context of the incident was interpreted. Their claims were the typical interpretation after 1954. Such post-1954 framing will be discussed later. Of course, such discourse on the ATS-related problem might have existed already. However, such framing was not the main one, nor the typical one, as contemporary documents suggested. The problems were not caused by the effects of ATS but by the production, distribution and sale of it that provoked young people to commit crimes. *The Stimulant Control Law* was established in 1951 with legal backup to control activities like production, distribution and sales of ATS. The Toyama Chemical Incident gained more attention than the Saitama Incident. For this reason, just after the law was established, many newspaper articles on ATS contained reports on smuggling and illegal manufacture (e.g., Asahi Shinbun, 1951, November 26; Mainichi Shinbun, 1951, October 11 and 27, December 29; Yomiuri Shinbun, 1951, September 16, October 8 and 10).

One of the significant aspects of the new law was that prohibition of possession was stated explicitly in the provision. If the main problem was seen to lie in the effect of ATS, possession by users might also have been strictly controlled. However, it was not intended to punish the users of ATS but to maintain strict control on the smugglers. A government official clarified this fact in the Diet when discussing the establishment of the law:

> Clause number fourteen prohibits possession. One of the most difficult matters that official control bodies are faced with is the lack of a legal basis to control possession. They cannot prosecute those who possess stimulants to

sell in the town like Ueno. The Pharmaceutical Affairs Law is only for the companies and persons who manufacture and deal in medicine by occupation. Therefore, the Pharmaceutical Affairs Law cannot be administered to those who just possess stimulants. Even if a person possesses stimulants to sell, s/he cannot be arrested unless the crime is committed in the presence of an officer.

(National Diet, 1951, May 23, pp. 14–15)

The *Stimulant Control Law* was passed in June 1951. It prohibited possession of ATS. However, this clause in the beginning was also intended to arrest the smugglers and not ATS users.

New factors emerged leading to the amendment

The relevant question arises why many people today mistakenly believe that the law was established to control and even punish ATS users. This is because the retrospective interpretation of post-1954 has remained the dominant frame since then. In order to understand what happened in 1954, some other discourses need to be traced, which will reveal the political significance of stigmatisation of a particular group of people.

Discourses on law enforcement

Just after the *Stimulant Control Law* came into force on July 30, 1951, newspaper reports on ATS were almost fully preoccupied by issues of smuggling and illegal production. Asahi Shinbun reported that over 2,000 people were arrested in three months (Asahi Shinbun, 1951, November 26).

However, by the middle of 1952, some new factors were reported in the ATS-related news. A Korean village was reported to be the site for smuggling ATS and interestingly, one of the arrestees was reported to be an ex-member of the Communist Party (Asahi Shinbun August 25, 1952).[2] The question that comes to the mind is why did the news suddenly refer to 'Korean village' and a 'communist'? To answer this question, the process by which these words became significant in contemporary Japanese society should be traced: that was the background knowledge and the context for new framing.

Anti-communist movements in occupied Japan

After losing the War in 1945, Japan had been occupied by the General Headquarters/Supreme Commander for the Allied Powers (GHQ/SCAP) under the leadership of General Douglas MacArthur. During such occupation in Japan, the armed forces of the Communist Party of China gained superiority over the forces of the Chinese Nationalist Party on the Chinese Mainland. Further, some parts of GHQ/SCAP felt an impending crisis concerning the possible invasion of communism. Walter Crosby Eells, an advisor of the Civil Information and

Educational Section of GHQ/SCAP, advocated for suppression of communist influences and sentiments in Japanese universities in his speech in 1949. The speeches were interpreted to mean that GHQ/SCAP required the expulsion of communists out of the educational system, with the result that 2,000 teachers in primary, junior and senior high schools across the country were purged. Several months later, the People's Republic of China was founded by the Communist Party of China. By May in the following year (1950), General MacArthur argued that the Japanese Communist Party should be designated illegal. In July 1950, GHQ/SCAP urged the Japanese government to purge the communists and in September, 'Red Purge' was decided by the Cabinet in Japan. Over 10,000 people lost their jobs. Meanwhile, the Korean War broke out on June 25, 1950 and the menace of communism began to be talked about publicly even in the National Diet.

This kind of trend continued further in 1952 when large anti-government demonstrations and marches were organised on May Day in several big cities in Japan. Many people were arrested and 253 were prosecuted by January 1953 (Asahi Shinbun, 1953, January 28). The most infamous demonstration happened in the park in front of the Imperial Palace in Tokyo; 1,206 people were arrested. The Diet argued communists and their sympathisers were responsible for those incidents (National Diet, 1952, May 6, 7 and 9). The government also officially announced soon after that 'foreign communist countries' were causing the existing turbulences (National Diet, 1952, July 1).

That was the context in which new words like Korean village and communist could be found in the ATS-related news around 1952 (Sato, 2006, pp. 339–41). The implication was often tacit in the news because the Korean names of the suspects in the texts displayed their ethnicity. The illegal production and smuggling of ATS began to be interpreted as something connected with the communists through the Korean village.[3]

Recognising ATS-related problems within the new context

In the years afterwards, discourse containing the words 'communist' and 'Korean' were often found in texts that discussed matters related to the illegal manufacture and smuggling of ATS. However, the connection between the menace of communism especially from North Korea and the illegal activities connected with ATS was still unclear and almost always an ill-founded conjecture.

Such conjecture about the connection could be found in the comments of official bodies and even in discussion in the Diet. One representative of the Diet asked the head of the crime prevention department of the Metropolitan Police in October 1953 whether most of the smugglers of ATS were Korean people. He answered that 71 per cent of the arrests were Koreans and that the Metropolitan Police Forces were raiding Korean villages as their first priority.[4] He added that the suspects in the villages were so well organised that it was difficult to arrest all of them involved in such illegal activities. He alluded to some kind of supporting organisations behind the suspects (National Diet, 1953, October 30).

As the head of the department had said in the Diet, in October 1953, the Metropolitan Police conducted intensive inspections of Korean villages and other areas for suspected violations of the *Stimulant Control Law* and continued such inspections until the following month. As a result, there were 38,514 arrests in 1953, the second largest number of arrests in the history of the legislation. It accounted for the upward curve in the number of arrests in the 1950s (Figure 3.1). This trend continued till 1954 when the connection between communism and ATS was more explicitly referred to everywhere in spite of no evidence.

Youth problems caused by ATS

At the same time, youth problems related to ATS began to be debated more loudly than ever. Newspapers sometimes reported that the criminal behaviours of young people were often caused by the lack of money to purchase ATS. The lazy and violent lives of the young who craved ATS were also reported, featuring the murder of a son by his father (Yomiuri Shinbun, 1953, April 12). There was a report of a mother who complained that her son never worked but wasted money on ATS (Yomiuri Shinbun, 1953, March 7).

These kinds of troubles and movements against ATS merged into the social movement to 'protect' young people from the harm caused by ATS. In June 1953, the law for establishing the Council of Youth Problems was passed by the National Diet and the campaign to protect young people was launched in November 1953. In the campaign, ATS-related problems were designated as one of the major problems of youth. This movement officially defined young people as victims of ATS.

Movements against imagined invasion and for ATS control

The year 1954 can be considered as a landmark for ATS control in Japan. As already discussed, the *Stimulant Control Law* of 1951 was established to control illegal production and smuggling. ATS use itself was not the primary target of the law. However, one crucial incident happened in 1954 and the interpretation of the incident made another framing possible. Such framing was occasionally adopted but had never been the main or typical one. This time such framing intertwined with the context in which ATS became seen as one of the strategies underpinning an invasion by communism or foreign powers.

The Kyoko-chan incident

On April 20, 1954, an 11-year-old schoolgirl, Kyoko, was sexually assaulted and murdered in the restroom of a primary school in Tokyo. The incident seemed to be so shocking that the newspapers reported the proceedings of the investigation almost daily until the suspect was arrested. The suspect was a man named Sakamaki who was 20 years old. He had suffered from tuberculosis and started using Philopon. Before his arrest, the cause of the incident was often interpreted as the carelessness of the teacher of Kyoko's class. However, after the arrest, the cause began to be interpreted as the suspect's personality spoiled by his mother's nasty behaviours and the environment. Further, the discourse on the cause again took a turn towards the abnormal psychological and behavioural features of the suspect and the Philopon use that was thought to be responsible for his deeds.[5] Contemporary newspaper articles began to denounce Philopon and stressed the importance of eradicating ATS, advocating that ATS was forcing young people to lose their reasoning powers and commit crimes (Asahi Shinbun, 1954, May 7 and 8).

Confluence and the fight against the Koreans

This denunciation merged into the discourse that ATS was one of the means used by communists to invade Japan. In June 1954, the *Stimulant Control Law* was amended, in part to impose heavier punishment for violations of the law. However, the amendment was not meant to secure the eradication of addicts or users of ATS. In May 1954, in the discussion about the amendment of the law in the Diet, the chief of the Metropolitan Police, responding to one representative of the Diet who argued that addicts should be arrested and treated as criminals, said that addicts should be treated as patients unless they committed crimes (National Diet, 1954, May 20). The amendment was carried out to secure the eradication of smuggling and illegal production which provoked young people to commit crimes. A sort of traditional framing, in which the term 'young people' was interpreted as 'victims', still remained and functioned as a fulcrum to denounce the Koreans and communists.

Importantly, the objective of the amendment was to fight against the Koreans and communists. In a Diet debate regarding this amendment, the law was also discussed in terms of revising the Immigration Law, including the enforced repatriation of Korean people (National Diet, 1954, May 25). This was because of public perceptions that Korean people were smuggling ATS and many of them were communists or communist sympathisers who were engaged in an attack on Japan.[6] That is why the campaign for the eradication of ATS linked to a nationalist discussion was initiated following the amendment.

In October 1954, the government launched a campaign for the total eradication of ATS, which resulted in significant numbers of arrests; 55,664 people were arrested as shown by the peak of the curve in Figure 3.1. It is still the largest number of arrests in history by the *Stimulant Control Law* in Japan. The campaign was definitely against the assumed hostile forces, more explicitly the Koreans. When the campaign was launched, the head of the crime prevention department of the Metropolitan Police commented in a newspaper that the police would tighten controls over the smugglers even if Korean powers tried to interfere in their work (Asahi Shinbun, 1954, October 15).

The report of the Metropolitan Police on its 1954 campaign, which was published in the following year began as follows: 'In order to maintain the purity of Japanese ethnicity and especially to attempt to raise young people who will ensure our future generations, now is the time when we have to pluck up our courage to eradicate stimulants' (Metropolitan Police Headquarters, 1955, p. 1). The latter part of the report referred explicitly to the Koreans:

> 70 percent of these smugglers, illegal producers and bootleggers consist of Korean people and they gnaw at the bodies and spirits of approximately one million and five hundred thousand of our fellow countrymen. At its most extreme we seem to be living with a large crowd of people going insane and becoming brutal offenders. . . . Our fellow countrymen, especially young people, are the victims of Korean people pursuing their own interests and the result will be the destruction of our future generations, who will become sick and decline in health and finally turn into addicts who will destroy our entire social order. . . . Korean people who are well informed of the dangers of stimulants rarely use it themselves nor do they allow their children to use it.
> (Metropolitan Police Headquarters, 1955, pp. 19–20)

As these remarks show, the amendment and the resulting actions were undertaken to tighten control over smuggling and illegal production of ATS that were interpreted as one of the measures conducted for the profit of the Korean people. Interestingly, the police force had stopped referring to communism as a cause of ATS-related problems. They only referred to the Koreans and the Korean powers. That was because they could not find any evidence of communist invasion but only Korean people along with ATS. Of course, there is evidence to show that the search for the communist connection was continuing even during the campaign. However, no evidence was found to substantiate any such connection (e.g. Mainichi Shinbun, 1954, November 20). As a result, the explicit target of the campaign became the Koreans and the official voice of the campaign became nationalistic against them. The campaign against ATS became similar to the nationalist movement to protect Japanese youth against the Korean invasion. There were also lots of campaigns organised in many cities for the parents of young people who were addicted to ATS. Finally, the successful campaign resulted in maximum numbers of arrests in 1954 and 1955 (Figure 3.1).

After the campaign

The national movement against ATS successfully reduced the number of arrests in relation to the violation of the law. Many individuals who were involved in illegal production and smuggling were probably arrested and ATS black markets were shut down. Additionally, the newspaper reports on the campaign suggested that the arrest of people who used the drug was one of the means of reaching the smugglers and the illegal producers of ATS. Even many parents wished their children to be arrested, as they became violent and started spending money lavishly on the drug. This meant that the framing of young ATS users was changing. At the same time, the need for hospitalisation of users began to be discussed publicly. This led to the amendment of the Mental Health Law in the next year, 1955, making it possible to send ATS users to hospitals for treatment.

Table 3.1 Rate of prosecution (per cent)

Year	Number of newly registered suspects	Rate of prosecution (per cent)
1953	34,944	53.6
1954	53,352	63.6
1955	32,099	63.5
1956	6,645	58.0
1957	1,823	41.7
1958	609	37.1

Source: The White Paper on Crime 1960.

The statistics in the White Paper on Crime 1960 showed the scene afterwards (Table 3.1). As it shows, the rate of prosecution dropped dramatically from 63 to 37 per cent between 1955 and 1958. It signified that the circumstances surrounding crimes had changed and the ATS crisis ended.[7] The ATS crisis, which was assumed to be controlled by some foreign powers, was eradicated by the campaign, even if this kind of menace was imaginary and had never actually existed.

Conclusion: evil always comes from outside

In this last section, several points that are revealed through the description of the process of ATS control in Japan will be discussed.

The influence of control

It is now clear that the means by which ATS was controlled strongly influenced subsequent drug scenes in Japan. After the *Stimulant Control Law* was established in 1951 with the purpose only to control production and distribution, ordinary people stopped using ATS and the majority of users shifted from being busy workers to being delinquent youths who had access to underground markets. That might be one of the reasons why the connection between youth problems and ATS use was often paid much attention after the law was established. It became easier to keep stricter control over ATS users as well as smugglers and producers because the users already tended to be interpreted as delinquent. Busy workers had already left the drug scenes. There was no explicit objection to the measures taken to exercise control over delinquent youth because they became a risk to society. This is the reason why framing around young users of ATS changed around 1954. Even an imaginary foreign invasion accelerated the strict control of delinquent youths. The law when established was not primarily meant to exercise control over users of ATS. However, the framing of the problem was able to change later because the new drug scene and the new definition of the situation had already emerged because of the law itself.

These processes mean that the *Stimulant Control Law* and the enforcement of it along with specific framing of the issues functioned as a way to control other social problems beyond the original purpose and scope of the Law. It presumably worked as a way to maintain social order by the relevant authorities.

Framing and discourses

It is also clear that the framing processes of ATS control in Japan went through several stages. Methamphetamine use by immoral people was the trigger for the first control. Description of these immoral people was the key to evaluating the need for control. Such evaluation was inseparable from the very discourses on them as in Hirano's description of immoral people and in some medical doctors' accounts on them. Those discourses were available for Hirano and medical doctors to delineate the boundary of their moralistic world, which functioned as the frame through which a sort of mapping of the social order could be seen. This was framing. It means that there were some discursive devices available depending upon the situations. It was very close to an 'interpretative repertoire'. Interpretative repertoire is a set of statements and images with which people construct a version of reality. Repertoire originally means a performance in the ballet that can be interpreted as a set of actions. Similarly, interpretative repertoire can be thought of as a linguistic performance that is accomplished by a series of spoken words and images and it makes people understand what is going on and what the reality is. It also helps to maintain morality in interactions (Wetherell and Potter, 1992). As Van den Berg discussed, interpretative repertoire and framing are akin to each other with some difference in emphasis (Van den Berg, 2003). For example, in the first stage of ATS control, two typical framings for ATS use can be found. One framing depicts immoral novelists and performers. The cause of their drug use was interpreted as pathological and even addictive. Another framing describes responsible office workers and the cause was their working conditions. As such, each framing had its own discursive resources which constitute interpretative repertoires. In this example, when talking about ATS use, people had to use one of the two repertoires. At every stage of the framing process, some repertoires were available for several different frames. As mentioned, framing is sometimes multiple. Framing of young people shifted in accordance with the situation created by the new law as discussed earlier. We observed how framing and institutionalisation interacted with each other in the field of drug legislation in Japan. However, interestingly, those multiple framings converge at one point, as will be discussed later.

Othering and discourses

As the result of framing, 'othering' was accomplished through some specific discourses. As Spivak discussed with the example of the relationship between a British master and an Indian native, there are several dimensions to understanding othering (Spivak, 1985). One of them is concerned with knowledge that functions to create 'what will come to be perceived as a "natural" difference between the "master" and the "native"' (Spivak, 1985, p. 256). In the case of ATS, even though the relationship was not a racial one, after the war, medical doctors, as moral entrepreneurs, acted also as 'the subject of science or knowledge' (Spivak, 1985, p. 256). As mentioned, during the first stage of framing of the ATS problem, medical doctors indicated the problematic use of ATS by 'immoral people'. One medical paper discussed a comedy actor who abused ATS and was hospitalised. The paper analysed his script and concluded that the cause of the problem existed in himself: 'his association of ideas was superficial, but he was under the illusion that he enhanced his ability when using drugs. That is because he could entertain lowbrow audiences with such scripts' (Motoyoshi, 1949, p. 9). Medical analysis judged the value of the scripts and that was treated as the evidence for the cause of the problems. On the contrary, the same medical knowledge insisted that ATS use by 'healthy' busy workers was not problematic nor addiction. These descriptions reveal that scientific knowledge of drugs sometimes functioned as the 'othering' agency which delineated the boundary with one-sided values.

Attribution of the cause of the problem

The ATS-related problems in 1950s Japan were interpreted as some kind of attack by communism or foreign powers to invade Japan. After the menace was eradicated, Japan again experienced ATS-related problems in the 1970s and 1980s (Figure 3.1). It is referred to as the Second Wave of Stimulant Abuse Epidemic. During the Second Wave, the cause of the problem was attributed to the Japanese violent gang 'Bouryokudan' that was thought to import and smuggle ATS all over the country. Bouryokudan has always been marginalised in Japanese society. In the Second Wave, ATS-producing countries were suspected to be Korea and Taiwan.

The Third Wave of Epidemic began around 1994. As per the official documents, the Iranian people who visited Japan to work as migrant workers were thought to commit ATS smuggling during the Third Wave. North Korea was again designated as an ATS-producing country during the Third Wave.

As such, discourses related to ATS and framing of ATS problems have almost always identified some causes as related to factors from the fringe or outside Japanese society, sometimes coming from marginalised violent groups and sometimes from foreign people.

Many people consider that drug-related problems are closely connected only to some people living at the edge of, or outside, society. This typical notion and discourse about drug-related problems is still very popular in Japan even today. For example, the result of an opinion poll on the policy against drug abuse by the Cabinet Office in 1999 revealed that 80.9 per cent of people thought that the most desirable measure to solve the problems is strict law enforcement against smugglers who consisted of Bouryokudan and delinquent foreign people. Even in 2006, polls showed that 78.5 per cent of people held a similar opinion.

As these results show, drug-related problems have always been thought to arise from the border or outside of Japanese society. This might be the primary cultural framing that has been supported by many nationalist discourses. Evil always comes from outside and appears in the form of foreigners as others. This notion might act as an obstacle against a pertinent drug policy in Japan, because actual users are not others. They are always in the society.

Notes

1 In this chapter, all the news items related to ATS which appeared in three major newspapers in Japan during the 1940s and 1950s have been examined: *Asahi Shinbun, Mainichi Shinbun* and *Yomiuri Shinbun*. Additionally, all the minutes of the National Diet related to ATS in the same period, including the records of all committees of the National Diet, have been examined. However, only the materials referred to are listed in the references.
2 The newspaper *Yomiuri Shinbun* was the first one that referred to 'communist' when reporting the illegal production of ATS in November 1951 (Yomiuri Shinbun, 1951, November 22). However, there was no mention of the word Korean in it.
3 It is well known that there has been discrimination on the basis of ethnic origins, especially towards the Korean people in Japanese society. However, the words 'communist' and 'Korean village' were not used in the context of traditional discrimination.
4 The proportion of the Koreans in all arrests was 71 per cent, which might be a result of the prior investigations in the Korean villages.
5 Those interpretations about the harm of ATS had already been reported in some newspaper articles based on different people's experiences and also talk by psychopathologists. It means that those discourses became public and salient when some crucial incident happened in connection to ATS use.
6 The clause provided for enforced repatriation was not included in the final bill of the amendment because of the disagreement with South Korea.
7 The White Paper on Crime 1960 also showed that the proportion of categories of violation of the Stimulant Control Law had dramatically changed since 1954. In 1959, illegal ATS production led to only 1 per cent of all arrests for violation of the law.

References (all the Japanese titles are translated by the author)

Entman, R.M. 1993. Framing: Toward clarification of a fractured paradigm. *Journal of Communication* 43 (4), pp. 51–8.
Goffman, E. 1974. *Frame Analysis: An Essay of the Organization of Experience*. New York: Harper and Row.
Hirano, I. 1949. Philopon disaster: Modes of lives of postwar novelists. *Sekai Hyoron*, December, pp. 68–71.
Horimi, T. 1947. Additional comment. *The Journal of the Japanese Society of Internal Medicine* 36 (5/6/7), p. 99.
Ikuta, B. 1951. On stimulants. *Kagaku to Sousa* 4 (2), pp. 28–53.
Iwata, S. 1947. Precaution for continues use of Philopon. *The Journal of the Japanese Society of Internal Medicine* 36 (5/6/7), pp. 98–9.
Japan Medical Association. 1950. Editorial: Where does Philopon go. *The Journal of Japan Medical Association* 24 (2), p. 141.
Kasamatsu, A., and Kurino, R. 1950. Intoxication of Analeptic Amin. *The Journal of Japan Medical Association* 24 (2), pp. 92–101.
Kondo, K. 1955. Retrospective and prospective consideration on the offenders of stimulant control law. *The Journal of Police Science* 8 (1), pp. 40–51.

Metropolitan Police Headquarters. 1955. *The Harm and Evil of Stimulants (Philopon) and the Measures to Cope with It*. Metropolitan Police Headquarters.

Ministry of Justice. 1960. *The White Paper on Crime 1960*, Tokyo: Research and Training Institute, Ministry of Justice.

Ministry of Justice. 2016. *The White Paper on Crime 2016*, Tokyo: Research and Training Institute, Ministry of Justice.

Motoyoshi, I. 1949. On the hallucinosis of Philopon. *Japan Medical Journal* 1337, pp. 8–10.

Nagai, N. 1893. Results of the research on the contents of Chinese medicine Maou. *Journal of the Pharmaceutical Society of Japan* 139, pp. 901–33.

Nakazaki, T., and Mori, H. 1947. One case of acute intoxication of Philopon. *The Journal of the Japanese Society of Internal Medicine* 36 (5/6/7), p. 98.

Sato, A. 2006. *Drug and Discourse: Methamphetamine in Japan*. Tokyo: Toshindo.

Sato, A. 2009. Methamphetamine use in Japan after the Second World War: Transformation of narratives. *Contemporary Drug Problems* 35 (Winter/2008), pp. 717–46.

Shukan, A. 1949. *The Boy Addicted to Philopon*. 16 December, pp. 19–20.

Spivak, G.C. 1985. The Rani of Sirmur: An essay in reading the archives. *History and Theory* 24 (3), pp. 247–72.

Tamura, M. 1982. Methamphetamine epidemic and law enforcement. *Japanese Journal of Sociological Criminology* 7, pp. 4–32.

The National Council of Youth Problem (NCYP). 1950. *Minutes of the National Council of Youth Problem*. 9, 10 December, Tokyo: Chuo Seishonen Mondai Kyogikai, The Prime Minister's Office.

Van den Berg, H. 2003. Contradiction in interview discourse. In: Van den Berg et al. (Eds.), *Analyzing Race Talk: Multidisciplinary Approaches to the Interview*. Cambridge: Cambridge University Press, pp. 119–37.

Vlegenthart, R., and Van Zoonen, K. 2011. Power to the frame: Bringing sociology back to frame analysis. *European Journal of Communication* 26 (2), pp. 101–15.

Wetherell, M., and Potter, J. 1992. *Mapping the Language of Racism: Discourse and the Legitimisation of Exploitation*. New York: Columbia University Press.

Asahi Shinbun 1949, March 29th, November 22nd

1951, November 26th, August 25th

1952, August 25th

1953, January 28th

1954, May 7th, May 8th, October 15th

Mainichi Shinbun 1951, October 11th, October 27th

1951, December 29th

1954, November 20th

Saitama Shinbun 1950, Oct 1st, October 20th, October 23rd

Yomiuri Shinbun 1951, September 16th, October 8th, October 10th

1953, March 7th, April 12th

The Minutes of the National Diet

1949, Committee of Health and Welfare No. 7, the 5th Upper House, October 24th

1949, Plenary Session No. 18, the 6th Upper House, November 24th

1950, Committee of Health and Welfare No. 3, the 9th Upper House, December 5th

1951, Committee of Health and Welfare No. 29, the 10th Upper House, May 23rd

1952, Plenary Session No. 38, the 13th Lower House, May 6th
1952, Committee of Local Administration No. 38, the 13th Lower House, May 7th
1952, Committee of Law No. 47, the 13th Lower House, May 9th
1952, Plenary Session No. 59, the 13th Lower House, July 1st
1953, Committee of Health and Welfare No. 1, the 17th Upper House, October 30th
1954, Committee of Health and Welfare No. 48, the 19th Lower House, May 20th
1954, Committee of Health and Welfare No.45, the 19th Upper House, May 25th

4 Dangerous drugs, dangerous women

Declassé women, drugs and sapphic sexuality in 1930s London

Christopher Hallam

Introduction

This chapter explores a group of mostly upper-class women in interwar London who were consumers of illicit drugs. In accordance with the 1920 Dangerous Drugs Act, these drugs were known as 'dangerous drugs' and those who used them were often known by the Home Office, the Metropolitan Police and the courts as 'vicious addicts': unlike those who were prescribed such substances for medical reasons, these consumers used them for pleasure and entertainment – or, in the language of morality and media, for 'vice'.

The chapter begins with reference to what Richard Overy terms the 'morbid age', which provides the setting for an analysis of twentieth-century modernity and social modernism. It unpicks the complex social and cultural strands which formed the opiate and cocaine culture and points to the ambivalence of the interwar years in Britain: for some these represented a cultural pathology and the erosion of social, sexual and gender standards while for others a new social space in which freedoms and pleasures could be explored.

The chapter traces the emergence of social modernism in the aftermath of World War I ('the Aftermath'), along with the impact of war and other social changes on the upper classes out of which came the drugs bohemias of the 1920s and 1930s. The role of upper-class women in exploring the sexual and narcotic pleasures of this period was especially important; the bohemian women of the transitional aristocracy were key to broader shifts in gender and female sexuality. These women were profoundly symbolic both of 'morbid' culture and modernity and its freedoms. Their symbolic status led to intense attention from the Police and the Home Office Drugs Branch; while subject to continuous surveillance and searches for drugs, detectives appeared preoccupied by the lifestyle and sexual relationships they encountered in these groups. Diverse male authority figures cooperated with Police enquiries in providing lifestyle information.

Drugs were used for illicit pleasure by a tiny minority of the population, yet they provoked disquiet and sometimes outright panic beyond all proportion to their numbers and prevalence. The anxieties we shall examine here were, fundamentally, not about drugs; rather, drugs symbolised young women, who in turn symbolised modernity, in a process of potentially endless internal reference. The public health concerns surrounding dangerous drugs notwithstanding, drugs were in the interwar period a stand-in/substitute for a range of anxieties connected with young women, whose consumerism, desires, dreams and, it was feared, loss of control could drag down the edifice of British civilisation and the British race with it. Pursued by the Police and the courts, marked as pathological by the medical profession, represented in fearful terms by newspapers on a national, local and international scale, these vicious addicts were a new and surprising iteration of the old term 'dangerous classes'. Despite their wealth and glamour, and largely because of their connotation of modernity, they were objects of fear and loathing, as well as eroticised subjects of desire.

Modernity and morbid culture

British historian Richard Overy has characterised Britain's interwar period as 'the morbid age'. According to Overy's provocative thesis, the UK's intellectual culture was permeated by discourses heralding the demise of civilisation, of the nation and its empire, and of the British 'race'. These were the peak years of the eugenics movement, which saw in racial decline the looming crisis of a civilisation, drawing on an analogy between the life cycle of the individual and the race, which was born, matured, degenerated and died. Overy argues that this biological metaphor lent the eugenic discourse and the morbid culture more generally a scientific foundation (Overy, 2010).

As we will see in the course of this chapter, eugenics was highly influential in the medical and related professions and prominent in the thinking and practice of addiction specialists such as those who conducted the Royal College of Physicians Committee on Drug Addiction in 1938. Addicts were amongst a broad set of subgroups of the population that were considered degenerate and which threatened to bring down the entire social and racial order. At the annual Galton lecture of 1928, the speaker professed that 'the real factors which determine the rise and fall of nations and civilizations are the racial qualities and innate capacities of the citizens themselves' (Overy, 2010, p. 100). The eugenicist Austin Freeman, writing in 1921, listed the degenerate classes as comprising 'habitual criminals, the inmates of reformatories and industrial homes, tramps, vagrants, chronic inebriates, prostitutes, the subjects of drug habits, sexual perverts and the sufferers from various congenital neuroses' (Overy, 2010, pp. 111–12).

Morbid culture spread out from intellectual circles and permeated popular discourse, providing a context for the disquiet associated with recession, war and rapid social change. The consumers of dangerous drugs were viewed through the prism of this morbid culture, and upon them and the broader deviant population were focused the anxieties of the interwar era. The argument here is that these were linked to a profound sense of ontological unease – anxiety and panic surrounding the experience of self, identity, social roles – that accompanied modernity and the growth of social and cultural modernism.

The term modernism usually refers to the late-nineteenth- and early-twentieth-century movement in literature and the arts, at the core of which lay a critique of representation and a radical break with traditional materials and forms of expression (Cocks, 2007, pp. 26–41). This movement peaked in the years after World War I – the Aftermath. Along with this shift in cultural expression went what I will term here 'social modernism', which also involved a rupture with the past and traditional social forms. It was characterised by changes in sexual behaviour and attitudes to gender, to the internal governance of families, divorce, and for upper-class women an escape from the system of the chaperone, access to education and employment, greater freedom for children and youth, ethnic mixing, fashion and individuality. While the world of cultural criticism was riven with conflict over the merits or otherwise of literary and artistic modernism, the social aspects of modernism were of greater significance for people in society at large. By way of example, short dresses, bare backs and arms, lipstick and other cosmetics, cigarette smoking, dancing and access to the spaces of metropolitan night-time entertainment marked the young women of the Aftermath, to the shock and alarm of their parents' generation (Tinkler, 2006; Dyhouse, 2013, pp. 76–9). Promiscuity, bisexuality and drug use pushed the process still further and led the police, doctors and other authorities to act.

The dangerous (upper) classes

The 'dangerous classes' of the nineteenth century were viewed by the authorities as existing outside the ordered hierarchy of British society; they were beyond the reach of industrial work discipline and immune to the values that embedded individuals within the social structure. It was a category that would be reincarnated in the discourse of the 'underclass' in the sociology of the late-twentieth-century political right (Welshman, 2013).

The interwar years, however, saw the appearance of a different group to whom the epithets 'dangerous' or, more commonly, 'vicious' were applied. They were the inhabitants of the 'dangerous drugs' scene of interwar Britain, and especially London – what the Home Office, the Metropolitan Police and various doctors termed 'vicious addicts'. Perhaps the most striking characteristic of these individuals was their class origin: far from the impoverished residuum that haunted the class relationships of Victorian London, this group was largely drawn from the elite ranks of the upper classes and extended down as far as the middle classes but not much further (Hallam, 2018). Its representatives were primarily young women. Many were wealthy, glamorous and celebrated figures, the very antithesis of the residual poor, those criminals and prostitutes who inhabited the rookeries and slums of the nineteenth-century metropolis. What marked out their dangerousness were two key elements: their use of dangerous drugs (as these materials were defined in law in 1920) and their dissident sexualities. They were also associated with what the press signified as dangerous spaces – nightclubs and bottle parties, the consulting rooms of marginal doctors and even certain private flats, studios and residences in Chelsea, Mayfair and Soho. This collection of upper-class women represented a new form of peril, as the dangerousness of the drugs they consumed leaked into their minds and bodies, rendering them vicious and déclassé. It was a phenomenon of circulating menace and multiple, interwoven modes and sites of risk that the women embodied.

The British upper classes had entered a period of crisis prior to World War I, with several factors challenging its centuries-old pre-eminence in wealth, social position and political power at the dawn of the era of mass democracy. Between 1880 and 1930, wealth and power shifted from the British-landed classes to a new, international plutocracy (Cannadine, 1996). Moreover, the growth of the state during the war years and after proved difficult for the aristocracy to negotiate. Nonetheless, they adapted to new circumstances, mixing and merging with the plutocracy, establishing marriages that exchanged titles for money, lending their ancient charisma to the new glamour of America (Balfour, 1933). By the 1920s and 1930s, the gilded sons and daughters of the upper classes were clashing with state authority figures, especially the police, over their leisure pastimes, including the policing of private motor cars, restrictive drug control and the regulation of medicine, and the limits imposed on the night-time economy – which comprised licensing hours in night clubs and the confines placed upon public dancing and live music.

This golden youth, coming of age since the end of the unprecedented carnage of the Great War, were moreover in conflict not only with the state but with the older generation who had allowed the war to happen. The 'Bright Young People' was the press term for an aristocratic and bohemian youth culture that emerged in the 1920s, indulging in treasure hunts and 'freak parties' where guests dressed up, according to a prearranged theme, as babies, sailors, Mozarts, Peter Pans and the like (Taylor, 2007). This conduct may be viewed as infantile but was arguably part of a reaction against the alleged maturity of business, war and politics. It produced a sensibility summarised by literary critic Martin Green:

> The war had roused great anger against the fathers, as well as guilt amongst them, and great pathos and love for the fallen sons, and the new dandies were able to appeal to those feelings in support of their cult of youth. They refused to grow up into men of responsibility, fathers of families, and of the state, soldiers.
>
> (Green, 1992, p. 152)

These perceptions also fed into the powerful strand of homosexuality amongst the aesthetic movement and the Bright Young People. However, homosexuality in the latter group is often emphasised at the expense of the equally strong presence of the feminine within this micro-culture, which may be understood as part of the feminisation of wider English culture in the interwar years. Alison Light has written of the years between the wars as featuring

> a move away from formerly heroic and officially masculine public rhetorics of national identity . . . to an Englishness at once less imperial and more inward looking, more domestic and more private – and, in terms of pre-war standards, more "feminine".
>
> (Light, 2013, p. 8)

The feminisation of London's high bohemian culture, while it bore a family resemblance to the culture pictured by Light, followed a different trajectory: these were modern, metropolitan women, and their inward focus and privacy owed more to morphine and hashish, opium and cocaine than it did to conservatism and rural nostalgia.

The forbidden pleasures of the Aftermath

Historians such as Paul Fussell have located the birth of the modern sensibility in the traumatic experience and gallows humour of World War I (Fussell, 1975). The scepticism, hostility to tradition, irony and detachment this entailed were certainly a fit with the attitudes and lifestyle of the Bright Young People of the 1920s, the youth culture from which London's white drug scene emerged ('white' drugs being those powders containing alkaloids extracted from plant-based drugs such as morphine, heroin and cocaine). Sexual experimentation was a key characteristic of these groups as was the leading role played by young women. What some saw as the 'lost generation', cast adrift from the certainties of the Victorian and Edwardian years, was experienced by others as a space in which new freedoms and pleasures could be identified and developed. Many of these revolved around sexuality and gender.

Homosexual acts between men (or acts of 'gross indecency') had been illegal in Britain since the Labouchere amendment to the Criminal Law Act of 1885 (Hall, 2012). A subsequent debate over the Criminal Law Amendment Bill took place in 1921. Conservative MP Frederick Macquisten sought to add a clause stating that 'any act of gross indecency between female persons shall be a misdemeanour and punishable in the same manner as any such act committed by male persons under Section 11 of the Criminal Law Amendment Act, 1885'.[1] Macquisten argued that such a measure was 'long overdue' in Britain and claimed professional knowledge of numerous 'calamitous cases' of sapphism. 'These moral weaknesses', he claimed,

> dated back to the very origin of history. . . . [W]hen they grew and became prevalent in any nation or in any country it was the beginning of the nation's downfall. The falling away of feminine morality was to a large extent the cause of the destruction of the early Grecian civilisation, and still more the cause of the downfall of the Roman Empire.[2]

Macquisten saw the same trend in the Britain of the Aftermath, believing that only if criminal law was introduced could such practices be limited or even eradicated. He invoked what was a familiar theme in the period, linking sexual degeneracy with the consumption of dangerous drugs and invoking scientific authority to do so. 'Neurologists would tell them how largely the spread of the use of cocaine and other drugs was due to the dreadful nerve deterioration which beset many of the idle part of the population', and that he had seen 'happy homes wrecked in this way'.[3]

Sir Ernest Wild spoke in support, informing MPs that he had spoken to many asylum doctors who told him that 'the asylums were largely peopled by nymphomaniacs and people who indulged in this vice. . . . It debauched young girls and produced neurasthenia and insanity' (Lancet, 1921). Major Farquhason – speaking, as a physician – called upon the House to adopt the clause as 'a physical protection to the race'.[4]

While the move received some vocal support in the House, other MPs were wary. Josiah Wedgwood, for example,

> could not believe that the House would pass the clause, which would advertise a beastly subject. To call in the policeman to suppress a vice was the best way to encourage the knowledge of that vice and the spread of it.
>
> (Lancet, 1921)

Ultimately, Macquisten's clause was removed from the amendment, parliament voting it down by approximately two to one, largely on the grounds elaborated by Wedgwood. It would be safest if the topic remained confined to whispers in the consulting rooms and laboratories of medical men. Nonetheless, the discursive cluster settling on the concept of the lesbian is clear: threats to civilisation, racial degeneration, and dangerous drugs. All of these would be associated with the white drug culture that emerged alongside the media tarnishing of the Bright Young People in the late 1920s.

Sapphic relationships were prevalent amongst the high bohemian sets inhabiting the Aftermath. Women of the new celebrity culture that accompanied the rise of international (especially American) plutocracy enjoyed sexual encounters with their own or both sexes. From actresses Tallulah Bankhead and Marlene Dietrich to painter Tamara de Lempicka and entertainer Josephine Baker, all made the most of the varied menu of sexual experiences available to them in the new modern erotic landscape that was forming in the 1920s and 1930s (Mackerell, 2015). The lives of such women were endlessly covered by the popular press and were played on the 'silver screen' by famous actresses such as Greta Garbo and Louise Brooks; they were, consequently, highly influential. Moreover, the fact that such women played the parts of flappers on screen made 'every fashionable young woman . . . part of a larger modern narrative' (Gundle, 2008, p. 160).

The Chelsea white drug scene

Drug use was also a fashionable component of the bohemian lifestyle, with cocaine probably being the most widely consumed drug. The drug culture discussed here was initially based in Chelsea, emerging amongst a group of well-known Bright Young People, including Brenda Dean Paul, Anthea Carew, Brian 'Napper' Dean Paul, Olivia Wyndham, Ruth Baldwin, Dolly Wilde, Leonie Fester and David Plunket Greene. Many of those making the transition from the Bright Young People to the Chelsea white drug scene began their relationships with intoxicants by using alcohol – cocktails in particular were *de rigueur* – along with a range of 'pick-me-ups' and nostrums available over the pharmacy counter.

The central figure in this group was Brenda Dean Paul. Paul was a celebrity before she began using drugs, a society 'it-girl' whose presence was a permanent feature at the most widely publicised 1920s parties (Hoare, 2004). Born in Kensington in 1907, her father was Sir Aubrey Dean Paul, the 5th Baronet, and her mother Lady Irene Dean Paul, who went by the stage name of Poldowski; she was the daughter of a celebrated Polish violinist. Brenda was very close to her mother, a musician and composer who introduced her to modernist culture and the circles of continental high bohemia. Her parents separated in 1922, and she barely saw her father after this date; he would have nothing to do with her following her first court cases involving drugs and the notoriety that followed her thereafter. According to Dr Thomas Creighton, house physician at the Park Lane hotel, Paul was already a morphine addict when he treated her for abdominal pain in 1928.[5] There are several versions in existence of Paul's first encounter with morphine – her memoirs suggest that she was initially given the drug at a party at a Parisian artist's studio (Dean Paul, 1935). What is certain is that by the beginning of the 1930s, her habit was fully established. Brenda's preference was for morphine, though she sometimes used heroin and other opioids, and later in her drug career was prescribed vast quantities of cocaine. By 1931, she was being monitored closely by the Metropolitan Police, who were aware of her drug use and were seeking to identify her sources of supply.

Although she made use of illicitly acquired drugs from time to time, Brenda's regular source was the lawful medical prescribing of doctors, which was possible owing to Britain's regulatory system. In 1926, following a period of flux during which the British government was uncertain in its responses towards drug use and addiction, the *Departmental Report on Morphine and Heroin Addiction* was published (Departmental Committee on Morphine and Heroin Addiction, 1926). This document was the outcome of the deliberations of a Committee of doctors appointed by the Ministry of Health to advise the government 'as to the circumstances, if any, in which the supply of morphine and heroin (including preparations containing morphine and heroin) to persons suffering from addiction to those drugs may be regarded as medically advisable' (Departmental Committee on Morphine and Heroin Addiction, 1926, minute of appointment of the committee). Under the chairmanship of Sir Humphry Rolleston, President of the Royal College of Physicians and the King's Physician-in-Ordinary, the Committee examined the problem of addiction and whether it could be treated by recourse to morphine or heroin. In the report which still bears Rolleston's name, the Committee decided that in certain circumstances, it could. According to the Report:

(8) There are two groups of persons suffering from addiction to whom administration of morphine or heroin may be regarded as legitimate medical treatment, namely:

    (a) Those who are undergoing treatment for cure of the addiction by the gradual withdrawal method;

(b) Persons for whom, after every effort has been made for the cure of the addiction, the drug cannot be completely withdrawn, either because:

(i) Complete withdrawal produces serious symptoms which cannot be satisfactorily treated under the ordinary conditions of private practice; or

(ii) The patient, while capable of leading a useful and fairly normal life so long as he takes a certain non-progressive quantity, usually small, of the drug of addiction, ceases to be able to do so when the regular allowance is withdrawn.

This pattern of prescribing gave rise to a relatively small number of doctors, based mostly in the capital, who made the supply of addicts the cornerstone of their practice. These were known by the Home Office and by Scotland Yard as 'script doctors', regarded as dubious physicians who were ready to prescribe drugs to addicts for purposes that were almost entirely pecuniary (Spear and Mott, 2002, pp. 42–3). Over the ensuing decades, Brenda developed an uncanny ability to locate and identify these practitioners and used them to support her addiction to opiates and cocaine.

Scotland Yard's pursuit of Brenda Dean Paul

Police surveillance of Brenda Dean Paul and Anthea Carew began in 1931. A visit by officers to the two women's shared house in Godfrey Street, Chelsea, revealed that 'alleged drug addict' Brenda had been treated in a Nursing Home in October 1930 and was still 'taking injections'.[6] When detectives visited the premises shortly afterwards, they found Napper Dean Paul, Brenda's brother and fellow drug user, dressed in his pyjamas (it was 1 p.m.) and 'lying on a couch whilst his legs were being massaged by a masseur', who beat a hasty retreat from the house before his name could be ascertained.[7] Napper was described in police files as 'an effeminate young man', and the officers were highly suspicious of the homosexual undercurrents of these goings on.[8] The Godfrey Street premises were kept under observation, and the occupants' cab journeys around London were followed up by detectives. These investigations highlighted the preoccupation of the police with the social aspects of the women's behaviour.

Many of the places to which Brenda and Anthea went were celebrated spaces in the history of cultural modernism, such as the Eiffel Tower Hotel and Restaurant (pre-war capital of the Vorticist movement[9] and still a watering hole for smart bohemia), the Blue Lantern and Uncles (two of the night clubs at which the Bright Young People gathered) and the Gargoyle Club (the hangout of artistic and literary bohemia in the 1930s). There were also numerous visits to various doctors' consulting rooms, often followed by stops at pharmacies. The police were attempting to trace Brenda's supplies of morphine and would interview pharmacists and staff concerning the young woman and her doctors. These interviews, conducted by male detectives with male pharmacists, are significant. Inspector Barker of the Yard made enquiries at Boots Cash-Chemist shop in South Audley

Street, and 'ascertained that Miss Dean Paul purchased some "Coty" perfume and face powder'. She then 'proceeded, in the shop, to "make up" her face, which I was informed occupied her for nearly half an hour'.[10] Brenda's cosmetic practices are, on the surface, entirely unrelated to the object of this police enquiry. However, the uncomprehending tone and the focus on such details clearly demonstrates the attitudes towards modern young women held by these police and medical professionals, and the fact that the driving force behind the drug enquiry was social and cultural rather than criminal as such, or rather that the criminality primarily provided a pretext.

In April 1931, Anthea Carew booked a room at the Park Lane Hotel. Brenda called on her that evening and stayed the night. According to Scotland Yard files:

> A night porter was called to their room during the night and he reported that he found both of them apparently intoxicated and one of them was sitting on the bed in almost a nude condition. The other one was in bed. They were, in consequence, not regarded as suitable guests and were informed . . . that their room was required.[11]

Again, it is the erotic and gender association of the women's behaviour that is of paramount interest to the Scotland Yard detectives who assembled materials for these files.

In November 1931, Sir Aubrey Dean Paul called at Scotland Yard to ask the Met what they could do to stop Brenda gaining access to dangerous drugs. According to Inspector Barker, Sir Aubrey 'stated that his daughter was not living with him and she was not under his control'.[12] He informed the Inspector that 'he was anxious that something should be done to cure his daughter of the habit taking these drugs as he feared that she might become a confirmed drug taker and bring disgrace upon herself and her family'.[13] Barker responded, however, that the licit supply of drugs to Brenda was a matter of medical judgement and was in the hands of doctors rather than those of the Police. In fact, though her father was not told, a summons had been issued for her two days previously. She had broken the law by receiving supplies of morphine and heroin from several doctors at once and was summoned to appear at Marlborough Street Police Court.

The magistrate at this famous central London court was Frederick Mead, born in 1847 and a thoroughgoing Victorian in his social and cultural attitudes. The court was told that Brenda had acquired her addiction as the result of medical treatment undergone in France and was unconnected with her social-modernist lifestyle (Playfair, 1969, p. 170). Mead had presided over the trial of Ada Lau Ping, the opium cook in the Billie Carleton case, calling her 'the high priestess of these unholy rites' and sending her to Holloway (Kohn, 1992, p. 88). In the present case, however, perhaps won over by the high social standing of the defendant and the culpability of gallic physicians, he bound Brenda over for three years on condition that she undertake a residential cure.[14]

While the Police attitudes towards social modernism and bohemia were in some ways confined to their institutions and internal discourses, the outcome of their investigations in prosecutions and court cases led to enormous public-ity for some of the women of the Bright Young People and for the antagonism felt towards them by the Police. Brenda Dean Paul, one of the most famous and celebrated of the group, found her unhappy court experiences spread across the national press and syndicated around the globe. These views would also issue in spells in Holloway.

According to her memoirs, Brenda Dean Paul was made subject to a number of restrictions by the court:

> (a) I was not to live with or near anyone my own age; (b) I was not to live near or with anyone belonging to the set I had known and mixed with in the past; (c) that I must be under the supervision of someone older than myself, in a reliable and respectable position.
>
> (Dean Paul, 1935, pp. 204–5)

Her court-mandated period of 'cure' was passed in a number of medical set-tings, including the family home of one Dr A. H. W. Fleming of Regents Park. Dr Fleming had called on the Police, saying that he 'feels convinced that it is essential that Miss Paul should have a holiday abroad as this is the only means of removing her from her present circle of friends'. Fleming felt that she could only be cured if he could 'rebuild her character'.[15] Visited at the house by her close friend Anthea Carew, she was alleged to have received morphine ampoules and was compelled to appear again before Frederick Mead for breaking the conditions of her bail. The charge could not, however, be proven.

Anthea Carew and 'Those Beastly Police'

Anthea Rosemary Carew (nee Gamble) was sister to another Bright Young per-son, Patrick Gamble, who hosted one of the first 'Blackbird Parties' for the all black cast of the 1926 revue 'Blackbirds', a great London stage success (Dean Paul, 1935). Growing up in Belgravia, Patrick and Anthea were the children of the Dean of Exeter. Anthea married *Times* journalist Dudley Carew in 1928, though the marriage was a brief affair, he later describing it as a 'whirlwind romance . . . (that) had an air of unreality about it' (Carew, 1974, pp. 80–1). The relationship of Brenda and Anthea was an extremely close one, which may have included a sexual element. Such friendships were a striking characteristic amongst this group of women and were an element of social modernism, with elective relationships being held in much higher esteem than those resulting from family ties. Many were divorced and/or living apart from the families that sought to regulate their conduct, and the police, doctors and courts invariably sought to separate them from their network of friends as part of the strategy to cure them of their drug habits.

In 1932, Brenda and Anthea Carew were involved together in two highly pub-licised court cases related to their drug use. In the first, Anthea, who was staying in Devon for a short period, posted a small quantity of morphine to Brenda in

London. The arrangement was for her to pick up the parcel at Waterloo station, but it was intercepted by Police, who arrested both women, charging Brenda with possession. Anthea had written to Brenda on Marylebone Police court notepaper, an ironic touch that doubtless went down poorly with the detectives. 'Darling', she wrote, 'I think these beastly police are probably going to stop me having ANY more',[16] in which case Brenda was supposed to send some back to Anthea in Exeter.

The case was heard at Tower Bridge Police Court, with Mr Morgan Griffiths-Jones the presiding magistrate. Griffiths-Jones did not take kindly to Brenda's lifestyle, telling her that

> You have got to pull yourself together. What is required in your case is discipline. But you are a lady by birth, and therefore I am inclined to trust you to help yourself. I have convicted you, but I am not going to sentence you. I am going to remand you for one month to see that you behave yourself properly and obey the doctor's orders, and I may go on remanding you month by month for six months; and if I get any unsatisfactory reports I shall be quite satisfied that Holloway will be the best place for you.[17]

Brenda was committed to the Norwood Sanatorium, a well-known institution treating addicts and alcoholics, and was reported to be recovering well. However, shortly before her next court attendance was due, she underwent an emergency dental procedure, and in combination with the symptoms of opiate withdrawal and the hyoscine treatment she had been receiving, this rendered her unable to attend. The magistrate was furious, and despite the statements of her doctors attesting that she was too ill to attend, Brenda was sentenced to six months imprisonment. Her solicitor asked the attending physician, 'In your view as a medical man is she in a fit state to come here today?'[18] The medical man – the customary term at this time – was further questioned as to the likely effect of attending court on Brenda's health. He replied that 'She would have had to come on a stretcher, and she could not have answered questions'[19] (Davenport Hines, 2001, pp. 294–7). None of this had any impact on Mr Griffiths-Jones, despite medical advice and the pleading of Brenda's counsel. The sentence was, however, overturned on appeal, though only after Brenda had spent several weeks in Holloway. Upon winning her appeal and being released from this grim Victorian institution, her response was – 'Oh the joy of a Camel and some lipstick once more; the joy of kind, loving and attractive people each side of me' (Dean Paul, 1935, p. 254).

Following his sentencing of Brenda, the magistrate received an anonymous postcard, clearly from a supporter of Brenda and her opiate consumption. Addressed to 'Griffith-Jones, Arch fiend devil monster', it went on to say that

> morphine is a product of nature's wild flowers – the Poppy – nature is feminine and 'Men' like you do all you can to cut women off from their Divine Mother Nature – by denying them the soothing remedies SHE provides for suffering – millions use these remedies.[20]

The message anticipates a kind of eco-feminism and perhaps gives an indication of the views held by some of the drug-using women involved in interwar English bohemia. It is, of course, impossible to estimate how prevalent such views were.

The second court case involving Brenda and Anthea around this time featured a French countess, Marie de Flammerecourt, who was found in possession of a small amount of cocaine while staying at the Hotel Somerset, Orchard Street in the West End. Acting on information received from a certain Dr Ripman, the Met visited Countess Flammerecourt in her hotel room to search for drugs; while Police were undertaking the search, Anthea Carew and Brian Dean Paul showed up, followed shortly afterwards by Brenda.

It appeared that Anthea had been trying to purchase cocaine for her friend, who, she alleged, was suffering from opiate withdrawal sickness. She had written to the countess asking for drugs, saying the only thing that would help Brenda in this condition was 'Coc', and including a cheque in her letter.[21]

The hotel manager was very helpful to the Police, reporting to Detective Sergeant Griffey that the Countess's lifestyle was 'highly suspicious'. 'It was learned that she received frequent visits from men of effeminate appearance and very frequently did not return to the hotel until 3 or 4 in the morning'. Detectives decided to maintain close contact with Mr Davies, the hotel manager, 'who was also anxious to know exactly what mode of life the woman was living'.[22] The relationship between these professional men even extended to the hotel manager accompanying Griffey to the Police station, where the Countess was arrested on suspicion of possessing dangerous drugs. She denied, meanwhile, that the drugs, which had been found in a drawer, were hers.

The Paris Police supplied further information on Countess de Flammerecourt. Met officers learned that she was a drug trafficker who had been prosecuted after 1 kg of unspecified drugs was located in her luxurious Paris apartment. She had divorced her husband, the Count, in 1921, but had continued to use the title. The report went on:

> It is not known exactly whence this woman obtains her means of existence. Her life is very animated; she frequents night halls and night clubs in Paris with a view to meeting an occasional lover. . . . Upon the whole the information received concerning Marie Lefranc is unfavourable from every point of view. She is considered an adventuress capable of anything to gain money.[23]

Her brother also appeared to have been involved in trafficking, each having links to the Marseilles underworld, which was where their drug connections lay. The Met undertook thorough investigations, and the Countess's confiscated address book was passed to Sir Malcolm Delevingne at the Home Office Drugs Branch. However, nothing significant was uncovered, and even the possession charge had to be dropped, the Countess denying ownership of the cocaine and the Police being unable to prove otherwise.

Anthea Rosemary Carew appeared in court in September 1932, charged with attempting to procure cocaine for Brenda Dean Paul, with an additional charge of supplying Brenda with morphine. The advent of another West End drug case provoked great interest amongst the newspapers. Anthea appeared before Frederick Mead, who sent her to Holloway for a week while he pondered what to do with her. In the event, she was fined one shilling and bound over for three years, on condition that she reside at Mowbray House, a private nursing home near her mother's home in Exeter, where she would be under the care of Dr Andrew, a noted local physician. Her mother felt strongly that she would benefit from being away from London and subject to a different set of influences – she would be amongst 'friends of the right kind'.[24]

Medical men and drug-using women

As already noted, the regulations based on the Rolleston Report provided the context for the medical treatment of 'drug addicts'. These gave to medical practitioners a great deal of flexibility; a group of medical men known to the Home Office and the Police as 'script doctors' provided drugs to addicts on a generous scale and with few restrictions. Although the Rolleston Committee devised a system of tribunals under which those doctors considered to be merely pandering to their clients' vicious habits could in theory be brought under control, in practice the tribunals were not used. The Metropolitan Police, the Home Office and large numbers of medical men were thoroughly dissatisfied with the actual day-to-day treatment that addicts received under the Rolleston regulations. The clash of views led to tensions manifesting in court cases and were reported in the newspaper coverage.

Dr Frederick Stuart, a Mayfair physician and 'man of a certain age' who was involved in the Billie Carleton case spoke for Brenda in court, claiming that for a successful cure 'it is essential she should have pleasant surroundings, fresh air, good and proper food and good influence'.[25] He believed that if she were sent to prison, she might lose her mind. During her appeal against her six-month prison sentence, which 'fashionably dressed women were in court' to hear, the prison physician Dr Morton judged that 'she is in an institution where, as Kipling might have said, "Neither foes nor loving friends can hurt"'.[26] Morton defended prison treatment for addicts and argued that it was the only setting in which they were unable to obtain drugs.

Dr Morton was fairly typical of prison doctors in holding these views; however, dissatisfaction with the Rolleston apparatus among medical men was not restricted to those working in a carceral setting. There was a strong and growing feeling across the 1930s that the regulations were not sufficiently restrictive, which peaked in the 1938 Royal College of Physicians Committee on Drug Addiction[27] (Royal College of Physicians, 1938). There was a powerful eugenics component in the makeup of this committee, which was in fact initiated by a eugenics organisation, the National Council for Mental Hygiene (Hallam, 2018, pp. 123–34). Dr R. D. Gillespie, Honorary Secretary to the Council, argued in 1933 that 'the present custom of allowing drug addicts to live in the outside world with a permitted daily allowance of morphia is repugnant to the medical mind'.[28]

In 1937, the National Council for Mental Hygiene approached the Royal College of Physicians proposing they set up a Committee to examine this issue, which they did. The eugenicists on the Committee included Lord Dawson of Penn (the King's physician) and Sir William Willcox (senior medical consultant to the Home Office), each of whom had been involved at various points with the treatment of Brenda Dean Paul. The eugenicists advocated rapid withdrawal, compulsion and institutional confinement. Dawson of Penn, their lead speaker, argued that they were dealing with a population that had 'one foot in crime and one in pathology'.[29]

Addicts were viewed as a part of the unfit, a 'standing army of biological misfits', and these views were represented in the national press, again mediating expert discourses of drugs and drug users. One aspect debated by the Committee was whether to focus solely on addicts or to extend their proposals to the entire population of biological misfits. Those seeking the confinement of addicts wished to incarcerate solely on the ground of addiction – the subject of this process would not need to have committed any crime under the law. This was what rendered the programme legally controversial. Russel Brain, who would later chair Committees on drugs in the 1960s, emerged as the leading dissenter on the 1938 Committee and submitted a minority report contesting the views in the official Report.[30]

More broadly, medicine did much to associate women with drugs. Young women were the symbolic focus of American consumerism, another facet of modernity that drove anxieties in interwar Britain; the drug scene may be understood as a monstrous form of consumerism, associated with its dreams and desires and the loss of control it perpetually threatened. As noted by Dr Robert Armstrong Jones:

> It is also known that women yield more readily to the love of luxury, excitement, and pleasure, than men do, thus becoming more self-indulgent, and in consequence flying to sedatives in order to cope more readily with the artificial pleasures of social life.
>
> (Armstrong Jones, 1915)

And, according to Sir William Willcox:

> In some cases, especially amongst women of the underworld, cocaine and heroin are taken commonly as snuff, with the idea that transitory mental brilliance and attractiveness are produced. Prostitution and sexual vice are closely associated with drug addiction. Thus, cocaine may in the early stages of addiction have an erotic effect, and there is evidence that it is an important factor in the causation of unnatural sexual vice.
>
> (Willcox, 1923, p. 1015)

'Addiction of the vicious type', he added, 'is a canker to be stamped out' (Willcox, 1923, p. 1015).

Conclusion: panic and the modern girls

The dangerous class of young women among the vicious addicts of the 1920s and 1930s became representatives of oncoming modernity, and in multiple ways engendered and embodied the anxieties of the years between the twentieth century's two global wars. Symbolic of multifaceted social change and the ontological insecurity it produced, they shared destabilising characteristics with the dangerous drugs the young women consumed. It was a heady mixture, drugs already possessing associations with the oriental, the dark, the promiscuous mixture of races and cultures that established authorities found so disconcerting.

What Overy identifies as 'morbid culture' represents, I argue, the anxieties and tensions provoked by the social changes involved in the advent of twentieth-century modernity – the manifestation of insecurities concerning the self and society, which were changing in unforeseen ways. These included a new confidence and assertiveness amongst young women, especially around sexuality and dress; the growth of the use of drugs, the immigration of foreigners, particularly of the dark variety; the emergence of jazz and new musical forms alongside modernism in art and literature. This was enough to initiate fear and alarm amongst those who supported, and were supported by, the old order in terms of class, race, sexuality, gender, age and culture.

This ontological insecurity can be seen in the archive evidence of the Metropolitan Police and the Home Office deployed in the foregoing text. The focus of detectives on the lifestyles and choices of these people is clear and, despite the law, drugs appear to be subsidiary aspects of Police enquiries. Women were the focus of Police action and prosecutions – specifically young women – and were the representatives of the drug culture in newspaper reporting. The discursive mechanisms that established them as dangerous, vicious and declassé were primarily the police and court authorities, the medical profession (especially addiction specialists) and the newspapers, which mediated the phenomena into popular narrative, threat and glamour. Drugs have continued to occupy this symbolic role, and amidst the play of representation have connoted and distributed images of social risk into our own time.

Notes

1 Parliamentary intelligence. *The Lancet*, August 13th, 1921, p. 368.
2 Ibid.
3 Ibid.
4 Ibid.
5 The National Archives. MEPO 3/2579 Brenda Dean Paul Drug Addict: Activities and Associates, 1931–1963.
6 The National Archives. MEPO 3/2579, February 16th, 1931.
7 Ibid.
8 Ibid.
9 Vorticism was a short-lived modernist movement in British art and poetry of the early twentieth century, partly inspired by Cubism.
10 The National Archives. MEPO 3/2579, May 23rd, 1931.

11 Ibid.
12 The National Archives. MEPO 3/2579, November 18th, 1931.
13 Ibid.
14 Miss Paul's drug mania: Three years' supervision. *Daily Mail*, December 7th, 1931.
15 The National Archives. MEPO 3/2579 CID Memorandum, May 10th, 1932.
16 The National Archives. MEPO 3/2579 letter from AC to BDP, August 20th, 1932.
17 Drug charges: Miss Brenda Paul convicted: Remands without imprisonment. *The Times*, September 6th, 1932.
18 Brenda Dean Paul sentenced: Girl fails to appear in court: Sentence of six months imprisonment. *Daily Express*, October 4th, 1932.
19 Ibid.
20 The National Archives. MEPO 3/2579 Postcard to Mr Griffith Jones.
21 The National Archives. MEPO 3/2579, CID Memorandum, April 4th, 1932.
22 Ibid.
23 The National Archives. MEPO 3/2579, 'Paris 15 October 1932 NOTE'.
24 Brenda Dean Paul's friend: Fined one shilling; mother's undertaking to magistrate. *Yorkshire Post*, September 9th, 1932.
25 Brenda Paul – Another chance. *Daily Mirror*, September 6th, 1932.
26 New life for Brenda Paul: From prison to Surrey nursing home. *Daily Mirror*, November 12th, 1932.
27 Royal College of Physicians. 1938 MS5911, *Minutes of the Committee on Drug Addiction*.
28 Mental hygiene: Doctor critics of legal procedure. *Edinburgh Evening News*, November 25th, 1933.
29 Royal College of Physicians. *Minutes of the Committee on Drug Addiction* meeting held on January 18th, 1938.
30 Minutes of the Committee on Drug Addiction memorandum from Dr Russell Brain undated.

References

Armstrong Jones, R. 1915. Drug addiction in relation to mental disorder. *British Journal of Inebriety* 12 (3), January.

Balfour, P. 1933. *Society Racket: A Critical Survey of Modern Social Life*. London: John Lang.

Cannadine, D. 1996. *The Decline and Fall of the British Aristocracy*. London: PaperMac.

Carew, D. 1974. *A Fragment of Friendship: Evelyn Waugh as a Young Man*. London: Everest Books Ltd.

Cocks, H. 2007. Modernity and modernism. In: Carnevali, F., and Strange, J.M. (Eds.), *20th Century Britain: Economic, Cultural and Social Change*. Harlow: Pearson, pp. 26–41.

Davenport Hines, R. 2001. *The Pursuit of Oblivion: A Global History of Narcotics 1500–2000*. London: Weidenfeld and Nicholson.

Dean Paul, B. 1935. *My First Life: A Biography*. London: Dent.

Departmental Committee on Morphine and Heroin Addiction. 1926. *Report*. London: HMSO.

Dyhouse, C. 2013. *Girl Trouble: Panic and Progress in the History of Young Women*. London: Zed Books.

Fussell, P. 1975. *The Great War and Modern Memory*. Oxford: Oxford University Press.

Green, M. 1992. *Children of the Sun: A Narrative of English Decadence After 1918*. London: Pimlico (first published 1976).

Gundle, S. 2008. *Glamour: A History*. Oxford: Oxford University Press.

Hall, L.A. 2012. *Sex, Gender and Social Change in Britain Since 1880*. London: Palgrave Macmillan.

Hallam, C. 2018. *White Drug Cultures and Regulation in London 1916–1960*. London: Palgrave Macmillan.

Hoare, P. 2004. Paul, Brenda Irene Isabelle Frances Theresa Dean (1907–1959). *Oxford Dictionary of National Biography*. Oxford: Oxford University Press.

Kohn, M. 1992. *Dope Girls: The Birth of the British Drug Underground*. London: Lawrence and Wishart.

Light, A. 2013. *Forever England: Femininity, Literature and Conservatism between the Wars*. London: Routledge.

Mackerell, J. 2015. *Flappers: Six Women of a Dangerous Generation*. London: Palgrave Macmillan.

Overy, R. 2010. *The Morbid Age: Britain and the Crisis of Civilisation 1919–1959*. London: Penguin.

Playfair, G. 1969. *Six Studies in Hypocrisy*. London: Secker and Warburg.

Spear, B., and Mott, J. 2002. *Heroin Addiction, Care and Control: The British System*. London: Drugscope.

Taylor, D.J. 2007. *Bright Young People: The Rise and Fall of a Generation 1918–1940*. London: Chatto and Windus.

Tinkler, P. 2006. *Smoke Signals: Women, Smoking and Visual Culture*. Oxford: Berg.

Welshman, J. 2013. *Underclass: A History of the Excluded Since 1880*. London: Bloomsbury.

Willcox, W. 1923. Norman Kerr memorial lecture on drug addiction: Delivered before the society for the study of inebriety October 9. *British Medical Journal* 2 (3283, December 1, 1923), pp. 1013–18.

5 Drinking in pregnancy
Shifting towards the 'precautionary principle'

Betsy Thom, Rachel Herring and Emma Milne

Introduction

Debate rages both in academic circles and in the media over communicating messages to the public regarding alcohol consumption during pregnancy. Do women need accurate information enabling them to decide about the risks of alcohol consumption or is it better to send simple messages that tell them what they must do? This chapter considers how research-based evidence is translated into risk communications through three key mechanisms: 'official' publications and guidance issued by government departments or health authorities; websites run by advocacy groups and midwives at the front line in delivering advice to women. The focus is on the UK, and, to a lesser extent, other countries (the United States, Australia, New Zealand), where the 'risk narrative' around drinking in pregnancy and pressures towards adopting the 'precautionary principle' have emerged and strengthened over recent decades. Used initially in the context of environmental risk, there is no one definition of the 'precautionary principle'. It is generally applied in situations where there is uncertainty or lack of clarity regarding the evidence for policy action and is intended to avoid policy stagnation (ILGRA, 2002).

The chapter is based on literature sources, on analysis of policy documents in the UK and on an analysis of the website of one major international advocacy group. We recognise the value of adopting a feminist critique to examine issues around drinking in pregnancy; but this is available elsewhere (e.g. Ettorre, 1992, 1997). Rather we draw on framing theory as our conceptual framework as this allows us to examine how different strands of action and different groups of stakeholders have increasingly come together to create a 'risk narrative' around alcohol consumption in pregnancy that sits uneasily with available evidence but, through the adoption of the 'precautionary principle', has gained a dominant position in informing policy and practice.

Concern over drinking in pregnancy is not new. In past centuries there was awareness of the possible effects of alcohol consumption on reproduction (Sclare, 1980). Alcohol consumption has frequently been seen to threaten women's traditional gender roles and the social status quo or to result in a declining birth rate, unhealthy children and the 'degeneracy of the race' (Warner, 2003; Ziegler, 2008). By the mid-twentieth century, amid changing social conditions and rapid changes in women's social roles, increasing drinking problems were seen as 'the ransom of emancipation' (Shaw, 1980, p. 19). At this time, understanding of the possible effects of heavy drinking during pregnancy was still uncertain although improving; but 'Such uncertainty has not deterred some individuals with a sense of evangelical purpose from engaging in petulant political campaigns for instantaneous governmental action regarding this hazard' (Sclare, 1980). Moreover, as Jessup and Green (1987) pointed out, the most stigmatised female user was the pregnant woman. So, women were again the focus of activist attention. By the end of the twentieth century, evidence for the existence of foetal alcohol syndrome (FAS) was generally accepted, but by now a debate had emerged around the wider concept of foetal alcohol spectrum disorders (FASD). Crowe's *Fatal Link* (2008) presented the 'undeniable connection' between brain damage from prenatal exposure to alcohol and school shootings while on the opposite side, Emily Oster (*Expecting Better*, 2013), part of an emerging group of (largely middle class) critics, argued that gardening was more dangerous than food or alcohol consumption, due to an increased risk of toxoplasmosis which could be contacted from cat faeces. Thus, examination of FAS and FASD must be seen within the context of wider gender- based discourses on alcohol consumption at any particular historical period and with regard to the different ways in which 'risk' is framed and communicated.

From FAS to FASD

Knowledge of FAS is generally traced back to a publication by Jones and Smith (1973), who coined the term 'foetal alcohol syndrome'. But there had been prior observation and discussion concerning the possible deleterious effects of maternal transmission of viruses such as herpes, of syphilis, of the effects of maternal rubella in pregnancy, of the use of drugs such as heroin and of prescribed medication – fuelled by the thalidomide tragedy in 1961 (Sclare, 1980). As Saunders (2009) notes, there was also some work on the transmission of alcohol to the foetus; a study by Lemoine and colleagues in France provided a clinical description of 127 children born to predominantly alcoholic mothers (Lemoine et al., 1968). But it was the work of Jones and Smith that opened a wave of interest and research on the effects of alcohol consumption in pregnancy. Reviewing knowledge on FAS, Sclare documented the following essential features: growth deficiency, abnormalities of the head and face, brain deficiency, associated features (a range of physical abnormalities) (Sclare, 1980, p. 60) and concluded that 'A substantial body of evidence from clinical sources and animal experimentation has now accumulated to suggest that a characteristic set of physical and mental defects, known as the foetal alcohol syndrome (FAS), may occur in the infants of alcoholic mothers' (Sclare, 1980, p. 64). However, he also pointed out that there were still uncertainties regarding what quantity of alcohol, over what time period and at what point in the pregnancy it might be harmful.

Following the work of Jones and Smith, the concept and diagnosis of FAS underwent rapid refinement and enlargement (Benz et al., 2009). 'Foetal alcohol effects' were introduced to describe behavioural and cognitive effects in the absence of full FAS symptoms but its clinical imprecision meant that it was not adopted for longer term. By 1996, five separate classes of prenatal alcohol effects had been distinguished by the United States Institute of Medicine; but Benz et al. (2009) comment that the IOM guidelines consisted of vague categories that did not clearly define the diagnostic criteria used and led to an inconsistent approach across clinics. Subsequent amendments to the classification in 1997, 1999, 2004 and 2005 and the development of the Canadian diagnostic criteria in 2005 attempted to improve diagnostic precision (Benz et al., 2009). By 2004, extensive discussion and collaboration resulted in a consensus definition of FASD:

> FASD is an umbrella term describing the range of effects that can occur in an individual whose mother drank alcohol during pregnancy. These effects include physical, mental, behavioral, and/or learning disabilities with possible lifelong implications. The term FASD encompasses all other diagnostic terms, such as FAS, and is not intended for use as a clinical diagnosis.
>
> (Williams et al., 2015, p. e1396)

As the quotation highlights, FASD is not a discrete category and is not intended as a clinical diagnosis; it remains, therefore, open to interpretation and debate.

There is little disagreement with the message that 'heavy' drinking during pregnancy carries a significant risk of FAS or a degree of harm to the foetus, especially during the first nine weeks of pregnancy (Striessguth and O'Malley, 2000; British Medical Association, 2007). But, as is seen in the following sections, opinions differ regarding consumption of low to moderate amounts of alcohol during pregnancy and there is no consensus on what constitutes a low risk. In the absence of conclusive evidence on the effects of low to moderate alcohol consumption on the foetus, the 'precautionary principle' is adopted by many health and advocacy organisations. Women are advised to abstain from alcohol when pregnant and, in some cases, abstinence is also advised when trying to conceive. In the following sections, we will look at three examples of how the evidence on drinking in pregnancy is interpreted and conveyed to the public – in 'official' policy and guidance documents, in advocacy group advice and by midwives in their day-to-day encounters with pregnant women.

Framing 'risk': from moral to medical to public health model?

It is only within recent decades that the rationale for advice on drinking in pregnancy shifted from a predominantly moral or Eugenic model towards an evidence-based, medical model and then a public health model (Lowe and Lee, 2010). This is reflected in recent advice to women on drinking during pregnancy. O'Leary and colleagues (2007), for example, examined policy in seven English-speaking countries, including guidelines from relevant medical, nursing and non-professional sources. They found that policies could be grouped into three categories: those that recommend abstinence alone; those that recommend abstinence as the safest choice but also indicate that small amounts of alcohol are unlikely to cause harm; those that advise that a low alcohol intake poses a low risk to the foetus. Most of the guidelines stated that they were based on evidence from literature reviews. Despite the variation in advice documented by O'Leary et al., the perception that there is insufficient evidence to conclude that any level of alcohol consumption during pregnancy is low risk has led to the wider application of the 'precautionary principle' and the message that pregnant women (in some sources including women intending to become pregnant) should abstain from alcohol. As Low and Lee (2010) among others argue, given that the evidence base for the advice to pregnant women is unclear and contested regarding the consumption of low/moderate levels of alcohol, messages based on the 'precautionary principle' reflect a new construction of 'risk' because it formalises a connection between uncertainty and danger. Thus, alcohol consumption during pregnancy has become framed in terms of risk and danger to the foetus – a frame that is promoted through some channels and contested in others. When we look more closely at these shifts – as we do in the following – we see that the moral model persists, in some form or other, across frame shifts.

Framing the issue: what the scientific research tells us

The evidence for risk from drinking during pregnancy that is cited as the basis of policy and public health communication derives from research that uses a range of study designs and measures to investigate the possible short-term and longer-term effects of maternal alcohol consumption on the foetus and the development of the child. These studies reflect a particular construction of 'risk', which is not necessarily shared even within the research community. Indeed, for many years, feminist researchers have argued that whether or not women are at risk during pregnancy, they are stigmatised and pathologised by the body of literature on the foetal alcohol syndrome (Gomberg, 1979; Ettorre, 1992). Moreover, how 'risk' is constructed and interpreted from research findings may not reflect how it is interpreted and acted upon by pregnant women, by different social groups, by relevant health professionals and by the general public.

There is a large literature on the effects of alcohol on the foetus; but in this chapter we will focus on findings from reviews and longitudinal studies, on the assumption that the latter are the best way to research longer-term effects.

Reviews and longitudinal studies

A main finding from the existing body of work is that there is little evidence of harm from maternal low/moderate levels of alcohol consumption.

In a review of 24 prospective studies and two quasi-experimental studies, Mamluk et al. (2017) concluded that evidence of harm arising from drinking 32 g a week or less (up to two UK units of alcohol up to twice a week) compared with no alcohol was sparse. The review found some increased risk of babies being born SGA (small for gestational age) but little direct evidence of any other detrimental effect. The authors also noted the lack of research and evidence regarding possible benefits of light alcohol consumption versus abstinence. Considering the implications of the review findings, the authors suggest that

> The recently proposed change in the guidelines for alcohol use in pregnancy in the UK to complete abstinence would be an application of the precautionary principle. . . . For some, the evidence of the potential for harm – mostly coming from animal experiments and human studies of effects due to higher levels of exposure will be sufficient to advocate that guidelines should advise women to avoid all alcohol in pregnancy, while others will wish to retain the existing wording of guidelines.
>
> (Mamluk et al., 2017, pp. 11–12)

An earlier systematic review by Henderson et al. (2007) of research conducted between 1970 and 2005 also found no significant effects of drinking up to 12 g a day on miscarriage, stillbirth, intrauterine growth restriction, prematurity, birth weight, SGA at birth or birth defects including FAS.

The risk of long-term effects appearing as the child grows older has been much debated. But again, the results from prospective studies have not established a clear link between maternal alcohol consumption in pregnancy and problems emerging up until the child is 7 years old. For instance, two large, longitudinal follow-up studies, one from the UK and one from Denmark, found no increased risk of socio-emotional difficulties, cognitive deficits or executive functioning in children at age 5 and when followed up at age 7.

In the UK study (Kelly et al., 2010, 2013), women were grouped into five categories: never drinker (teetotallers); not in pregnancy; light, not more than 1–2 units per week or per occasion; moderate, not more than 3–6 units per week or 3–5 units per occasion; heavy/binge, 7 or more units per week or 6 or more units per occasion. At age 5 years (Kelly et al., 2010), children born to mothers who drank up to one to two drinks per week or per occasion during pregnancy were not at increased risk of clinically relevant behavioural difficulties or cognitive deficits compared with children of mothers grouped as not-in-pregnancy. These results were confirmed at 7 years old. Kelly et al. (2013) reported that low levels of alcohol consumption during pregnancy are not linked to behavioural or cognitive problems during early to mid-childhood.

The Danish study (Skogerbø et al., 2012), which also examined a large cohort of women and children, found no significant effects of low to moderate alcohol consumption on executive functioning at the age of five years. The definition of 'a drink' followed the definition from the Danish National Board of Health, with one standard drink being equal to 12 g of pure alcohol. Low drinking was defined as the consumption of between one and four drinks per week, and moderate drinking was defined as the consumption of between five and eight drinks per week. Despite the results of the study, the authors concluded that

> Even though this study observed no consistent effects of low to moderate levels of prenatal alcohol exposure on executive functioning at the age of

5 years, and only unsystematic and insignificant associations were found for binge drinking, alcohol is a known teratogen, and safe levels of alcohol use during pregnancy have not yet been established. Consequently, women should be advised that it is safest to abstain from using alcohol when pregnant.

(Skogerbø et al., 2012, p. 9)

It is, perhaps, not surprising that this public health caveat was proposed in the conclusion of the Danish paper because the research was supported by the US Centers for Disease Control and Prevention (CDC) and the authors were based in public health institutions. Researchers, especially those in the public health field, tend to adhere to the zero risk frame in their conclusions even though they report mixed attitudes and behaviours among their study respondents and a lack of evidence for harm from low levels of consumption. It is, however, but one example of how the 'precautionary principle' has succeeded in becoming a dominant influence in conveying academic findings into the public arena. Risk continues to be present even in the absence of evidence. As Brown and Trickey (2018, p. 4) note with respect to the UK guidelines, the precautionary principle 'contrasts with the informed choice approach that underpins alcohol advice for the general population', and they conclude that, 'it does appear that the underpinning rationalisation in relation to pregnancy is values-based rather than evidence-led' (Brown and Trickey, 2018, p. 14). In the next section, we look at how this is manifest in official policy and guidelines.

Frames in official guidance and policy

Two key themes can be identified from an assessment of the official guidance and policy issued by the British Government, medical councils and health authorities between 2000 and 2018: (1) risk and uncertainty, and movement from foetus to baby and (2) employment of the ideology of the 'good' mother.

Risk and uncertainty

Guidance from all sources begins from the basic principle that there is risk and uncertainty attached to drinking in pregnancy. All sources acknowledge that the impact of low-level drinking on the foetus is generally unknown or believed to be limited. Nevertheless, the guidance remains that women should not drink any alcohol while pregnant. For example, the National Institute for Clinical Excellence (NICE) who provide guidance, advice and information services for health, public health and social care professionals produced the following guidance in 2008, which continues to be their advice as of October 2018:

Pregnant women and women planning a pregnancy should be advised to avoid drinking alcohol in the first 3 months of pregnancy if possible because it may be associated with an increased risk of miscarriage.

If women choose to drink alcohol during pregnancy they should be advised to drink no more than 1 to 2 UK units once or twice a week (1 unit equals half a pint of ordinary strength lager or beer, or one shot [25 ml] of spirits. One small [125 ml] glass of wine is equal to 1.5 UK units). Although there is uncertainty regarding a safe level of alcohol consumption in pregnancy, at this low level there is no evidence of harm to the unborn baby (National Institute for Health and Care Excellence).

(NICE, 2008, p. 15)

A similar message is communicated by the British Medical Association (BMA) who have advocated since 2007, when they first published guidance about foetal alcohol spectrum disorder, that 'Women who are pregnant, or who are considering a pregnancy, should be advised not to consume any alcohol' (British Medical Association [BMA], 2007, p. 12). In their updated guidance, the BMA recognised that the evidence for harm from low-to-moderate levels of alcohol consumption is inconclusive. Nevertheless, it is advised that the safest option for women is abstinence from any alcohol (BMA, 2016, p. 21).

Significantly, within sources of guidance, a shift towards advocating abstinence can be witnessed. At the turn of the millennium, the official guidance provided by the Chief Medical Officer (CMO) was that in order

to minimise risk to the developing fetus, women who are trying to become pregnant or are at any stage of pregnancy, should not drink more than 1 or 2 units of alcohol once or twice a week, and should avoid episodes of intoxication.

(Department of Health [DoH], 1995, p. 27)

Such guidance was provided with recognition 'that alcohol consumption (other than at very low levels) is associated with particular risks to fetal and early infant development' (DoH, 1995, p. 24). This guidance was overhauled in 2016, with the publication of new guidelines from the CMO. The new guidance acknowledged that the risks were low if only small amounts of alcohol had been consumed before the pregnancy was known, but stated:

If you are pregnant or planning a pregnancy, the safest approach is not to drink alcohol at all, to keep risks to your baby to a minimum.

Drinking in pregnancy can lead to long-term harm to the baby, with the more you drink the greater the risk.

(DoH, 2016a, p. 27)

Such 'shifts' in guidance can also be seen in medical bodies (with the exception of the BMA who have always advocated abstinence). For example, the Royal College of Obstetrics and Gynaecology (RCOG) stated in 1999:

There is no conclusive evidence of adverse effects in either growth or IQ at levels of consumption below 120 gms. (15 units) per week. Nonetheless, it is recommended that women should be careful about alcohol consumption in pregnancy and limit this to no more than one standard drink per day.

(RCOG, 1999, p. 3)

By 2006, the guidance was modified to advise that 'The safest approach in pregnancy is to choose not to drink at all', but that 'Small amounts of alcohol during pregnancy (not more than one to two units, not more than once or twice a week) have not been shown to be harmful' (RCOG, 2006, p. 1).

A similar message was presented in 2015 (RCOG, 2015), but this guidance was removed from the public domain following the updated guidance from the CMO and was replaced in 2018 with the following message:

> The safest approach is not to drink alcohol at all if you are pregnant, if you think you could become pregnant or if you are breastfeeding.
> Although the risk of harm to the baby is low with small amounts of alcohol before becoming aware of the pregnancy, there is no 'safe' level of alcohol to drink when you are pregnant.
>
> (RCOG, 2018, p. 1)

The key element across the guidance is that while there is uncertainty about the impact of low-level drinking on pregnancy and the development of the foetus, no risk is acceptable, and thus a woman should not drink any alcohol while pregnant.

From 'foetus' to 'baby' and the 'good' mother

Language is an important mechanism in how issues are framed and communicated. A notable development in the guidance across time is the movement from talking about the impact of drinking alcohol on the 'foetus' to discussion of impact on the 'baby'. Such developments can be seen to happen in conjunction with the movement from talking about 'pregnant women'/'women who are pregnant' to 'mothers'. The clearest example of this development can be seen in the Government guidance. The CMO guidance published in 1995 advocated 'women who are trying to get pregnant or are at any stage of pregnancy' should drink no more than 1 or 2 units of alcohol once or twice a week 'to minimise risk to the developing *fetus*' (emphasis added, DoH, 1995, p. 27). The guidance published in 2007 was that 'Pregnant women or women trying to conceive' should not drink alcohol, but if they do, they should not drink more than 1–2 units once or twice a week 'to protect the *baby*' (emphasis added, HMG, 2007, p. 3). Between these publications, there is a change from 'foetus' to 'baby', but the woman continues to be referred to as a woman who is pregnant. In the latest guidelines published in 2016, the subject that the advice is targeted at (women who may be pregnant) is presented in direct connection to her foetus, who is now referred to as 'your baby':

> If *you* are pregnant or planning a pregnancy, the safest approach is not to drink alcohol at all, to keep risks to *your baby* to a minimum.
>
> (emphasis added, DoH, 2016a, p. 27)

This subtle shift in language frames a woman who is pregnant as having a direct impact on the foetus, with the suggestion being that she would want to avoid drinking alcohol, as this is the motherly thing to do in order to ensure protection for the child. The guidance is now framed by talking specifically to her, rather than general guidance for the population.

Such a message became even more prominent in the final version of the guidance approved by the Government:

> If *you* are pregnant or think *you* could become pregnant, the safest approach is not to drink alcohol at all, to keep risks to *your baby* to a minimum.
>
>   (emphasis added, DoH, 2016b, p. 26)

Here, the focus has moved from women planning to become pregnant to any woman who thinks she could become pregnant. In reality, this is any woman who is of reproductive age, as public health messages, rightly, advise that no contraception is 100 per cent reliable (National Health Service, 2017), unless she knows that she is unable to get pregnant, such as due to undergoing a hysterectomy. The message also has the impact of advocating that women choose between drinking alcohol and having sex – a choice that is not asked of men, despite suggestions that alcohol impacts the quality of sperm and thus potentially the health of the foetus (Ouko et al., 2009). Thus, framing alcohol consumption as a 'risk' can be seen as a mechanism for exercising control over women's autonomy.

More pronounced connection between not drinking and being a 'good' mother is evident in presentation of advice on the National Health Service (NHS) website, which provides a 'comprehensive health information service' that 'help[s readers] make the best choices about [their] health and lifestyle' (NHS, 2018). The guidelines are, expectedly, in line with the Government's publication in 2016: 'the safest approach is not to drink alcohol at all to keep risks to your baby to a minimum' (NHS Choice, 2017). However, as the guidance goes on to discuss the impact on the foetus if a woman has drunk alcohol in the early stages of pregnancy before knowing she was pregnant, the framing of the message changes:

> Women who find out they're pregnant after already having drunk in early pregnancy should avoid further drinking.
>
>   However, they should not worry unnecessarily, as the risks of their baby being affected are likely to be low.
>
>   (NHS Choice, 2017)

By shifting from referring to the pregnant woman in the second person when suggesting abstinence to referring to her in the third person when advising not drinking alcohol, there is an implicit message that the 'good' woman/mother will know she was pregnant or might be pregnant and will not have consumed alcohol. It is only 'other' women, and thus 'bad' women/mothers, who would have consumed alcohol and thus put *their baby* at risk.

Increasingly, therefore, official advice has moved towards the 'precaution-ary principle' framing while recognising that the evidence base for the advice is unclear. The question arises – how did this happen and what influenced this shift? Advocacy action is one source of influence on government and in the next section we look at the work of the National Organisation on Foetal Alcohol Syndrome (NOFAS) as an example of how an advocacy group frames research evidence and conveys it to the public and how this may be one important influence on the government response. There are other advocacy groups and they do not all frame women's alcohol consumption in the same way; for example, National Advocates for Pregnant Women (NAPW) in the United States (Ettorre and Campbell, 2011; NAPW, n.d.) and British Pregnancy Advisory Group in the UK (BPAS n.d.) take a very different approach to that of NOFAS. However, we have chosen NOFAS as it is perhaps the most prominent and internationally influential organisation and it has successfully promoted its particular message on alcohol consumption in pregnancy.

The National Organisation on Foetal Alcohol Syndrome (NOFAS): an advocacy frame

Framing the issue and the solution

The US-based NOFAS is a not-for-profit organisation which declares its mission:

> NOFAS works to prevent prenatal exposure to alcohol, drugs, and other substances known to harm fetal development by raising awareness and sup-porting women before and during their pregnancy, and supports individu-als, families, and communities living with Fetal Alcohol Spectrum Disorders (FASDs) and other preventable intellectual/developmental disabilities.
>
> (NOFAS, 2017)

NOFAS advocates abstinence in the preconception period and throughout the pregnancy, with this message encapsulated in the strap lines on their digital and written materials: 'Prenatal Alcohol Exposure. No safe amount. No safe time. No safe alcohol. Period' and 'Play it Safe. Alcohol & Pregnancy Don't Mix' (NOFAS, n.d., a). This clear abstinence message is also delivered by the numerous affiliate organisations throughout the world. NOFAS-UK states:

> The best thing a woman can do for her unborn baby is to avoid alcohol at all stages of pregnancy and whilst trying to conceive.
>
> (NOFAS-UK, 2018a)

Thus, the message that NOFAS wants organisations to unify around and spread is one of abstinence in the preconception period and throughout the pregnancy.

NOFAS also suggests reasons why women continue to drink in pregnancy. In an undated position statement, on the EU FASD Alliance website, entitled 'Drinking during pregnancy – who is responsible?' it is claimed that 'up to 50% or more of women may drink during pregnancy' (EU FASD Alliance n.d., a). A range of reasons are offered, including confusion due to inconsistent and conflicting advice given by health professionals or contained in media articles, unawareness of pregnancy in the early stages particularly if unplanned ('many' pregnancies are described as unplanned), 'addiction' to alcohol and alcohol advertising which portrays fun and friendship as intricately linked with drinking alcohol (EU FASD Alliance, n.d., a). The appropriate response is seen as provision of awareness and education and support for those who have consumed alcohol before the pregnancy was known, but also action to counter advertising alcohol as fun and to ensure that messages on the harm associated with alcohol consumption are clearly conveyed. Coalitions and networks are crucial to national and international advocacy organisations in order to disseminate a unified message – in this case that no alcohol should be consumed during pregnancy. A strong advocacy network has evolved around this framing of the issue.

The advocacy network

NOFAS was established in 1990 with the aim of promoting research and awareness of FAS by Patti Munter whose interest was rooted in her work with Native American people living on reservations (NOFAS, 2014, 2017). NOFAS was established during what Armstrong and Abel (2000, p. 276) describe as a period in the United States when FAS went from being 'an unrecognised condition to a moral panic', with the high level of concern not reflecting the evidence on prevalence or impact. They suggest that FAS rapidly became seen as a 'social problem' as it resonated with broader social concerns about the harmful impact of alcohol on American society and a perceived increase in child neglect and abuse. The NOFAS Affiliate Network was established in 2002 in order to 'unite organisations in an international coalition with the purpose of preventing FASD and meeting the needs of people living with the disorders while each member organization maintains its identity and autonomy' (NOFAS, n.d., b). The stated objectives are 'to open lines of communication among FASD organizations, share resources, unify core values, messages and priorities, and increase advocacy for FASD recognition and investment' (NOFAS, n.d., b).

With three types of membership Affiliates, FAS Resource Organisations and NOFAS Partners, the network reaches across a large number of organisations. Affiliates are autonomous, independent organisations that are described as 'usually the most familiar with FASD resources in their state or location' (NOFAS, n.d., b), they are primarily US based; only 3 of the 34 Affiliate organisations are not American (Australia, the UK and Ukraine). FASD Resource Organisations have an interest in FASD and offer resources such as information but are not active members of NOFAS and currently all are US based. NOFAS Partners are organisations with which NOFAS has 'official and unofficial' partnerships and includes government agencies, practitioners and societies – for example, the Centers for Disease Control and Prevention (CDC), National Institute on Alcohol Abuse and

Alcoholism (NIAA) and American College of Obstetricians and Gynaecologists (ACOG) (NOFAS, n.d., b).

The European (EU) FASD Alliance, which is a non-profit international member organisation registered in Sweden, was founded in February 2011 'to meet the growing need for European professionals and NGOs concerned with FASD to share ideas and work together' (EU FASD Alliance, n.d., b). The impetus to establish the EU FASD Alliance came from the First European Conference on FASD held in the Netherlands in 2010 and organised by the FAS Foundation of Netherlands (EU FASD Alliance, 2012). There were 160 delegates from 23 countries; since then conferences have been held every two years, with 275 people attending the 2016 conference in London (EU FASD Alliance, 2018). The Alliance's stated aims are to support its member associations to improve the quality of life for all people with FASD and their families/carers; to increase awareness of the risks of drinking alcoholic beverages during pregnancy; to act as a 'liaison centre' through the dissemination of information, encouragement of knowledge exchange and transfer between national associations; the development of new national FASD Associations; and by fostering international collaboration on research studies (EU FASD Alliance, n.d., b). The EU FASD Alliance is governed by a Board comprising members from across Europe, supported by a Scientific Advisory Council (experts from across Europe) and a Council of Lifelong Experts (adults with FASD). Membership has grown from 9 members to at least 25 members (latest available report is the 2015–2016 Annual Report, EU FASD Alliance, 2016).

These networks operate, therefore, at all spatial levels – local, regional, national and international – and key players within the FASD advocacy networks include a wide range of stakeholders – parents (adoptive, birth and foster) of children with FASD, professionals working with individuals with FASD, in particular psychologists, child and adolescent psychiatrists, intellectual disability psychiatrists, special needs educationalists and practice- and policy-relevant organisations. The activity of NOFAS-UK is illustrative of how a consistent framing of the issue and its solution is disseminated and used to gain policy attention both through working with relevant stakeholder groups such as professionals and parents and by direct action aimed at policy-makers.

NOFAS-UK: conveying the message and stimulating action

NOFAS-UK is a registered charity, founded in 2003 by Susan Fleischer, an American living in the UK and the adoptive mother of a child with FAS (NOFAS-UK, 2018b). Susan Fleischer was Chief Executive Officer (CEO) of NOFAS-UK until 2016 and her successor Sandra Butler is a foster carer of a child with FAS. NOFAS-UK are a founding member of the FASD UK Alliance which is a coalition of support groups for those affected by FASD (birth and adoptive parents, carers, individuals living with FASD, families) and of interested individuals. FASD UK Alliance and NOFAS-UK co-administer a closed Facebook group (FASD UK Facebook Support) and also one for professionals.

NOFAS-UK undertakes three distinct strands of activity, which are illustrative of the overall approach of the network.

Firstly, they provide training and educational materials for professionals (e.g. health, social care, teachers), the general public (in particular, pregnant women) and for carers of individuals with FASD (e.g. foster, birth and adoptive parents). Awareness and training are delivered to different target groups in a number of ways:

- films and leaflets targeting specific audiences (e.g. midwives, GPs, pregnant women) – highlighting that the information leaflets for midwives and GPs have been 'reviewed' by the Royal College of Midwives, thereby 'legitimising' the outputs;
- Continual Professional Development (CPD) courses and conferences, including an online FASD course, adapted from the American 'FASD – The Course' using a grant from the then Alcohol Research Council (AERC, UK);
- a UK wide programme of study days for midwives which was funded by Diageo (alcohol producer) in 2011 for five years and caused considerable controversy (Mooney, 2011; IAS, 2011). All the materials and training state that there is no 'safe' level of alcohol consumption and that women should not drink alcohol when trying to conceive and throughout pregnancy. Mooney (2011) noted that the advice that midwives were being trained to give to women differed from the Department of Health's advice at the time[1] (no more than 1 or 2 units of alcohol once or twice a week and should not get drunk);
- use of the media and social media. For instance, NOFAS, NOFAS-UK and the EU FASD Alliance are all members of the 'International Campaign to Raise Awareness of the Risks of Drinking in Pregnancy'. The campaign – 'Too Young to Drink' (TYTD) – was first launched on September 9, 2014. September 9 has been declared International FAS Day and September FASD Awareness Month. A key aim is to harness social media (Facebook, Twitter and Instagram) and the Internet to 'spread coherent and univocal health messages via all media involved' (TYTD, n.d.). The campaign which is launched each year on September 9 uses strong imagery, with all campaigns featuring various images of foetuses either in alcohol bottles (wine, champagne, beer, spirits) or alcoholic drinks (with ice, bubbles, lime slice) to promote a message of 'zero alcohol in pregnancy'. The network extends across the globe and the materials are produced in seven languages.

Secondly, NOFAS-UK offers support to those affected by FASD (families, parents/carers, individuals) through the operation of a national helpline and a network of support groups for families and carers of individuals with FASD.

The third strand of activity seeks to engage and influence policy-makers more directly, in particular the British government.

One example of this is a report of a roundtable discussion, 'Our Forgotten Children: The Urgency of Aligning Policy with Guidance on the Effects of Antenatal

Exposure to Alcohol' (NOFAS-UK, 2018c). The discussion was held with FASD stakeholders, including FASD UK Alliance, in the Houses of Parliament in May 2018. It was co-chaired by Prof. Sheila the Baroness Hollins (Emeritus Professor of the Psychiatry of Disability, St George's University, London) and Bill Esterson (Member of Parliament, Chair, All Party-Parliamentary Group on FASD, set up in June 2015) and included representatives of national, regional and local support organisations, clinical and educational experts. The report makes a series of recommendations, including an urgent review of Government policy on FASD and increased training of front-line practitioners on FASD (NOFAS-UK, 2018c).

While scientific evidence is often cited as the basis for policy action, the use of experiential evidence is equally valued and well used in framing how the issue is presented and in arguing for policy attention. On behalf of the FASD UK Alliance, NOFAS-UK produced a briefing paper for policy-makers based on the experiences of FASD stakeholders. In contrast to other publications from advocacy groups, *Hear Our Voices* (FASD Alliance & NOFAS-UK, 2018) does not draw on scientific evidence; indeed, it categorically states: 'It is not scientific, it is anecdotal precisely because stakeholders are rarely brought into discussions that impact their lives and futures' (FASD Alliance & NOFAS-UK, 2018, p. 2). *Hear Our Voices* petitions the UK Parliament to ensure that the 2016 CMO guidance on alcohol and pregnancy (no alcohol) is consistently delivered across the health service and also embedded into the Personal, Social, Health and Economic (PHSE) and sex education curricula in schools (FASD Alliance & NOFAS-UK, 2018, p. 2).

Advocacy approaches are therefore consistent and widespread, framing the issue and the solution in much the same way as public health policy and guidance. As Entman suggests, the advocacy frame is employed intentionally as a tool to promote a particular definition and interpretation of reality (Entman, 1993). This is in contrast to frames that emerge and change as a result of interactions and conflicts between social actors and that are dependent on a range of different factors and contexts. We see examples of a more dynamic and shifting framing process in the findings of qualitative studies investigating how midwives and pregnant women perceive the issue of alcohol consumption in pregnancy.

Delivering the message – caught between professional 'dictates' and real life

There are a number of small qualitative research studies looking at the attitudes, beliefs and reported behaviour of midwives and other stakeholders towards alcohol consumption in pregnancy. This section considers how midwives, key figures in pregnancy care, respond to the expectation that they will deliver messages according to national guidelines on alcohol consumption during pregnancy.

Midwives tend to support the contention that women are 'confused' by messages from different sources providing variable advice and that a clear, unambiguous message is the preferred option However, very often midwives are reluctant to advise total abstinence as they are aware of the lack of good evidence for that message or feel that small amounts do no harm (Van der Wulp, 2013; Schölin et al., 2018; Crawford-Williams et al., 2015):

> I really think that *a* drink won't hurt. . . . These days everything is very extreme, they say no coffee, no alcohol etc. with limited evidence.
>
> (midwife #3, in Crawford-Williams et al., 2015, p. 332)

> When you drink two glasses of wine at Christmas or on New Year's Eve, well, that really will not do any harm.
>
> (Midwife 7, in van der Wulp, 2013, p. e94)

Although trained and expected to convey official messages, not all midwives report doing so, particularly after the first consultation (Crawford-Williams et al., 2015; Jones et al., 2011; van der Wulp et al., 2013). As individuals, they are also subject to personal frames of reference and lay understanding of appropriate behaviour when pregnant. In one study, some midwives held a different personal opinion compared to the professional advice they dispensed:

> In the back of your mind you go 'one's not gonna kill ya' but I prefer to say 'no, no drinking'.
>
> (English midwife 5, quoted in Schölin et al., 2018, p. 4)

The dilemmas faced in conveying official advice in the real world of everyday practice are also highlighted in discussions on how to respond when women say they have been drinking before they knew they were pregnant (van der Wulp, 2013). The message that drinking anything at all is a potential risk to the foetus is recognised as worrying for some women and linked to fear of being seen as a 'bad' mother (Meurk et al., 2014). Anxiety about how others will judge them is not unfounded when we consider the views of midwives regarding women who drink when pregnant. In a study comparing English and Swedish midwives, it was generally felt that, 'we should all be singing from the same hymn sheet' regarding delivering an abstinence message (Schölin et al., 2018, p. 5), and that any drinking during pregnancy could indicate an underlying alcohol problem. Comparing the risk discourses of the nine Swedish and seven English midwives interviewed, Schölin et al. (2018) reported that English midwives' views were quite nuanced and the uncertainty around the risk of drinking small amounts was mentioned. By contrast, Swedish midwives' risk discourse was binary: either women stop drinking or they continue because they have an underlying drinking problem. Similar attitudes emerged from an Australian study where some practitioners, including midwives, were of the opinion that drinking during pregnancy indicated possible mental health issues, drug use and other co-morbidities that had to be addressed (Crawford-Williams et al., 2015).

Attitudes also differ towards different segments of the target group. Pregnant teenage women were marked out in one instance as 'high risk' because they were seen as more likely to binge drink (Jones et al., 2011). In particular, midwives have been found to believe that the provision of simple messages is especially important for women with lower educational attainment and with mental health or substance use problems. This view is shared by at least some of the public. In one study, safeguarding 'vulnerable' groups featured in discussions among new parents – who did not include themselves as 'vulnerable' and were protective of their own autonomy (Brown and Trickey, 2018). A class-based interpretation of risk behaviours is not new. In the United States, for example, it is reported that even many feminists supported early-twentieth-century eugenic compulsory sterilisation laws for 'defectives' as part of a programme of class-based social control (Ziegler, 2008). Furthermore, current perceptions of risk from alcohol consumption are part of a much wider shift towards 'safeguarding' the foetus from a range of possible harms while in the womb, especially among some social groups. Lowe et al. (2015) have shown how UK policies have focused increasingly on concerns over pregnancy and the 'developing brain' and have identified 'disadvantaged women' as most at risk of suffering from stress and depression, thereby causing neurological damage to the foetus resulting in anti-social behaviour as adults. Interestingly, UK longitudinal studies (Kelly et al., 2010, 2013) suggest that women in less advantaged socio-economic situations are more likely to abstain when pregnant. They found that mothers in the 'not in pregnancy' group were more advantaged than the 'never-drinker' group but less advantaged than the 'light' drinking group. Schölin et al. (2018) also report midwives mentioning that women of higher socio-economic status disputed the abstinence advice.

These studies help to illuminate how individuals draw on evidence from different sources, apply value judgements and use cost-benefit assessments in framing the risk incurred from alcohol consumption in pregnancy and how they balance that risk against other perceived priorities. The complexity and nuances of the issues emerge well from the research and illustrate the existence of conflicting and flexible frames around both the behaviour (drinking alcohol when pregnant) and the pregnant woman.

Conclusion

This chapter has focused on how the evidence on alcohol consumption during pregnancy, in particular regarding low to moderate levels of consumption, has been interpreted and conveyed to women through three major sources of information – government policy and guidelines, online advice from advocacy sources and advice from midwives. We have shown how a strong 'risk narrative' has been created, how the framing of risk has shifted through successive versions of official communication in Britain and how advocacy and public health communication based on the 'precautionary principle' has become increasing consistent and dominant in the messages given to women.

This frame shift did not take place in a vacuum; it was closely linked to other political and social trends coming, initially, from the United States. Armstrong and Abel (2000, p. 277) locate the origins of FAS within a 'new temperance zeitgeist' and 'concern about the victimisation of children' prevailing in America in the 1970s. They argue that preventing FAS became 'an American crusade' resulting in 'moral panic' and 'biomedical entrepreneurship' that included the expansion of the diagnosis to FASD and the rise of new groups of experts. Among them were doctors and researchers with new opportunities for research funding and 'a pragmatic interest in framing the issue in terms of low thresholds' (Armstrong and Abel, 2000, p. 279). In the UK, the rise of policy and public concern over alcohol consumption in pregnancy came later. Early studies on drinking in pregnancy among 'normal' women were led by Moira Plant (1985, p. 102) who concluded that 'alcohol in moderate doses (*one or two units once or twice a week*) does not appear to cause harm' (brackets added) and advised against alarmist messages. Ten years later, the conclusion was much the same (Plant, 1997, p. 173). But the political climate in the UK was changing. The Blair–Brown's New Labour government (1997–2010) had brought in a 'puritanical, almost Cromwellian streak' (MacGregor, 1998, p. 251) which signalled the return of religion to public life, intertwined, in particular, with social welfare policy, and the moral values that activated welfare state developments (Jawad, 2012). In the alcohol field, the rise of a strong public health perspective was accompanied by increased research on public health aspects of alcohol use, the emergence and growth of advocacy activity (Thom et al., 2016) and a growth in researchers sympathetic to the public health framing of alcohol issues and public health aims regarding the necessary policy responses. Against this background, the precautionary principle fitted well within prevailing perspectives on alcohol use and alcohol-related harms (ILGRA, 2002).

The increasing normalisation of the precautionary principle regarding drinking in pregnancy reinforced perceptions of a link between alcohol consumption, other problem behaviours and health issues, and women who drink anything at all during pregnancy risk being seen as deviant and in need of care and control. Along with the 'official' drive to provide consistent messages advocating abstinence, informal forms of control and sanctions – such as enlisting partners and the general public to reinforce abstinence messages – are frequently part of research studies' recommendations for policy and practice (Crawford-Williams et al., 2015a; van der Wulp et al., 2013). As in the past, risk messages have become closely aligned with moral judgements on motherhood and the image of the 'good' mother, while the language changes noted earlier in policy documents – towards personalised, emotive messages – reflect the ethos of wider social policy towards individualised interventions and individual assumption of responsibility. At the same time, as Lee (2017) has argued, interpretation of evidence on alcohol consumption in pregnancy has spawned the belief that simple messages are needed and are in women's 'best interests'. In other words, women are required to follow the rules and their rights to choice and autonomy are denied while the responsibility for possible harm to their children rests on their shoulders alone.

Note

1 The advice was changed in January 2016 to advise women that if they were pregnant or planning a pregnancy, they should not drink alcohol at all following a review of alcohol guidelines by the UK Chief Medical Officers' (DoH, 2016a).

References

Armstrong, E., and Abel, E. 2000. Fetal alcohol syndrome: The origins of a moral panic. *Alcohol and Alcoholism* 35 (3), pp. 276–82.

Benz, J., Rasmussen, C., and Andrew, G. 2009. Diagnosing fetal alcohol spectrum disorder: History, challenges and future directions. *Paediatric Child Health* 14, pp. 231–7.

BPAS. n.d. Alcohol in pregnancy–What are the issues? *BPAS Briefing*. Available at: www. bpas.org/get-involved/campaigns/briefings/alcohol-in-pregnancy/.

British Medical Association [BMA]. 2007. *Fetal Alcohol Spectrum Disorders: A Guide for Healthcare Professionals*. June. Available at: http://bmaopac.hosted.exlibrisgroup. com/exlibris/aleph/a23_1/apache_media/3UQ4QIHNR25DH7623BMFDY45UIK7LH. pdf (Accessed February 28, 2018).

British Medical Association [BMA]. 2016. *Alcohol and Pregnancy: Preventing and Managing Fetal Alcohol Spectrum Disorders*. June 2007 (updated February 2016). Available at: www.bma.org.uk/collective-voice/policy-and-research/public-and-population-health/alcohol/alcohol-and-pregnancy (Accessed February 28, 2018).

Brown, R., and Trickey, H. 2018. Devising and communicating public health alcohol guidance for expectant and new mothers: A scoping report. *Alcohol Concern/Alcohol Research UK*. Available at: https://alcoholchange.org.uk/publication/communicating-public-health-alcohol-guidance-for-expectant-mothers-a-scoping-report-1 (Accessed November 2018).

Crawford-Williams, F., Steen, M., Esterman, A., et al. 2015a. 'If you can have one glass of wine now and then, why are you denying that to a woman with no evidence': Knowledge and practices of health professionals concerning alcohol consumption during pregnancy. *Women and Birth* 28, pp. 329–35.

Crawford-Williams, F., Steen, M., Esterman, A., et al. 2015b. 'My midwife said that having a glass of red wine was actually better for the baby': A focus group study of women and their partner's knowledge and experiences relating to alcohol consumption in pregnancy. *BMC Pregnancy and Childbirth* 15 (79). doi:10.1186/s12884-015-0506-3.

Crowe, J.A. 2008. *Fatal Link. The Connection Between School Shooters and the Brain Damage from Prenatal Exposure to Alcohol*. Parker, CO: Outskirts Press.

Department of Health [DoH]. 1995. *Sensible Drinking: The Report of an Inter-Departmental Working Group*. December. Available at: http://webarchive.nationalarchives.gov.uk/20130105043158/www.dh.gov.uk/prod_consum_dh/groups/dh_digitalassets/@dh/@en/documents/digitalasset/dh_4084702.pdf (Accessed February 28, 2018).

Department of Health [DoH]. 2016a. *Alcohol Guidelines Review – Report from the Guidelines Development Group to the UK Chief Medical Officers*. January. Available at: www. gov.uk/government/uploads/system/uploads/attachment_data/file/545739/GDG_report-Jan2016.pdf (Accessed February 28, 2018).

Department of Health [DoH]. 2016b. *How to Keep Health Risks from Drinking Alcohol to a Low Level*. August. Available at: http://gov.wales/docs/dhss/publications/160825governmentresponseen.pdf (Accessed March 5, 2018).

Entman, R. 1993. Framing: Towards clarification of a fractured paradigm. *Journal of Communication* 43 (4), pp. 51–8.

Ettorre, E. 1992. Women and alcohol. In: Ettorre, E. (Eds.), *Women and Substance Use*. Basingstoke: Palgrave Macmillan, ch. 2, pp. 32–51.

Ettorre, E. 1997. *Women and Alcohol. A Private Pleasure or Public Problem?* London: The Women's Press.

Ettorre, E., and Campbell, N. 2011. *Gendering Addiction. The Politics of Drug Treatment in a Neurochemical World*. London: Palgrave Macmillan.

European FASD Alliance. n.d., a. *Drinking During Pregnancy – Who Is Responsible?* Available at: www.eufasd.org/pdf/drinking_during_pregnancy – who_is_responsible. pdf (Accessed September 29, 2018).

European FASD Alliance. n.d., b. *The Alliance*. Available at: www.eufasd.org/alliance_2. php (Accessed September 29, 2018).

European FASD Alliance. 2012. *First Annual Report EU FASD Alliance 2011–2012*. Available at: www.eufasd.org/pdf/ann_rep_2011_2012.pdf (Accessed October 10, 2018).

European FASD Alliance. 2016. *European FASD Alliance Annual Report 2015–2016*. Available at: www.eufasd.org/pdf/ann_rep_2015_2016.pdf (Accessed October 10, 2018).

European FASD Alliance. 2018. *Report of European Conference on FASD 2016 12th-15th September – Royal Holloway, University of London*. Available at: www.eufasd.org/pdf/ EUFASD_2016_report.pdf (Accessed October 10, 2018).

FASD Alliance and NOFAS-UK. 2018. *Hear Our Voices: FASD Stakeholders Share their Experiences with Policy Makers*. Available at: www.nofas-uk.org/WP/wp-content/ uploads/2018/05/HearOurVoicesPublication_FINAL2_ForWebsite.pdf (Accessed November 7, 2018).

Gomberg, E.S. 1979. Drinking patterns of women alcoholics. *Women Who Drink*. Springfield: Thomas.

Henderson, J., Gray, R., and Brocklehurst, P. 2007. Systematic review of the effects of low-moderate prenatal alcohol exposure on pregnancy outcome. *BJOG* 114 (3), pp. 243–352.

HM Government. 2007. *Safe. Sensible. Social. The Next Steps in the National Alcohol Strategy*. 5 June. Available at: http://webarchive.nationalarchives.gov.uk/20130123192107/ www.dh.gov.uk/en/Publicationsandstatistics/Publications/PublicationsPolicyAnd Guidance/DH_075218 (Accessed March 5, 2018).

ILGRA Inter-Departmental Liaison Group on Risk Assessment. 2002. *The Precautionary Principle: Policy and Application*. UK Health and Safety Executive. Available at: www. hse.gov.uk/aboutus/meetings/committees/ilgra/pppa.pdf.

Institute of Alcohol Studies. 2011. *Responsibility Deal Under Pressure, Alcohol Alert, 2 Institute of Alcohol Studies*. Available at: www.ias.org.uk/What-we-do/Alcohol-Alert/ Issue-2-2011/Responsibility-deal-under-renewed-pressure.aspx (Accessed September 24, 2018).

Jawad, R. 2012. Religion, social welfare and social policy in the UK: Historical, theoretical and policy perspectives. *Social Policy and Society* 11 (2), pp. 553–64.

Jessup, M., and Green, J.R. 1987. Treatment of the pregnant alcohol-dependent woman. *Journal of Psychoactive Drugs* 19 (2), pp. 193–203.

Jones, K.L., and Smith, D.W. 1973. Recognition of the fetal alcohol syndrome in early infancy. *Lancet* 302 (2), pp. 999–1001.

Jones, S.C., Telenta, J., Shorten, A., et al. 2011. Midwives and pregnant women talk about alcohol: What advice do we give and what do they receive? *Midwifery* 27, pp. 489–96.

Kelly, Y.J., Sacker, A., Gray, R., et al. 2010. Light drinking during pregnancy: Still no increased risk for socioemotional difficulties or cognitive deficits at 5 years of age? *Journal of Epidemiology and Community Health*. doi:10.1136/jech.2009.103002.

Kelly, Y.J., Iacovou, M., Quigley, M.A., et al. 2013. Light drinking versus abstinence in pregnancy – behavioural and cognitive outcomes in 7-year-old children: A longitudinal cohort study. *BJOG* 120, pp. 1340–7.

Lee, E. 2017. Alcohol abstinence advice and the manipulation of evidence. *Talk Delivered at: Policing Pregnancy: Who Should be a Mother?* Canterbury Christchurch University May 2017. Available at: www.youtube.com/watch?v=1HELABu4K_Q&feature= youtu.be.

Lemoine, P., Harousseau, H., Borteyru, J.P., et al. 1968. Children of alcoholic parents: Anomalies observed in 127 cases. *Quest Medical* 25, pp. 476–82.

Lowe, P.K., and Lee, E.L. 2010. Advocating alcohol abstinence to pregnant women: Some observations about British policy. *Health, Risk & Society* 12 (4), pp. 301–11, doi:10.1080/13698571003789690.

Lowe, P.K., Lee, E., and Macvarish, J. 2015. Growing better brains? Pregnancy and neuroscience discourses in English social and welfare policies. *Health, Risk and Society* 17 (1), pp. 15–29.

MacGregor, S. 1998. A new deal for Britain? In: Jones, H., and MacGregor, S. (Eds.), *Social Issues and Party Politics*. London: Routledge, pp. 248–72.

Mamluk, L., Edwards, H.B., and Savović, J. 2017. Low alcohol consumption and pregnancy and childhood outcomes: Time to change guidelines indicating apparently 'safe' levels of alcohol during pregnancy? A systematic review and meta-analyses. *BMJ Open* 7 (c015410). doi:10.1136/ bmjopen-2016-015410.

Meurk, C.S., Broom, A., Adams, J., et al. 2014. Factors influencing women's decisions to drink alcohol during pregnancy: Findings of a qualitative study with implications for health communication. *BMC Pregnancy and Childbirth* 14 (246). https://doi. org/10.1186/1471-2393-14-246 (Accessed September 2018).

Mooney, H. 2011. Women told that they must abstain from alcohol in pregnancy, in campaign financed by drinks industry. *BMJ* 342, p. d3762.

NAPW. n.d. *About NAPW.* Available at: www.advocatesforpregnantwomen.org/main/ about_us/about_us.php.

National Health Service. 2017. *How Effective Is Contraception at Preventing Pregnancy?* 20 June. Available at: www.nhs.uk/conditions/contraception/how-effective-contraception/ (Accessed October 14, 2018).

National Health Service. 2018. *About the NHS Website*. 17 September. Available at: www. nhs.uk/about-us/about-the-nhs-website/. (Accessed October 14, 2018).

National Institute for Health and Care Excellence [NICE]. 2008. *Antenatal Care for Uncomplicated Pregnancies*. 26 March. Available at: www.nice.org.uk/guidance/cg62/ resources/antenatal-care-for-uncomplicated-pregnancies-pdf-975564597445 (Accessed March 5, 2018).

NHS Choice. 2017. *Drinking Alcohol While Pregnant*. 14 January. Available at: www. nhs.uk/conditions/pregnancy-and-baby/alcohol-medicines-drugs-pregnant/ (Accessed February 28, 2018).

NOFAS. n.d., a. *NOFAS Website*. Available at: www.nofas.org (Accessed September 12, 2018).

NOFAS. n.d., b. *Affiliates Network*. Available at: www.nofas.org/affiliates/ (Accessed September 12, 2018).

NOFAS. 2014. *NOFAS 25th Anniversary*. Available at: www.nofas.org/nofas25/ (Accessed September 12, 2018).

NOFAS. 2017. *Mission and Objectives*. Available at: www.nofas.org/missionandobjectives/ (Accessed September 12, 2018).

NOFAS-UK. 2018a. *Alcohol and Pregnancy: Advice for Pregnant Women*. Available at: www.nofas-uk.org/?cat=24 (Accessed September 25, 2018).

NOFAS-UK 2018b. *The Beginning of NOFAS UK: Susan's Story*. Available at: www.nofas-uk.org/?cat=10 (Accessed December 9, 2018).

NOFAS-UK. 2018c. Our forgotten children: The urgency of aligning policy with guidance on the effects of antenatal exposure to alcohol. *Report of a Roundtable Discussion Held Houses of Parliament on 23rd May 2018*. Available at: www.nofas-uk.org/WP/wp-content/uploads/2018/06/20180523_Report_FIN.pdf (Accessed October 2, 2018).

O'Leary, C.M., Heuzenroeder, L., Elliott, E.J., et al. 2007. A review of policies on alcohol use during pregnancy in Australia and other English-speaking countries. *Medical Journal of Australia* 186 (9), pp. 466–71.

Oster, E. 2013. *Expecting Better. Why the Conventional Pregnancy Wisdom Is Wrong and What You Really Need to Know*. New York: Penguin Books.

Ouko, L.A., Shantikumar, K., Knezovich, J., et al. 2009. Effect of alcohol consumption on CpG methylation in the differentially methylated regions of H19 and IG-DMR in male gametes – Implications for fetal alcohol spectrum disorders. *Alcohol Clinical and Experimental Research* 33, pp. 1615–27.

Plant, M. 1985. *Women, Drinking and Pregnancy*. London: Tavistock Publications.

Plant, M. 1997. *Women and Alcohol Contemporary and Historical Perspectives*. London: Free Association Books.

Royal College of Obstetricians and Gynaecologists [RCOG]. 1999. *Alcohol Consumption in Pregnancy Guideline No. 9*. Originally published November 1996. December (Accessed August 21, 2018 via email to RCOG).

Royal College of Obstetricians and Gynaecologists [RCOG]. 2006. *Alcohol Consumption and the Outcomes of Pregnancy*. RCOG Statement No. 5. March. Available at: www.alcoholpolicy.net/files/RCOG_Alcohol_pregnancy_March_06.pdf (Accessed June 26, 2018).

Royal College of Obstetricians and Gynaecologists [RCOG]. 2015. *Information for You: Alcohol and Pregnancy*. February (Accessed June 26, 2018 via email to RCOG).

Royal College of Obstetricians and Gynaecologists [RCOG]. 2018. *Information for You: Alcohol and Pregnancy*. 12 January (originally published February 2015). Available at: www.rcog.org.uk/globalassets/documents/patients/patient-information-leaflets/pregnancy/pi-alcohol-and-pregnancy.pdf (Accessed June 26, 2018).

Saunders, J. 2009. Were our forebears aware of prenatal alcohol exposure and its effects? A review of the history of fetal alcohol spectrum disorder. *The Canadian Journal of Clinical Pharmacology* 16 (9), pp. e288–e295.

Schölin, L., Hughes, K., Bellis, M.A., et al. 2018. 'I think we should all be singing from the same hymn sheet' – English and Swedish midwives' views of advising pregnant women about alcohol. *Drugs: Education, Prevention and Policy*. doi:10.1080/096876 37.2018.1478949.

Sclare, A.B. 1980. The foetal alcohol syndrome. *Camberwell Council on Alcoholism Women & Alcohol*. London: Tavistock Publications, ch. 3, pp. 53–66.

Shaw, S. 1980. The causes of increasing drinking problems amongst women: A general etiological theory. *Camberwell Council on Alcoholism Women & Alcohol*. London: Tavistock Publications, ch. 1, pp. 1–40.

Skogerbø, A., Kesmodel, U.S., Wimberley, T., et al. 2012. The effects of low to moderate alcohol consumption and binge drinking in early pregnancy on executive function in 5-year-old children. *BJOG*. doi 10.1111/j.1471-0528.2012.03397.x.

Striessguth, A.P., and O'Malley, K. 2000. Neuro psychiatric implications and long-term consequences of fetal alcohol spectrum disorders. *Seminars in Neuropsychiatry* 5, pp. 177–90.

Thom, B., Herring, R., Thickett, A., and Duke, K. 2016. The alcohol health alliance: The emergence of an advocacy coalition to stimulate policy change. *British Politics* 11 (3), pp. 301–23.

TYTD. n.d. *About the Campaign*. Available at: www.eufasd.org/awareness/tytd2015.html (Accessed October 10, 2018).

van der Wulp, N.Y., Hoving, C., and de Vries, H. 2013. A qualitative investigation of alcohol use advice during pregnancy: Experiences of Dutch midwives, pregnant women and their partners. *Midwifery* 29, pp. e89–e98.

Warner, J. 2003. *Craze. Gin and Debuchery in an Age of Reason*. London: Profile Books.

Williams, J.F., and Smith, V.C., and The Committee on Substance Abuse. 2015. Fetal alcohol spectrum disorders. *American Academy of Pediatrics Clinical Report*. doi:10.1542/peds.2015-3113.

Ziegler, M. 2008. Note, eugenic feminism: Mental hygiene, the women's movement, and the campaign for eugenic legal reform, 1900–1935, 31 *Harvard Journal of Law & Gender* 211. Available at: h p://ir.law.fsu.edu/articles/339.

6 Creating safe spaces in dangerous places

'Chicks Day' for women who inject drugs in Budapest, Hungary

Camille May Stengel

Introduction

This chapter frames understandings of danger and safety by drawing on experiences from clients and staff of 'Chicks Day' (*Csajnap* in Hungarian), which was the only women-exclusive needle and syringe exchange programme (NSEP) in Budapest, the capital of Hungary. Located in a socio-economically deprived area of Budapest, Chicks Day provided once weekly harm reduction services for women who injected drugs from 2010 to 2014. Harm reduction interventions like NSEP aim to address the potential adverse effects of injecting drug use based on public health evidence-informed principles and practices, ideally grounded in non-judgement and drug users' autonomy. Chicks Day primarily provided new needles and syringes for self-identified women who injected drugs, as well as a secure deposit place for Chicks Day clients to safely dispose of used syringes. The rationale behind NSEP is to facilitate safer injecting practices and prevent the spread of blood-borne diseases like HIV and hepatitis C by discouraging the reusing and sharing of needles and syringes when injecting drugs. For staff of Chicks Day, the NSEP was the entry point to provide a range of other services and supports for women who inject drugs that were otherwise disregarded in Hungarian society.

Clients of the Chicks Day were primarily ethnically Roma women, most of whom lived in poverty and many who engaged in sex work. As stated by one Chicks Day staff, the intersecting label as 'the junkie Gypsy prostitute' meant clients were constructed as a triple threat to the norms of mainstream Hungarian social and moral values. However, clients were not only framed as a 'threat' to societal norms: Chicks Day clients also experienced danger through their precarious physical, emotional, financial and sociocultural conditions. Chicks Day clients navigated their day-to-day lives with the threat and reality of stigmatisation, racism, misogyny and violence as reaction to these overlapping 'othering' labels. Chicks Day staff aimed to offer some respite from this barrage of harms through the delivery of the women-only day as a 'safe space'. This goal was constrained by precarious funding and a hostile political backdrop in Hungary that ultimately led to the centre which housed Chicks Day closing in August 2014.

This chapter contributes to feminist and visual scholarship by examining how a sample of women clients and workers at a harm reduction centre often understood contrasting yet overlapping experiences of danger, safety, harm and harm reduction through digital and analogue photographs. The data discussed in this chapter were generated using ethnographic methods and qualitative interviews in combination with the visual method known as photovoice, where participants become photographers and document their understandings of the research phenomena in question. Chicks Day clients and staff took photographs about their experiences of harm production and harm reduction and participated in focus groups and individual interviews about their and others' photographs.

Overlapping dimensions of harm

This chapter first contextualises the overlapping identities of perceived risk that Chicks Day clients faced in their day-to-day lives: as people who inject drugs (PWID), as women and as Roma 'gypsies'. This first section outlines some of the ways in which these groups both experienced danger and were perceived as dangerous, as well as the philosophy underpinning a harm reduction response for PWID. In this context, harm, whether real or imagined, is connected to the fear of danger and risk.

Intertwined with such various understandings of risk in this context is the impact of stigmatisation of Chicks Day clients. People who deviate from perceived dominant sociocultural norms and values, such as PWID, or people who engage in sex work are heavily stigmatised, in part because of their perceived abnormal behaviours related to injecting drugs or selling sex, which is deemed illegal or heavily regulated (Benoit et al., 2018; Campbell and Ettorre, 2011; EHRN, 2010). The process of stigmatisation can result in negative health outcomes for the individual or group being stigmatised (Link and Phelan, 2001, 2006). Taboos surrounding hygiene, uncleanliness and disease transfer have long been associated with people who use drugs, especially PWID, as well as sex workers (Douglas, 1966; Fitzgerald and Threadgold, 2004; Parkin, 2014; Simmonds and Coomber, 2009). These taboos result in further 'spoiled identities' and social marginalisation of groups of people already deemed to be 'tainted' because of the association with some aspect or feature of that group with negative stereotypes (Goffman, 1963). Such spoiled identities can perpetuate the fear of the 'other' and construct groups of people as divergent from the normative society of 'us' (Lupton, 1993). The process and impact of stigmatisation is strongly evident among so-called at-risk populations – i.e. PWID and sex workers, due to the higher increased risk of contracting and transmitting HIV. Injecting drug use and by extension PWID are largely framed within a public health context as a population that needs to be managed. Widespread incorporation of harm reduction policies and practices developed primarily as a global public health response to the human immunodeficiency virus (HIV) epidemic in the 1980s and continued to prioritise the reduction of other blood-borne viruses, including hepatitis C (Friedman et al., 2001).

'Dangerous' people: women who inject drugs

Women who use drugs, and especially women who inject drugs, are depicted in popular imagination as either out of control addicts or highly emotional victims who need to be controlled (Du Rose, 2015; Ettorre, 2004; Measham, 2003). In both instances, they are dangerous. Women who use drugs are not only immersed within the societal rules of cultural femininity: the intrinsically *female* act of pregnancy (or potentially pregnant bodies) and motherhood (or the potential to *be* mothers) further adds pressure to conform to gender norms (Boyd, 1999). Violation of these norms through the act of perceived dangerous activities such as injecting drug use is a threat to gendered and societal expectations and cultural scripts (Boyd, 2004; Stengel, 2014).

One response to such disruption of social norms is stigmatisation and marginalisation. Stigmatisation can hinder women who inject drugs from accessing services they need. The health and social risks for women who inject drugs are multitudinous. Women who inject drugs have reported being 'second on the needle' when sharing syringes with other people who inject drugs, therefore putting women at greater risk for developing abscesses by using blunted needles or contracting blood-borne viruses from infected syringes (Csete, 2006; El-Bassel et al., 2012; Iversen et al., 2015). The pervasiveness of various forms of violence towards women who inject drugs is well documented (EHRN, 2010; Kensy et al., 2012; Pinkham et al., 2012; Roberts et al., 2010; Stoicescu et al., 2018). Many women who inject drugs are embedded in systemic poverty and social instability (Levy, 2014; UNODC, 2014). This contributes to the day-to-day dangers in the lives of women who inject drugs.

There is a variety of evidence that suggests an overlap between women who inject drugs and women who engage in sex work, and that with this overlap is an increased risk factor for sexually transmitted infections and blood-borne diseases, as well as the aforementioned risks of violence and difficulties accessing services (Móró et al., 2013; Platt et al., 2018; Rekart, 2005; Stoicescu et al., 2018). However, there are estimated to be significantly fewer women than men who inject drugs worldwide, and women's status as a minority within a marginalised population risks a continuation of gender-blindness in the development of harm reduction delivery (El-Bassel and Strathdee, 2015; UNODC, 2014). This means that the development of women-only harm reduction initiatives such as Chicks Day is significant and needed.

Situating harm reduction among PWID

Harm reduction is an approach to drug use that acknowledges that some people do not want to or are not able to stop taking drugs and aims to help people consume substances more safely (International Harm Reduction Association, 2010). While abstinence from drug use may be a goal for some people who use drugs, a harm reduction approach views abstinence as one choice on a spectrum of responses rather than the only alternative to drug use (Marlatt, 1996). The primary goal of different harm reduction initiatives is to reduce drug-related harms to people who use drugs, as well as any community or societal public harms related to drug use (Lenton and Single, 1998). Reducing drug-related harms is often part of a public health response to drug use. A public health-oriented approach to harm reduction emphasises evidenced-based outcomes rather than strategies which stigmatise people who use drugs (EMCDDA, 2010).

Harm reduction philosophy embraces a non-judgemental attitude towards drug use, so that those delivering harm reduction services do so without placing moral judgement on people who use drugs or furthering stigmatisation (O'Hare et al., 1992; Stimson, 1998). Reducing dangers for PWID means implementing various public health initiatives without furthering stigmatisation, such as providing new syringes and injecting equipment for users and safely disposing of used syringes in the form of a NSEP, as well as testing for HIV and hepatitis C to monitor the risk of blood-borne viruses spreading to the general public. Depending on the drug-related legislation in each country, services also include opioid substitution clinics for opioid (i.e. heroin) injectors and safe consumption rooms for people to inject and/or smoke in a sterile environment under medical supervision (HRI, 2018). Such initiatives are provided through 'low-threshold' services, meaning there are minimal requirements or restrictions for use (Melles et al., 2007). A low-threshold approach aims to accept anyone who needs to use harm reduction services and help them gain access with as few barriers as possible.

The Chicks Day programme was held within a low-threshold harm reduction centre that primarily operated as a needle and syringe exchange programme (NSEP). NSEP are a central component of harm reduction theory and practice (O'Hare et al., 1992). NSEP usually provides injection-related equipment, which can include but is not limited to new syringes, clean water, filters, cookers, disinfectant skin wipes, tourniquets, body lotion and ascorbic acid. Furthermore, syringe exchange programmes often facilitate a safe space to dispose of used syringes in some form of biohazards bins. The goal of NSEP is to reduce the physical harms of drug use and provide a first point of contact for harm reduction outreach workers to interact with PWID (Bluthenthal et al., 2000; Strathdee and Vlahov, 2001). The thought is that this also reduces some of the public health risks related to injecting drug use; harm and risk are often used interchangeably, or more accurately, risk can lead to harm. Indeed, PWID are known in the public health language as 'at-risk' populations for developing and spreading HIV and other blood-borne diseases such as hepatitis C. This can be extrapolated into understanding a 'risk environment' in which drug-injecting behaviour and surrounding circumstances are dangerous and need to be contained or managed (Rhodes, 2009).

A criticism of harm reduction is that the overemphasis on risk assessment and disease prevention ignores gendered factors relating to drug use and gendered risk environments (Malinowska-Sempruch and Rychkova, 2015; Pinkham et al., 2012; Kensy et al., 2012). When gender is factored into harm reduction interventions, it is commonly done through quantitative epidemiological comparisons of men versus women as a risk-related factor rather than qualitative explorations that aid an understanding of women's and men's lived experiences, or, even better, a combination of the two methods (Campbell and Ettorre, 2011). The Chicks Day programme aimed to incorporate gender-sensitive practices into the harm reduction centre's service delivery. Also, the harm reduction programme in general was aware of the added layer of stigma faced by their clients who were primarily of a Roma ethnic background.

'Dangerous' people: Roma gypsies

Roma are far from a homogeneous group, even within those Roma communities that live in Hungary. In Hungary, Roma as a group are recognised as a distinct ethnicity from Hungarians, who are thought to be mainly descended from the Magyar tribe (Hancock, 2002). Roma is a socially and historically constructed ethnic group with unclear racial origins. Although Roma people are thought to have originated from India over a thousand years ago, the contemporary Hungarian population is rich with a variety of racial compositions. The 1993 Minorities Act was established to grant groups such as Roma people protection from harms and to promote autonomous cultural rights and safety (Corsi et al., 2008).

However, in Hungary and other parts of Central and Eastern Europe, policy has not necessarily translated into practice. While Roma populations are diverse, their health indicators are all below other non-Roma Europeans' health outcomes (Földes and Covaci, 2012). Roma are historically stigmatised through the stereotype as carriers of disease (Masseria et al., 2010). This stigma is amplified for Roma people who inject drugs. Physical harms and socio-economic hardship disproportionately affect Roma people in part because they face cultural and ethnic discrimination by virtue of being Roma.

This has also resulted in the ghettoisation of geographically marginalised Roma populations, like those in the district where the Chicks Day programme operated, and has exacerbated poverty-based crime rates (e.g. theft) among the Roma population (Rácz et al., 2007). The district where the centre was located had a reputation as being one of the most impoverished districts in Budapest (Csák et al., 2013). Historically, the area has disproportionately high concentrations of reported crime, unemployment, low educational attainment of the residents and poor-quality housing when compared to the rest of Budapest (Kovács, 2009). The 'ghetto'-like conditions in parts of this district have fostered social segregation and marginalisation: those primarily affected are Roma people (Rácz et al., 2015). People of ethnic Roma origin have been discriminated against in Hungary and much of Europe for centuries (Hancock, 2002). This history includes social exclusion and ethnic persecution that has resulted in a disproportionate lack of educational attainment, exacerbated poverty and poor health outcomes among Hungarian Roma in comparison to the rest of the population (Hancock, 2002; Kende, 2000; Ladányi and Szelényi, 2005; Masseria et al., 2010).

Additionally, the district where the Chicks Day programme took place was 'well known' for sex work, both on the street and in brothels, although all forms of sex work are illegal in Hungary (Móró et al., 2013). Illicit drug use, including a considerable injecting drug use population, has been part of the social spatial composition of the district where the Chicks Day programme operated for decades (Csák et al., 2013; Rácz et al., 2015). Roma people, PWID and sex workers have all historically been associated with the stigmatising stereotype of carrying and transmitting diseases (Hancock, 2002; Masseria et al., 2010). This has been constructed as a public health danger, as well as a threat to social norms and behaviours. It was this trifecta of identities that made up the client population of Chicks Day.

Context of the Chicks Day programme

Although HIV rates have overall remained low in Hungary, hepatitis C among people who use drugs, and especially PWID, has steadily increased (Rácz et al., 2007, 2016). While this is worrying, the larger political context of Hungary has not fostered a harm reduction response to PWID specifically or socially marginalised people in general. The concept of harm reduction was slow to gain national understanding and acceptance as a legitimate public health response in Hungary and is still widely unknown or misunderstood among the general Hungarian population (Csorba et al., 2003; Rácz et al., 2016). Hungary currently has NSEP and opioid substitution therapy programmes in various parts of the country (but not in prisons) and does not have safe consumption rooms (EMCDDA, 2018). While on a global scale this is not unusual, the absence of these services signals that Hungary does not yet have comprehensive harm reduction practices. Also, NSEP have been in decline since 2014 (Gyarmathy et al., 2016). Indeed, the government is seemingly not interested in a harm reduction approach. The right leaning conservative *Fidesz* political party implemented their own national anti-drugs strategy for 2013–2020, titled 'Clear Consciousness, Sobriety and the Fight against Drug Crime'. (Parliament Resolution No.80/2013. (X.16)). Harm reduction is not one of the strategy's objectives, and harm reduction is only sparsely mentioned in conjunction with abstinence-based outcomes. Hungary's current anti-drugs strategy, in combination with other local and national changes to social and welfare policies, has arguably not resulted in a supportive environment for harm reduction–oriented policies and organisations.

Critics claim that Hungary's current punitive strategies and legislative acts surrounding issues of drug use and poverty maintain systemic societal inequalities for already marginalised groups such as PWID (Bence and Udvarhelyi, 2013; Human Rights Watch, 2013). This seems to be ideologically consistent with the curtailing of other citizens' freedoms and rights that have been a trend within the changing legislation in Hungary in recent years (Lendvai-Bainton, 2017). Although Hungary has not provided the most welcoming of environments for harm reduction interventions to occur, a Budapest-based NGO set up an outreach programme in 1996 and opened a NSEP in 2006 in one district in Budapest as a response to local need. After the NSEP opened, staff of the harm reduction centre found that clients who identified as women did not engage with the services as much when men were present, whether that was male clients or male staff. In order to address this disparity in client engagement, the centre created Chicks Day in conjunction with other women-only initiatives. Chicks Day began as a twice a month service in 2010, which eventually progressed into a once a week programme after a grant from an international donor in 2012. In addition to the standard NSEP providing clean syringes and paraphernalia, computer access with Internet and hepatitis C and HIV testing, Chicks Day also provided free second-hand clothing, shoes, and children's toys; a female hepatologist and female lawyer for one-on-one consultation; condom distribution; pregnancy tests and light snacks. During the field research described in this chapter, an average of 40–50 clients entered Chicks Day every week. In 2013, women made up 35.6 per cent of the client base of the larger harm reduction centre (Rácz and Csák, 2014).

Methodology

To gain an understanding of clients and staff of the Chicks Day programme located at the harm reduction centre in Budapest, the methodological tools of photovoice and photo-elicitation were used alongside ethnographic observations and participation. Photovoice enables participants to document their own understandings of a research topic by recording their issues, experiences and observations through photographs (Wang, 1999; Wang and Burris, 1997). The method of photovoice allows participants to document their surroundings in a way that holds personal meaning and representation, contextualises the photographs and assists in identifying the main codes, themes and issues relevant to them (Baker and Wang, 2006). Images such as photographs can be used as a tool to communicate and a medium to facilitate discussion on issues that underlie people's everyday experiences. In order to capture the photographer's understanding of their own photographs, participant interviews are a key element of the photovoice research process in order for the researcher to situate images within the photographer's intended meaning (Pink, 2007). But a photograph is not only interpreted as the photographer intended; the signs and symbols in the photograph will be connoted with meaning based on the context of those viewing the image (Rose, 2016).

Photovoice also often involves some manifestation of an action-based output, such as a photo exhibition. Showcasing participants' photographs has the potential to be creative and empowering when using photovoice (Robinson, 2013). The action-oriented outcome of photovoice provides a space for visual representation and re-representation that has the potential to reach larger audiences beyond those in the research community or through conventional research outputs such as peer-reviewed journal articles (Fitzgibbon and Stengel, 2018). Sharing research not only provides a compelling platform to convey the outcome of a research project but can also act as a way to 'give back' to the community initiatives that were involved in photovoice research (Mitchell et al., 2017). As with any research method, photovoice has the potential to succumb to researcher bias. The collaborative approach of photovoice arguably lessens this potential through photographer (i.e. research participant) and researcher engagement in analytic dialogue about the visual data. While the write-up of the analysis that follows is ultimately the work of the researcher, arguably the methodological conditions provided for the co-creation of knowledge and data that have been used in this chapter.

Methods

Over an eight-month period, Chicks Day clients and staff were given a combination of analogue and digital cameras to document their understandings of 'harm' and 'harm reduction' in the context of the women-only harm reduction programme. A total of 19 photo-elicitation interviews were conducted with 10 Chicks Day clients. Four Chicks Day staff also took part in a series of 16 photo-voice workshops throughout the data collection process, which involved exploring the photovoice method through activities, group interviews about photographs taken by staff and analysis of staff and client photographs. Participant-produced images then provided the basis for individual and group interviews with both clients and staff. With consent, interviews were also conducted about other participants' images. For example, client images were shown to the staff and their responses and interpretations framed group interviews. In addition, the author combined ethnographic observations and participation of Chicks Day dynamics of clients and staff by observing interactions and volunteering at the harm reduction centre, as well as assisting with outreach activities such as neighbourhood needle and syringe collection. Staff workshops culminated in an action-based output in the form of a public photo exhibition and fundraiser. The event raised 94,091 Hungarian Forints (about 300 euros) to support the operational costs of the Chicks Day programme.

The research study was approved by the University of Kent Research Ethics Committee prior to the start of data collection. Informed consent was sought prior to each interview and workshop, and the use and ownership of the photographs were agreed with participants prior to any public display. Participants are not identifiable in the images published in this chapter. To the author's knowledge, this was the first research project to use photovoice within a harm reduction context and with women who inject drugs in Hungary.

Data coding and analysis

All interviews were audio recorded, transcribed to English and were used as a guide to match comments with related participant-generated images. Comments from participant-generated notes that were physically created during individual and group interviews were also matched to the relevant photographs. Data analysis was in part co-constructed throughout the research process, particularly with Chicks Day staff, due to their more frequent involvement in the research through the regular workshops. Elements of grounded theory, semiotic analysis and thematic analysis guided the data interpretation (Grbich, 2007; Pink, 2007; Rose, 2016). Participant interviews were analysed in conjunction with the relevant photographs. Participant interpretation and analysis of their own and other participants' photographs were triangulated with ethnographic fieldnotes to create a thematic understanding of participant constructions of 'harm' and 'harm reduction'. These themes were revisited and reframed to conceptualise spaces and people associated with 'danger' and 'safety' within the context of this chapter.

Participant characteristics

Research participants included both clients and staff of the Chicks Day programme. All clients who chose to answer demographic questions were identified as Roma. Basic demographic questions were asked during the interview, although not all participants chose to answer in full. The youngest client interviewed was 19, and the oldest was 46 years old. All but one client said they had injected drugs at some point in their lives, and eight out of the ten clients said they currently injected drugs. Four out of ten clients were explicitly identified as sex workers. One client stated she had hepatitis C. The staff estimated that the number of Chicks Day clients who were sex workers and had hepatitis C was likely higher but suggested the clients chose not to disclose this information during data collection. Chicks Day staff were identified as white Hungarian, most with some level of higher education (either completed or in the process of completing during the research), between the age of 23 and 36, and none had ever injected drugs.

Participant-produced photographs

This chapter presents a selection of results from over 500 images that were generated during the field research. The images and the interpretation of these images presented here are primarily by Chicks Day staff. The staff occupied the unique position of both knowing the clients and their needs and day-to-day risks, as well as being aware (and experiencing) of the normative and political vitriol towards the client population constructed as a threat to the Hungarian status quo. All names used in this chapter are pseudonyms to protect anonymity.

Various configurations of risk, danger and safety

The images selected for this chapter articulate divergent and complicated narratives of danger and safety among different groups. Images produced by clients and staff of Chicks Day showcase the dangers for women who inject drugs, via the drugs they inject, the way they consume the drugs, as well as the life around their drug use (which included sex work, intimate partner violence and discrimination). Chicks Day staff attempt to mitigate such harms by creating Chicks Day as a 'safe space' from both a traditional harm reduction response and a gender-sensitive response to wider client needs. However, the 'spoiled identities' that Chicks Day clients occupied represented a danger to Hungarian society, and ultimately the Chicks Day programme was met with lack of support and hostility from external groups which led to the harm reduction centre being forced to close. The images and corresponding narratives around the photographs are indeed incomplete 'snapshots' that provide some insight into the complex lives of Chicks Day clients, primarily through the eyes of the harm reduction centre staff.

Injecting dangers for Chicks Day clients

Chicks Day clients experienced danger in their everyday lives. From a public health standpoint, the most explicit risk was the act of injecting drugs. Image 6.1 illustrates some of these risks.

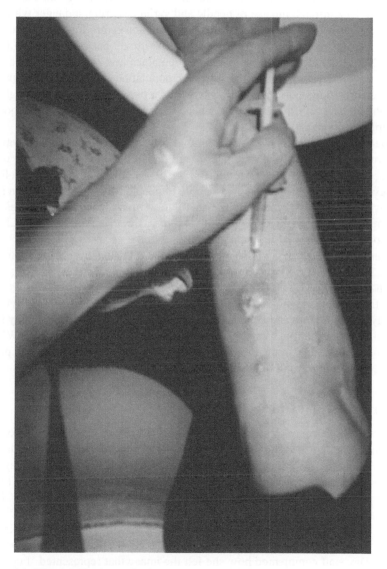

Image 6.1 'The drug is always first'

Source: Image taken by Chicks Day client Marianna.

The photograph shows Anita's arms shortly before injecting. Anita, a Chicks Day client, has a syringe in her left hand pointing towards an abscess on her right arm. A clear example of physical harm can be found in the signs of the abscesses in Image 6.1. Abscesses are a noted side effect of injecting drug use (Lloyd-Smith et al., 2005). Among Chicks Day clients, the most visible physical harms as a result of injecting were damaged skin in the form of sores and lacerations on clients' hands, arms and legs from injecting sites. These sores caused physical discomfort and sometimes became infected, as they appear to be in Image 6.1.

Other immediate risks were of contracting blood-borne viruses such as hepatitis C and HIV through the use of needle and syringe sharing, a danger which the NSEP explicitly aimed to reduce. The harm reduction centre found an increase in clients sharing syringes from 33 per cent in 2009 to 53 per cent in 2014 (Tarján et al., 2015; Rácz et al., 2016). HIV risk has remained low, but incidences of hepatitis C have increased among the injecting population in Hungary (Gyarmathy et al., 2016). Blood-borne viruses such as hepatitis C and HIV have a high rate of being transferred between people when syringes are shared for the purpose of multiple injections (HRI, 2018).

Clients from the harm reduction centre as a whole, including Chicks Day clients, reported needing 10–15 syringes a day due to the high frequency in which the substances were injected (Rácz and Csák, 2014). This rate is higher than found in previous research conducted on a sample of people who injected drugs in Hungary who had accessed NSEP and used similar new psychoactive substances such as pentedrone at a lower average rate of 5.4 times a day (Tarján et al., 2015). NSEP were originally designed to respond primarily to the needs of opioid users, who on average inject significantly less (2–3 times a day) than Chicks Day clients (up to 10–15 times a day) (Botescu et al., 2012; Csák et al., 2013; Péterfi et al., 2014; Tarján et al., 2015). This is likely because new psychoactive substance users inject more times a day and require a greater number of syringes. Using more syringes per day provides more daily chances where those injecting could physically harm their skin or veins through missed injections, share syringes with other PWID or take too much of one or a combination of substances and overdose. These potential instances could result in physical danger to Chicks Day clients.

Other dangers for Chicks Day clients

The risk of violence was an additional danger to the risk of blood-borne infections for Chicks Day clients. The title of Image 6.2 is an educational pamphlet that was displayed in the harm reduction centre. During Chicks Day, the Chicks Day staff displayed this and a variety of other informational pamphlets in the centre for the clients to read and take with them. Image 6.2 prompted a discussion by the Chicks Day staff about the prevalence of violence in the Chicks Day clients' lives.

The discussion was one of despair and hopelessness where the Chicks Day staff felt powerless to help Chicks Day clients escape violent relationships. One Chicks Day staff commented how she felt the image that represented 'I could be that fifth woman – you, me, everyone'. Milla's comment connotes the deeply

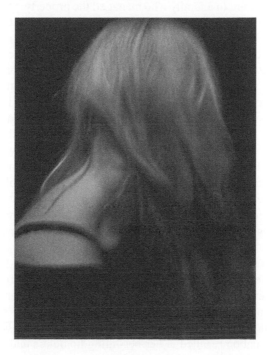

Image 6.2 'One in every five women is beaten regularly by their husband or partner'
Source: Image taken by Chicks Day staff Bora.

entrenched violence against women that resulted in a societal narrative that any woman is in danger of becoming a potential victim of violence, not just Chicks Day clientele. This comment signifies the potential everyday threat for women to be a target for violence because of their gender. Milla's comment can also be interpreted as implying that symbolic violence occurs from the threat of violence and causes women to self-monitor and take precautionary measures to avoid being victimised.

Throughout the fieldwork period, various Chicks Day clients entered the centre with visible injuries such as bandages and bruises. The following field notes describe an example of the multiple forms of violence one client experienced in her daily life:

> Yesterday at *Csajnap*, Anita, a client we had recruited for participation, came in to the centre with a black eye and a limp on her left leg. It visibly pained her to sit down. After one of the staff spoke with Anita to assess her physical and mental state, we [an interpreter and the researcher] approached her and asked how she was doing. She apologised for not bringing the disposable camera back, and proceeded to explain how she had come to have these injuries on her face and leg. Anita was living in an unfinished basement where

she paid daily rent to a family who managed the property. She told us she had paid the rent to someone else, and that the money was not passed on to the father of the household like it usually was. As retribution the daughter physically assaulted Anita. Anita was further subjected to violence when the father physically attacked her under the accusation that Anita's daughter was bullying this man's daughter online. Anita told us she consumed tranquilisers and a benzo[diazepine] called Rivotil because she was in pain. While she was high, the ex-wife of Anita's perpetrator trafficked her to two men. She told us that she woke up confused in a hotel, and the two men told her they were going to take her abroad to work. The interpreter assumed that by 'work' Anita meant working in the sex trade [likely assumed because Anita was a sex worker in Hungary and girls were known to work abroad]. Incredibly, Anita told the two men she didn't want to leave Budapest and they let her go without any trouble. Since her living situation was now unsafe she had moved to a shelter. Anita told us she slept in a large heated tent with other homeless people.

Anita's situation was rife with physical and emotional danger. In addition to the physical violence where she lived (and the precarity of her rough sleeping as a result), Anita experienced gendered symbolic violence in her involuntary and brief involvement in (allegedly) sex trafficking, although she also experienced long-term stigma due to her engagement with sex work. The risk environment in Anita's living situation resulted in her becoming homeless and exacerbating her experience of the everyday violence of abject poverty. The staff at Chicks Day tried to provide temporary refuge from some of these dangers and harms through the creation of the women's only programme.

Safe place: Chicks Day programme

Gender-responsive initiatives targeting 'vulnerable populations' such as women who use drugs have shown beneficial outcomes and measurable deliverables for the women accessing services in various parts of the world (El-Bassel and Strathdee, 2015). However, specific definitions of concepts such as 'safety' are needed to successfully develop and implement programmes that truly are gender responsive. Chicks Day facilitated a gender-sensitive environment that fostered a sense of cultural safety for Roma women who injected drugs. Outside of the NSEP, clients experienced danger in the form of violence, racism, sexism and stigmatisation. Inside the centre, women were temporarily relieved from these forms of danger. Harm reduction responses were situated in cultural and gender norms associated with the clientele of Roma women and their children.

The success of physical harm reduction initiatives depends on how 'success' is defined. The explicit purpose of Chicks Day was to provide a gender-exclusive space for women to exchange used syringes for new syringes. A tandem goal of Chicks Day was to encourage clients to return their used syringes for safe disposal. Most barometers used to measure the success of harm reduction interventions rely primarily on biomedical results that track and calculate risk reduction of infections and blood-borne viruses, including safe syringe disposal in designated containers, HIV and hepatitis C testing and sterile water. Chicks Day clients reported adhering to various harm reduction messages such as using the designated container to dispose of used syringes and never injecting alone so that someone could help them if they overdosed. According to this biomedical measurement, Chicks Day was successful at physical harm reduction initiatives for HIV prevention.

Image 6.3 depicts this success in action: Chicks Day clients queuing for the NSEP. Image 6.3 frames two women's legs as they stand in line to exchange their syringes during Chicks Day. The woman on the left leans against the syringe exchange counter where the harm reduction centre workers sat to count out used syringes and provide new syringes and other drug use equipment. The wood panelled door to the right of the woman features notices for the clients about steps for safe injecting. Another client with white trainers stands behind the first client, waiting for her turn to use the service. Image 6.3 was taken through one of the decorative holes in the back of a chair in the adjoining main room.

However, Chicks Day was not a purely public health operation; the gender-sensitive space provided an atmosphere of perceived safety for clients, including through the use of Roma music. The music provided a chance for Chicks Day clients to socialise and bond with other women who were dealing with similar

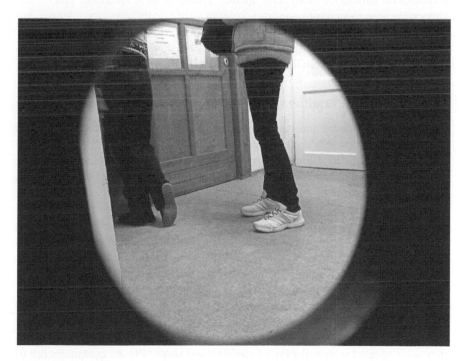

Image 6.3 'Peepshow'

Source: Image taken by Chicks Day staff Luzja.

overlapping harms in their daily lives. Music videos were sometimes the topic of conversation, but as the same Roma songs were usually played every week, they often became a backdrop for clients to peruse social media or engage in conversation with each other, often while looking through and trying on the second-hand clothes and shoes. The music of Chicks Day, and of the harm reduction centre more broadly, was symbolic of the atmospheric 'safe space' created for and with clients. Both the staff and some clients identified the music as 'Gypsy songs' and were accompanied by music videos produced by a particular Hungarian production company. These songs were catchy, and clients would often sing along. Music provided a platform for clients to express the harms and dangers that they were experiencing, whether it be to mourn a break-up with a lover or to use the cover provided by the music to speak with the Chicks Day staff about intimate partner violence more privately.

Recognising the threat and reality of violence in clients' lives, especially those who were sex workers, the Chicks' Day staff tried to develop and implement harm reduction responses for clients who were victims of violence. A peer group was created for clients who were sex workers with the hope of facilitating self-defence classes as well as a safe space to talk about their work experiences. During Chicks Day, the staff also provided the clients with information about shelters and hospitals women could go to if they were victims of domestic violence, and in some instances the Chicks Day staff accompanied clients to these locations. The Chicks Days were able to suggest temporary solutions for clients who faced danger, but ultimately could not change the structural issues surrounding gender-based violence. These issues were further complicated by the double stigmatisation statuses of PWID and Roma women that made up the majority of the Chicks Day clientele.

Dangerous place: funding and political environment

The context of creating and maintaining the 'safe space' within the Chicks Day programme was severely constrained due to the hostile local funding and political environments. The Chicks Day programme, and the harm reduction centre as a whole, aimed to respond to an array of needs without sustainable resources. Image 6.4 is symbolic of this point.

The client in Image 6.4 holds a burgundy top and marigold sweater in her hands. Positioned to the right of the client's hands is a black column of fabric shelving used to store and display the donated clothes. This was one of two shelves that were wheeled out by the Chicks Day staff once a week before Chicks Day opened. The Chicks Day staff would first sort through the clothing and shoes and discard any items that had visible stains or were of poor quality. They would then distribute a selection of clothing among two columns of fabric shelving and two tables and a plastic container of shoes underneath a table. These items were spread out over the far side of one wall of the centre so that when clients entered Chicks Day, they were greeted with a display of clothing and shoes. Plastic containers full of toys and children's books were kept in the staff-only area and were brought out

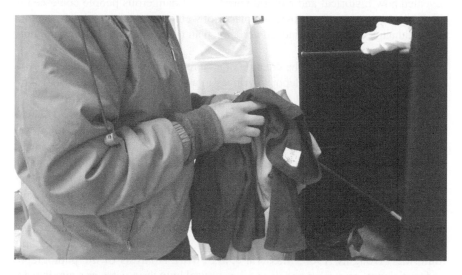

Image 6.4 'Four adults, four kids, three wheels'
Source: Image taken by Chicks Day staff Milla.

for clients to look through on request. The Chicks Day staff used the clothing and other items as incentives for clients to attend the gender-sensitive programme.

The Chicks Day staff joked that, similar to the 2007 political *Fidesz* slogan 'two children, three rooms, and four wheels', Image 6.4 should be called 'four adults, four kids, three wheels'. The slogan, which was used during *Fidesz* political strategy from 1998 to 2002, promised the 'capitalist dream' of family, housing and personal transport for Hungarian citizens. The title given to Image 6.4 is a satirical comment on the lives of Chicks Day clients. Most of the women who used the services at Chicks Day were living in dire poverty and relied on donations such as the clothing pictured in the image. These private donations from individuals and other charities to non-governmental organisations like the harm reduction centre were specifically crucial for Chicks Day clients because the Hungarian welfare state did not provide adequate care. Furthermore, state harms exacerbated danger to clients and ultimately the harm reduction centre as a whole. A mix of cuts to funding and political pressure forced the harm reduction centre to close in the second half of 2014, and with it, the Chicks Day programme was finished. As such, Chicks Day clients 'safe place' was lost.

Conclusion

The analysis presented in this chapter has been framed within the context of how clients and staff make sense of danger and harm, as well as the reduction of harm in their lives. Research conducted with and about Chicks Day clients and staff revealed how historical and cultural narratives of dangerous people coalesced to depict the harm reduction centre as a place not welcome in the perceived 'community', although clients were indeed very much an ingrained part of the community in a broader sense.

Response to danger was the creation of a 'safe place'. This safe place was two-fold: first, a 'safe place' to deposit syringes in a secure container and also a symbolic 'safe space' for PWID and identified as women to have a place of reprieve from the stigma and dangers they experienced in their day-to-day lives. Chicks Day was not an idyllic paradise in which clients could forget their life, but it was a pause in their harsh realities. The NSEP at the harm reduction centre provided a targeted public health intervention without the danger of stigma or judgement that clients feared from many other Hungarian medical services. Chicks Day clients experienced stigma and marginalisation because of both the societal discrimination of being Roma and the stigmatisation of drug use in general and injecting drug use in particular. Furthermore, clients were associated with pollution stigmas and taboos relating to injecting drug use, blood-borne diseases and ethnic minorities (Douglas, 1966; Masseria et al., 2010). Analysis of the photographs and participant interviews and discussions reveal how drug use was a signifier for overlapping sexist and racist constructions linked to power relations and structural inequality. This chapter also highlights the tenacity of the Chicks Day staff, who created a gender-sensitive safe space for a marginalised group of women who were deemed 'dangerous' to the Hungarian normative status quo.

Acknowledgements

Funding for the research presented in this chapter was provided by the Educational, Audiovisual and Culture Executive Agency of the European Union through an Erasmus Mundus Fellowship.

References

Baker, T., and Wang, C. 2006. Photovoice: Use of a participatory action research method to explore the chronic pain experience in older adults. *Qualitative Health Research* 16 (10), pp. 1405–13.

Bence, R., and Udvarhelyi, É.T. 2013. The growing criminalization of homelessness in Hungary – A brief overview. *European Journal of Homelessness* 7 (2), pp. 133–43.

Benoit, C., Jansson, M., Smith, M., and Flagg, J. 2018. Prostitution stigma and its effect on the working conditions, personal lives, and health of Sex workers. *The Journal of Sex Research* 55 (4–5), pp. 457–71.

Bluthenthal, R., Kral, A., Gee, L., Erringer, E., and Edlin, B. 2000. The effect of syringe exchange use on high-risk injection drug users: A cohort study. *AIDS* 14 (5), pp. 605–11.

Botescu, A., Abagiu, A., Mardarescu, M., and Ursan, M. 2012. *HIV/AIDS Among Injecting Drug Users in Romania – Report of a Recent Outbreak and Initial Response Policies*. Lisbon: EMCDDA. Available at: http://www/emcdda.europa/eu/attachements.cfm/att_192024_EN_HIV_outbreak_Romania_2012.pdf.

Boyd, S. 1999. *Mothers and Illicit Drugs: Transcending the Myths*. Toronto: University of Toronto Press.

Boyd, S. 2004. *From Witches to Crack Moms: Women, Drug Law, and Policy*. Durham: Carolina Academic Press.

Campbell, N., and Ettorre, E. 2011. *Gendering Addiction: The Politics of Drug Treatment in a Neurochemical World*. New York: Palgrave Macmillan.

Corsi, M., Crepaldi, C., Chiara, L., Lodovici, M.S., Boccagni, P., and Vasilescu, C. 2008. *Ethnic Minority and Roma Women in Europe: A Case for Gender Equality?* Luxembourg: Publications Office of the European Union.

Csák, R., Demetrovics, Z., and Rácz, J. 2013. Transition to injecting 3,4-methylene-dioxy-pyrovalerone (MDPV) among needle exchange program participants in Hungary. *Journal of Psychopharmacology* 22 (6), pp. 559–63.

Csete, J. 2006. 'Second on the needle': Human rights of women who use drugs. *HIV/AIDS Policy and Law Review* 11 (2/3), pp. 66–7.

Csorba, J., Dénes, B., Miletics, M., and Nyizsnyánszki, A. 2003. *Harm Reduction Programs in Hungary*. Budapest: Társaság a Szabadságjogokért [TASZ]. Available at: http://tasz.hu/files/tasz/imce/HCLU_-_Harm_Reduction_in_Hungary.pdf.

Douglas, M. 1966. *Purity and Danger: An Analysis of the Concepts of Pollution and Taboo*. London: Routledge.

Du Rose, N. 2015. *The Governance of Female Drug Users: Women's Experiences of Drug Policy*. London: Policy Press.

El-Bassel, N., and Strathdee, S. 2015. Women who use or inject drugs: An action agenda for women-specific, multilevel, and combination HIV prevention and research. *Journal of Acquired Immune Deficiency Syndrome* 69 (Suppl 2), pp. S182–S190.

El-Bassel, N., Wechsberg, W.M., and Shaw, S.A. 2012. Dual HIV risk and vulnerabilities among women who use or inject drugs: No single prevention strategy is the answer. *Current Opinion in HIV and AIDS* 7 (4), pp. 326–31.

Ettorre, E. 2004. Revisioning women and drug use: Gender sensitivity, embodiment and reducing harm. *International Journal of Drug Policy* 15 (5–6), pp. 327–35.

Eurasian Harm Reduction Network [EHRN]. 2010. *Women and Drug Policy in Eurasia*. Vilnius: EHRN.

European Monitoring Centre for Drugs and Drug Addiction [EMCDDA]. 2010. *EMCDDA Monographs: Harm Reduction: Evidence, Impacts and Challenges*. Rhodes, T., and Hedrich, D. (Eds.). Lisbon: EMCDDA.

European Monitoring Centre for Drugs and Drug Addiction [EMCDDA]. 2018. *Hungary: Country Drug Report*. Available at: www.emcdda.europa.eu/countries/drug-reports/2018/hungary_e.

Fitzgerald, J., and Threadgold, T. 2004. Fear of sense in the street heroin market. *International Journal of Drug Policy* 15 (5–6), pp. 407–17.

Fitzgibbon, W., and Stengel, C. 2018. Women's voices made visible: Photovoice in visual criminology. *Punishment and Society* 20 (4), pp. 411–31.

Földes, M.E., and Covaci, A. 2012. Research on Roma health and access to healthcare: State of the art and future challenges. *International Journal of Public Health* 57 (1), pp. 37–9.

Friedman, S.R., Southwell, M., Bueno, R., Paone, D., Byrne, J., and Crofts, N. 2001. Harm reduction – A historical view from the left. *International Journal of Drug Policy* 12 (3), pp. 3–14.

Goffman, E. 1963. *Stigma: Notes on the Management of Spoiled Identity*. New York: Simon and Schuster, Inc.

Grbich, C. 2007. *Qualitative Data Analysis: An Introduction*. London: SAGE Publishing.

Gyarmathy, V., Csák, R., Bálint, K., Bene, E., Varga, A., Varga, M., Csiszér, N., Vingender, I., and Rácz, J. 2016. A needle in the haystack – The dire straits of needle exchange in Hungary. *BMC Public Health* 16 (157). doi:10.1186/s12889-016-2842-2.

Hancock, I. 2002. *We are the Romani People*. Hertfordshire: University of Hertfordshire Press.

Harm Reduction International [HRI]. 2018. *The Global State of Harm Reduction*. Available at: www.hri.global/global-state-harm-reduction-2018.

Human Rights Watch. 2013. *Wrong Direction on Rights: Assessing the Impact of Hungary's New Constitution and Laws. United States of America*. Budapest: Human Rights Watch. Available at: www.hrw.org/sites/default/files/reports/hungary0513_ForUpload.pdf.

International Harm Reduction Association. 2010. What is harm reduction? Available at: www.ihra.net/what-is-harm-reduction.

Iversen, J., Page, K., Madden, A., and Maher, L. 2015. HIV, HCV and health-related harms among women who inject drugs: Implications for prevention and treatment. *Journal of Acquired Immune Deficiencies Syndrome* 69 (1), pp. S176–S181.

Kende, Á. 2000. The Hungary of otherness: The Roma (Gypsies) of Hungary. *Journal of European Area Studies* 8 (2), pp. 187–201.

Kensy, J., Stengel, C., Nougier, M., and Birgin, R. 2012. *Drug Policy and Women: Addressing the Negative Consequences of Harmful Drug Control*. London: International Drug Policy Consortium. Available at: www.grea.ch/sites/default/files/drug-policy-and-women-addressing-the-consequences-of-control.pdf.

Kovács, Z. 2009. Social and economic transformation of historical neighbourhoods in Budapest. *Tijdschrift voor economische en sociale geografie* 100 (4), pp. 399–416.

Ladányi, J., and Szelényi, I. 2005. The nature and social determinants of Roma poverty. *Review of Sociology* 8 (2), pp. 75–96.

Lendvai-Bainton, N. 2017. Radical politics in post-crisis Hungary: Illiberal democracy, neoliberalism and the end of the welfare state. In: Kennett, P., and Lendvai-Bainton, N. (Eds.), *Handbook of European Social Policy*. Cheltenham: Edward Elgar Publishing Limited, pp. 400–14.

Lenton, S., and Single, E. 1998. The definition of harm reduction. *Drug and Alcohol Review* 17 (2), pp. 213–19.

Levy, J. 2014. *Drug User Peace Initiative: A War on Women who Use Drugs*. London: International Network of People who Use Drugs. Available at: www.druguserpeaceinitiative. org/dupidocuments/DUPI-A_War_on_Women_who_Use_Drugs.pdf.

Link, B., and Phelan, J. 2001. Conceptualizing stigma. *Annual Review of Sociology* 27, pp. 363–85.

Link, B., and Phelan, J. 2006. Stigma and its public health implications. *The Lancet* 367 (9509), pp. 528–9.

Lloyd-Smith, E., Kerr, T., Hogg, R.S., Li, K., Montaner, J.S.G., and Wood, E. 2005. Prevalence and correlates of abscesses among a cohort of injection drug users. *Harm Reduction Journal* 2 (24). doi:10.116/1477-7517-2-24.

Lupton, D. 1993. Risk as moral danger: The social and political functions of risk discourse in public health. *International Journal of Health Services* 23 (3), pp. 425–35.

Malinowska-Sempruch, K., and Rychkova, O. 2015. *The Impact of Drug Policy on Women*. New York Open Society Institute. Available at: www.opensocietyfoundations.org/reports/impact-drug-policywomen.

Marlatt, G.A. 1996. Harm reduction: Come as you are. *Addictive Behaviours* 21 (6), pp. 779–88.

Masseria, C., Mladovsky, P., and Hernández-Quevedo, C. 2010. The socio-economic determinants of the health status of Roma in comparison with non-Roma in Bulgaria, Hungary and Romania. *European Journal of Public Health* 20 (5), pp. 549–54.

Measham, F. 2003. The gendering of drug use and the absence of gender. *Criminal Justice Matters* 53, pp. 22–3.

Melles, K., Márványkövi, F., and Rácz, J. 2007. Low-threshold services for problem drug users in Hungary. *Central European Journal of Public Health* 15 (2), pp. 84–6.

Mitchell, C., De Lange, N., and Moletsane, R. 2017. *Participatory Visual Methodologies: Social Change, Community and Policy*. London: SAGE Publications.

Móró, L., Simon, K., and Sárosi, P. 2013. Drug use among sex workers in Hungary. *Social Science and Medicine* 93, pp. 64–9.

O'Hare, P.A., Newcombe, R., Matthews, A., Buning, E.C., and Drucker, E. (Eds.) 1992. *The Reduction of Drug-Related Harm*. London: Routledge.

Parkin, S. 2014. *An Applied Visual Sociology: Picturing Harm Reduction*. London: Ashgate.

Parliament Resolution NO.80/2013 (X. 16) on the *National Anti-Drug Strategy 2013–2020: Clear Consciousness, Sobriety and the Fight Against Drug Crime*. 2013 (Vol. 2013). Budapest.

Péterfi, A., Tarján, A., and Horváth, C. 2014. Changes in patterns of injecting drug use in Hungary: A shift to synthetic cathinones. *Drug Testing and Analysis* 6 (7–8), pp. 825–31.

Pink, S. 2007. *Doing Visual Ethnography: Images, Media and Representation in Research* (2nd ed.). London: SAGE Publications.

Pinkham, S., Stoicescu, C., and Myers, B. 2012. Developing effective health interventions for women who inject drugs: Key areas and recommendations for program development and policy. *Advances in Preventive Medicine*. doi:10.1155/2012/269123.

Platt, L., Grenfell, P., Meiksin, R., Elmes, J., Sherman, S.G., Sanders, T, et al. 2018. Associations between sex work laws and sex workers' health: A systematic review and meta-analysis of quantitative and qualitative studies. *PLoS Medicine* 15 (12), p. e1002680. doi:10.1371/journal/pmed.1002680.

Rácz, J., and Csák, R. 2014. Új pszichoaktív anyagok megjelenése egy budapesti tűcsereprogram kliensei körében, [Emergence of novel psychoactive substances among clients of a needle exchange programme in Budapest]. *Orvosi Hetilap* 155 (35), pp. 1383–94.

Rácz, J., Csák, R., and Lisznyai, S. 2015. Transition from 'old' injected drugs to mephedrone in an urban micro segregate in Budapest, Hungary: A qualitative analysis. *Journal of Substance Use* 20 (3), pp. 178–86.

Rácz, J., Gyarmathy, V., and Csák, R. 2016. New cases of HIV among PWIDs in Hungary: False alarm or early warning? *International Journal of Drug Policy* 27, pp. 13–16.

Rácz, J., Gyarmathy, V., Neaigus, A., and Ujhelyi, E. 2007. Injecting equipment sharing and perception of HIV and hepatitis risk among injecting drug users in Budapest. *AIDS Care* 19 (1), pp. 59–66.

Rekart, M.L. 2005. Sex-work harm reduction. *Lancet* 366 (9503), pp. 2123–34.

Rhodes, T. 2009. Risk environments and drug harms: A social science for harm reduction approach. *International Journal of Drug Policy* 20 (3), pp. 193–201.

Roberts, A., Mathers, B., and Degenhardt, L. 2010. *Women Who Inject Drugs: A Review of Their Risks, Experiences and Needs*. Sydney: Reference Group to the United Nations on HIV and Injecting Drug Use. Available at: www.unodc.org/documents/hiv-aids/Women_who_inject_drugs.pdf.

Robinson, N. 2013. Picturing social inclusion: Photography and identity in down town eastside Vancouver. *Graduate Journal of Social Science* 10 (2), pp. 20–42.

Rose, G. 2016. *Visual Methodologies: An Introduction to Researching with Visual Materials* (4th ed.). London: SAGE Publications.

Simmonds, L., and Coomber, R. 2009. Injecting drug users: A stigmatised and stigmatising population. *International Journal of Drug Policy* 20 (2), pp. 121–30.

Stengel, C. 2014. The risk of being 'too honest': Drug use, stigma and pregnancy. *Health, Risk and Society* 16 (1), pp. 36–50.

Stimson, G.V. 1998. Harm reduction in action: Putting theory into practice. *International Journal of Drug Policy* 9 (6), pp. 401–9.

Stoicescu, C., Cluver, L., Spreckelsen, T., Casale, M., and Sudewo, A.G. 2018. Intimate partner violence and HIV sexual risk behaviour among women who inject drugs in Indonesia: A respondent-driven sampling study. *AIDS Behavior* 22 (10), pp. 3307–23.

Strathdee, S.A., and Vlahov, D. 2001. The effectiveness of needle exchange programs: A review of the science and policy. *AIDScience* 1 (16). Available at: http://aidscience.org/Articles/aidscience013.asp.

Tarján, A., Dudás, M., Gyarmathy, A., Rusvai, E., Tresó, B., and Csohán, Á. 2015. Emerging risks due to new injecting patterns in Hungary during austerity times. *Substance Use and Misuse* 50 (7), pp. 848–58.

United Nations Office on Drugs and Crime [UNODC]. 2014. *Women Who Inject Drugs and HIV: Addressing Specific Needs*. Available at: www.unodc.org/documents/hivaids/publications/WOMEN_POLICY_BRIEF2014.pdf.

Wang, C. 1999. Photovoice: A participatory action research strategy applied to women's health. *Journal of Women's Health* 8 (2), pp. 185–92.

Wang, C., and Burris, M. 1997. Photovoice: Concept, methodology, and use for participatory needs assessment. *Health Education and Behavior* 24 (3), pp. 369–87.

7 Risk factors and dangerous classes in a European context

The consequences of ethnic framing of and among Turkish drug users in Ghent, Belgium

Charlotte De Kock

Introduction

Dangerous classes and risk factors in the continental European context

Academic work and political (mis)use of 'dangerous classes' discourse differ considerably across continents. The deeply entrenched racialised segregation of American society as reflected in this discourse and the widespread use of race-based categories[1] of analysis cannot simply be transposed to a European context. Nevertheless, considerable similarities have emerged during the last two decades in Europe.

Over 20 years ago, Silver (1996) argued that the US- and UK-based 'dangerous classes' discourse depicted an 'underclass' category of predominantly 'black' citizens portrayed as 'unwilling' to participate in society. Contrarily, for example, French and Belgian public debates were, and are, much more dominated by the 'excluded' concept, argued to be less static and allegedly projecting the societal ideal of an inclusive post-ethnic (Martiniello, 2013) society. Exclusion then is a rupture of social bonds that needs fixing, whereas belonging to the dangerous underclass is simply a state of being, a choice and a static status (Morris, 1996, p. 162; Silver, 1996, p. 110). Nevertheless, French scholars such as Balibar (1992) also cautioned the use of the 'exclusion' concept, because 'no one is outside the society' (in Mingione, 1996, p. 115) and the use of this concept evades debates on class conflict, unemployment and exclusion from citizenship.

Indeed, notions of exclusion and integration that dominate Belgian public debate have similar societal consequences as the 'dangerous class' discourse in the United States. In Europe too, ethnicity and culture (rather than race) are lately more frequently presented as the root causes of societal problems. Subsequently, social policies are aimed at risk factors among, or problems 'caused by', specific migrant and ethnic minority populations (MEM in what follows), obfuscating the role of historical and contemporary structures that produce discrimination and disadvantage. Social policies, in other words, often focus on effects (i.e. drawing on religion or closer ethnic ties because of exclusion) rather than on the root causes (Moore, 1989, 2015).

In the domain of mental health and substance use treatment, culture and ethnicity are related to 'risk and protective factors' (i.e. religiousness, strong ethnic identity or network, etc.). Thus, 'dangerousness' in the form of 'risk factors' has influenced social work and the psy-disciplines too (Blackman, 1996; Castel, 1986). Since the beginning of the twentieth century, the 'dangerousness' of the 'mentally ill' has been gradually replaced by these 'risk factors' as 'characteristic' to individuals and groups.

Although specific groups (i.e. the poor, homeless and other 'aliens') are no longer presupposed to be 'dangerous', they are now attributed risk factors, potentially posing a threat to society (Castel, 1986) or themselves. In other words, the 'risky individual' became the individual at risk. A recent European study (Lemmens et al., 2017), for instance, suggests that 'coming from an alcohol culture, a khat culture or an opium culture' is a risk factor for problem use while 'being a devout Muslim' is considered a protective factor among some MEM.

Nevertheless, 'risk' still holds the potential imputation of 'being dangerous' and this is potentially harmful for the populations at hand. Madeira and colleagues (2018), for instance, found that perceiving migrants as a threat or risk to public health is indicative for health providers' self-reported bias in treatment, a bias directly related to lower-quality treatment.

European research on substance use and treatment among MEM

Even though most high-income countries (i.e. the United States, Canada, Australia) invested – be it with limited success – considerably in nationwide (mental) health equity programmes for MEM, Europe is lagging behind when it comes to both research and policy initiatives, especially in the domain of drug treatment. It seems as if the French sociological project to transcend Anglosaxon race discourse (see aforementioned discussion) and the European 'unity in diversity' discourse have had an opposite effect: we have neglected the needs and blatant disparities among MEM. There is surprisingly little evidence about (mental) health, let alone problem substance use and treatment, among these populations in the EU. A core impediment is the absence of standardised scientifically sound ethnicity-related proxies, indicators and variables in census (Farkas, 2017) and in European drug treatment data (De Kock, 2019b).[2]

Nordgren (2017, p. 43), in his study 'making drug use ethnic' argues that the topic 'has mainly been in focus in works considering drug policy in the United States, and to a certain extent in ethnographic research on street level dealing' (Bourgois, 1996; Bucerius, 2014; Lalander, 2017). European ethnographic studies have mainly argued that societal reactions to drug use among MEM have more to do with negative views about MEM than with the specific drugs (Nordgren, 2017) or the nature of participants' ethnic culture.

Indeed, evidence on the determinants of substance use and access to (mental) health suggests that culture is not the main issue in overcoming health disparities. In a study across 23 European countries, Missine and colleagues (2012) found that

European MEM experience more depressive symptoms compared to non-MEM counterparts due to socio-economic factors and discrimination. Dauvrin and Lorant (2012), Rechel et al. (2013) and Horyniak et al. (2016) in turn highlight that access restrictions, in Karl-Trummer and colleagues' words (2010), are increasingly 'used as a weapon' in restrictive immigration policies.

Nevertheless, culture and cultural competence are becoming buzzwords in European health care (see e.g. Hordijk et al., 2018; Sorensen et al., 2017). It was first introduced as a guiding principle in treatment and prevention by the American Substance Abuse and Mental Health Services Administration (SAMHSA) and has since influenced discourse on European health inequities. However, scholars have argued that evidence of the influence of cultural competence on disparities is insufficient (Horvat et al., 2014). Furthermore, little European research has attempted to understand culture and cultural competence in the drug treatment context and whether it is sufficient to deal with the roots of health disparities (Rechel et al., 2013).

The framing of treatment disparities in cultural contexts needs to be studied critically and scrupulously because 'irrespective of who is blamed [for health disparities], failure to recognise the intersection of culture with other structural and societal factors creates and compounds poor health outcomes' (Napier et al., 2014, p. 1607). The paucity of European research in this domain raises the question: should culture be a focus in improving substance use treatment for MEM and what does culture/ethnicity mean to specific MEM individuals? I intend to offer only a partial answer to this question by looking at the meaning and performative nature of culture and ethnicity, and experiences in treatment, among a purposive sample of recreational and problem users with a Turkish background in Ghent (Belgium)[3] and by comparing their perspectives to provider perspectives and the literature on cultural competence.

Building on our critique of the use of 'culture' and 'ethnicity' as static categories in epidemiology and the proposal to study problem use among MEM intersectionally at the micro-, meso- and macro-levels (De Kock et al., 2017), we will examine the grounds of 'being Turkish' and 'being Muslim' as ethnic constructions in the lived context of individuals and as perceived 'risk factors' among mental health providers and in cultural competence literature. We explore the grounds and fluidness of these constructs, the consequences of perceived negative framing in the community (because of drug use), in society (i.e. as 'Turkish' or 'Muslim') and its relation to help seeking and treatment.

Method

The analysis is based on interviews[4] with 47 individuals aged 18–65 with a Turkish migration background living in Ghent, Belgium. Participants were recruited by means of snowball and purposive sampling in a community-based participatory research study (De Kock and Decorte, 2017). All the respondents describe themselves as having a Turkish background and having experience with illegal substance use or episodes of excessive drinking during the last year. One participant

Table 7.1 Participants per user type and substance used

	Heroin (n = 13)	Cannabis (n = 14)	Alcohol (n = 12)	Prescription drugs (n = 11)	Speed (n = 2)	Hallucino-genics (n = 1)	Anabols (n = 1)	Gambling (n = 1)	Total
Users in recovery	9	5	4	2					20
Problem users	2	4	2	1				1	10
Recovered users	1				2		1		5
Recreational users		5	6			1			12

self-describes as a problem gambler. Participants self-described either as recreational or as problem users (Berger and Luckmann, 1966).[5]

Participants were further subdivided into four categories (see Table 7.1): users in recovery; problem users not in recovery (designated as 'problem users'); users who recovered and have not experienced a relapse in the past five years ('recovered users'); recreational users. Users in recovery have experienced at least one treatment episode. This categorisation is based on Best and colleagues' (2016) SONAR study on recovery capital. The majority of the interviews were conducted by trained community researchers with a Turkish migration background. The interviews with heroin users were conducted by a Belgian researcher without a migration background. The community researchers' specific attention to normative and religious frameworks that emerged during the primary analysis inspired the current secondary study. For in-depth descriptions of the interview guide, recruitment strategies and sample characteristics, I refer to previous publications from this study (De Kock and Decorte, 2017; De Kock et al., 2017).

For this secondary study, I analysed the following overarching thematic codes in qualitative research programme Nvivo12: ethnicity, the Turkish community, drug use, religion and treatment experiences. Before discussing these results, I will address (1) problem users' experiences in treatment and their experience with alternative treatment (by means of a secondary reading of 'substance use in the Turkish community in Ghent') (De Kock et al., 2017), (2) the frames applied by mental health providers as studied by Rondelez and colleagues (2018)[6] and (3) a literature review of the cultural competence (CC in what follows) concept in drug treatment (De Kock, 2019a). This integrated analysis allows us to describe how ethnicity interacts with problem use and treatment, to identify how provider views and CC discourse align with these needs or rather serve to frame culturalised 'risk factors' among these populations.

Rationale

Martiniello (2013) proposes studying the ethnicity construct at a micro-level (subjective feeling of belonging), meso-social level (ethnic group) and macro-level (structural constraints). Similarly, the eco-social health perspective (Krieger, 2012) posits that treatment barriers and causes of disease are located at the micro-level (client and provider), meso-level (service provision) and macro-level (health care policy and dominant theoretical scope) (see e.g. Andrade et al., 2014; Scheppers et al., 2006). This framework has been elaborated upon by Alegria who hypothesises that 'disparities in substance use services arise when disadvantages in the health care system interact with those in the community system' (Alegria et al., 2011, p. 377).

I add to the eco-social perspective of both ethnicity and health inequities the claim that access barriers as well as root causes for problem use are not only located at one or the other level but that the same 'barrier' and root cause should also be considered intersectionally at all three levels and both among (potential) clients and among providers. It follows that root causes for problem use will be located at intersections of client micro-, meso- and macro-levels and that access and quality in treatment can be located in these same intertwinements adding the actor of the treatment provider (micro), treatment service (meso) and broader health system (macro) (see Figure 7.1).

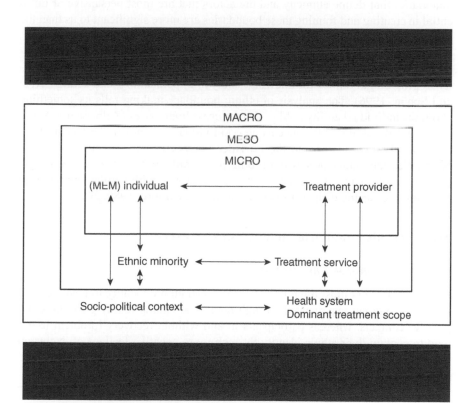

Figure 7.1 An eco-social perspective on substance use and treatment among migrants and ethnic minorities

Source: Adapted from Krieger and colleagues, 2013 (Epidemiology and the People's Health).

It goes without saying that the intertwinement of micro-, meso- and macro-levels is co-produced by subjective self-understanding and external framing of actors at all levels. In other words, the framing of ethnic minority and migrant clients among providers (as citizens), services and health systems will influence problem use, access and quality of care among (potential) clients.

Consequently, I intend to unpack the enactment of ethnicity as a subjective feeling of belonging among individuals and an ethnic group as well as its macro-consequences for the individual (among Turkish users in Ghent), but also the way it is constructed among professionals (working with Muslim clients) and in the literature on cultural competence in drug treatment. This will enable us to highlight the performative nature of ethnicity instead of 'the cultural stuff' enclosed within ethnic boundaries and examine the interaction with problem use, help seeking and treatment.

I depart from Weber's notion of ethnicity as the social construction of differences in social relations instead of objective differences between groups. This is in line with the idea that ethnicity is a means to create boundaries that enable groups to distance themselves from one another (Barth, 1969/1998). Consequently, the boundaries that define ethnicity and the actors that are most persuasive or influential in creating and framing these boundaries are more significant to us than the 'cultural stuff' perceived to be enclosed within them (Wimmer, 2013).

The ethnic boundaries or frames are conceived of as 'socially produced structures for selecting, organizing, interpreting, and making sense of a complex reality to provide guidelines for knowing, analysing, persuading, and acting' (Rein and Schön, 1996). The analysis of ethnic boundary making tells us something about the individual ability to blur, shift or cross boundaries (Zolberg and Woon, 1999) and about the – substance using – individual's agency in the face of these perceived boundaries.[7] From the provider perspective, the creation of ethnic boundaries can induce processes of 'othering' (Said, 1978) and frame seemingly static characteristics of populations as 'risk factors', with similar (moralising) consequences as the dangerous classes discourse (Moore, 1989, 2015).

Micro: ethnic boundaries among Turkish users

'I'm Turkish because I'm a migrant'

Recreational users most often link their personal ethnic identity to positive feelings of belonging, experienced through fasting, attending family gatherings and positive contacts, whereas participants in and without recovery (problem users) tend to explain their ethnic identity through more negative feelings of exclusion (by Belgians or by Turkish people).

> *Do you feel Belgian?*
>
> I do partly, partly not. I'm in between. I'm second generation. But being Belgian . . . I adapt to everything here. I can live like a Belgian. I live like that. But you remain a Turk, you've got tanned skin.
>
> (Mehmed, male, 44, in recovery, cannabis)

Do you feel Belgian?

Honestly, I don't. We can be Belgian on paper as much as we like, we will always be seen as . . . black people.

(Kaan, male, 35, recovered, steroids)

Recreational users tend to be more at ease with and clear about their ethnic identity, whether it means feeling wholly Belgian or Turkish or part Belgian and part Turkish. It is notable that, among problem users not in recovery, all but one feel more Turkish than Belgian. In contrast, among recreational users, all but one feel more Belgian.

What does it mean to you to be Belgian? Being Belgian . . . I can't be Belgian, I have the Turkish nationality. I belong to the Turkish people. I have contact with the Turkish people. The Turkish community . . . I feel more . . . I'm a Turkish person because I'm a migrant.

(Nezih, male, 42, in recovery, heroin and methadone)

What does it mean to be Belgian to you? It doesn't mean anything. **Why?** We live here. I'm Turkish but we have to integrate in this society. We have to adapt to their culture. . . . Being Belgian doesn't mean a thing to me. Being Belgian means not being an exception. I'm proud to be Turkish.

(Erol, male, 35, problem gambler)

'I am a junkie and that's how they look at me'

When participants are asked whether a Turkish community exists in Ghent, all answer that it does but explicitly clarify that there are subgroups and identities related to native villages, educational status and religion. Some participants note that a community exists because of the shared experience of exclusion from society and a shared migration history.

It used to be like one group, like one from Turkmentoy [village] . . . (doubts) well, let's say it was three groups, but today there's a lot more groups and they've all become smaller. In the past there was like one Diyanet mosque, the big mosque, and now there's the Suleymanci's and others that adhere to the bearded guys. There's all kinds of different groups.

(Derya, female, 38, in recovery, prescription drugs)

More than half of the participants state that they are different from most community members because they are not from the same village, are better educated or hold different values. The respondents who use these reasons for distancing themselves from the community are mainly recreational and, to a lesser extent, recovered users. They are creative about what they perceive of as ethnic boundaries and seem to be able to blur these boundaries in their personal lives by distancing themselves from the community regarding the aspects that they are not fond of.

I feel at home in that group, growing up, my whole life is associated with Turkey. But, on the other side, the Turkish communities in Belgium and Holland are more conservative.

(Eda, female, 22, recreational, cannabis)

Participants in and without recovery seem to experience the perceived ethnic boundaries as more static and restrictive and seem unable to blur, shift or cross (Zolberg and Woon, 1999) these perceived boundaries. All users in and without recovery describe the Turkish community negatively, and at least half state explicitly that they avoid contact with the community because they feel excluded and socially pressured because of their lifestyle and problem use. Some report that they are seen as 'junkies' and feel they are the subject of gossip. In other words, they feel the Turkish community frames drug users in a way that excludes them from this community.

There are bars and non-profit organisations that Turks visit and sit on their asses all day. And gossip about someone else's business and this and that. So I don't belong there. I am a junkie and that's how they look at me.

(Erhan, male, 55, in recovery, heroin and methadone)

Recreational and recovered users confirm this taboo on substance use. Four in five of the recovered users distance themselves from what they conceived of as 'the community'. One recovered heroin user rejoined the imagined Turkish community and incorporated an anti-drug discourse into his own discourse.

Look, it's users themselves that feel they are shameful. It's not like other people tell them, 'Oh we are going to gossip about you!' Users just say 'It's a shame I'm doing this. It's a shame I'm a dirty junkie'. That's what we think. We see it as a shame. We are not soft on users. We say: 'What bullshit is this?! Man up!' Actually I think that's a good thing. You are pushed into a corner – you have to be strong.

(Arda, male, 36, recovered, heroin and cocaine)

Two respondents mention they moved to another neighbourhood to avoid the stigma they were confronted with. Lastly, three participants mention that Turkish media – often watched by satellite – also mould the discourse on substance use.

You know, in the media in Turkey they report really badly on cannabis. They talk about it as if it were heroin, so you're seen as a . . . junkie.

(Cemil, male, 31, recreational, alcohol and cannabis)

'It's literally in the Koran that it [substance use] is forbidden'

All but three respondents state that they are Muslim. But being Muslim has very different meanings for the respondents. Similar to participants' feelings about the perceived community, recreational and recovered users more explicitly define their own position regarding the perceived values and norms of Islam, whereas participants in and without recovery feel pressured and ashamed towards the religious community.

> I'm a practising Muslim. But I'm also 22 in the twenty-first century. . . . I have my own ideas about the world. I can say, 'Okay, that's where religion comes from because of this or that reason', and that's how I take it.
>
> (Eda, female, 22, recreational, cannabis)

> It's literally in the Koran that [substance use] is forbidden, but it's my own choice. In theory I'm a good Muslim, but I don't practise. But I'm a good person, I work.
>
> (Bilal, male, 35, recreational, alcohol)

> I don't practise. I'm a Muslim, I should pray five times a day, do Ramadan. But I don't fast. I try my best to do the five prayers. But I believe in God.
>
> (Arda, male, 36, recovered, heroin and cocaine)

> I don't pray five times a day, but normally I should, but I don't do it. I should fast too. I can't because I drink methadone.
>
> (Ekrem, male, 47, problem user, heroin)

When participants are asked how they feel substance use is viewed within the Turkish community, half mention the notion of *haram* (opposite to *hallal*), referring to what is 'forbidden' in Islam and subsequently reflecting 'risk framing' by means of the perceived belief system. When probing what *haram* means to them, participants give remarkably different and a wide array of interpretations, demonstrating how individuals interpret religion differently. Participants mostly refer to the fact that the use of anaesthetising substances and mistreating the body is considered forbidden. Overall, mostly problem users seem to struggle with how to match their use with their beliefs, whereas recreational users take more individualist stances and interpret *haram* flexibly.

> I don't know the exact year, but heroin was invented in the 1940s. The rules of Islam date back way earlier. You can't just add new rules. So you can do [heroin], but it might be considered 'rather don't do it'.
>
> (Yaser, male, 18, recreational, cannabis)

> It's really difficult, you know, you struggle with your faith and your conscience: you know that you're not allowed to [drink alcohol] and you still do it anyway! . . . You're fighting your own conscience because you know you're doing the wrong thing by using alcohol. You don't want it, but you still do it, you have no control over it!
>
> (Elif, female, 45, problem user, alcohol)

'They will all look at me, like, "Oh there's that junkie"'

Only 3 out of 47 participants go to a house of prayer regularly. Similar to feelings of shame regarding Islam and the Turkish community, more than half of the participants in and without recovery explain that they do not feel accepted in the religious community. Their shame about substance use is the main reason for not going to a mosque. One person in recovery goes to a Moroccan mosque to avoid stigma.

> I don't go to the mosque. . . . You have to be clean, take a shower. Wearing the same dirty clothes and socks, you won't go. For prayer you can't have dirty socks.
>
> (Erhan, male, 55, in recovery, heroin and methadone)

> When I'm clean [I can go to a mosque]. When I drink, I can't go there for 40 days.
>
> (Adil, male, 21, problem user, cannabis)

> They will all look at me, like, 'Oh there's that junkie', that's how they'll look at me. I'll get angry with myself, while I'd want to do something good, it wouldn't turn out well. I won't feel good. Better to stay at home, pray at home and ask God for forgiveness.
>
> (Ekrem, male, 47, problem user, heroin)

Recreational users in turn feel less attached to the religious communities and seem more at ease with not going to a mosque.

> I've been to a mosque, and it has a large impact on me. The prayer really goes through my whole body. But I think, praying, for me, it doesn't have to be in a mosque.
>
> (Eda, female, 22, recreational, cannabis)

Some participants mention that they know about lectures in (some) mosques about drug prevention, but maintain that it is not the place to deal with continued problem use. Also, these lectures are, in some cases, interpreted as reinforcing the taboo and risk framing about substance use.

> The imam reads verses from the Koran and there are obviously a few things in there about addiction and what it's like, but I feel like it just says that it's punishable and why it's forbidden.
>
> (Evren, female, 18, recreational, cannabis)

'What will the imam say? Pray a bit?'

When asked if it is possible to discuss problem use with imams or hojas,[8] a large majority of participants answered negatively. The reason participants give is that imams or hojas are not the right people to help with such problems because they do not possess the skills needed to help problem users. Problem users also fear that an imam would judge their behaviour and gossip in the community, which in turn confirms problem users' feeling of being perceived as deviant in the religious community.

> It's a big taboo. For example, if you want to talk to a hoja about it you are totally dependent on what this person knows about it. Some time ago I got ill and I really wanted to talk to a hoja. You know what the first thing was that the hoja asked? 'Did you do something wrong in the face of Allah?' as if it would have been Allah who had punished me!
>
> (Derya, female, 38, in recovery, prescription drugs)

> Psychiatric problems . . . what will the imam say? Pray a bit? It's kind of limited. It's more the life questions they can help you with.
>
> (Fatih, male, 50, in recovery, heroin and methadone)

Nevertheless, two people dealing with psychosis did report good experiences of help from an imam.

> When I was in the hospital once [for psychosis], I asked an imam because I was having difficulties. He came and we recited Koran together, it relieves you.
>
> (Fatih, male, 50, in recovery, heroin and methadone)

Meso: treatment

All users in recovery by definition made use of treatment services. Half attended therapeutic communities, specialised and crisis units in hospitals several times. Participants describe treatment mismatch, waiting lists, blacklists and the lack of follow-up as the main issues in treatment.

The majority of participants argue that treatment models differ substantially across centres, and consequently their stories often reveal a treatment mismatch between personal treatment preferences and available treatment. This is exemplified by participants not agreeing with medication-based treatment (in crisis units, psychiatric wards and as prescribed by general practitioners), being in treatment with users with other types of dependencies and receiving treatment based on the 'breaking down – and building up' principle (De Kock et al., 2017, p. 111). Most participants report that they stayed for longer periods of time in centres that were less restrictive about visiting regulations and clients' freedoms.

Five out of 20 users in recovery mention frustration because of waiting lists for residential treatment. Being on a waiting list inhibits them from fully engaging at a crucial moment in the personal recovery process: the decision to have treatment. It also adds to treatment mismatch because the type of centre they are sent to is dependent on availability. Additionally, at least four participants report that they have been expelled and 'blacklisted' for what could be described as minor rule-breaking behaviour (De Kock et al., 2017, p. 114). They are barred from entering other treatment centres in the future, which in turn contributes to an increased chance that they will relapse.

All users in recovery explain that they began using again less than three months after successful treatment because they found it hard to retain their housing and easy to rejoin their old user networks (De Kock et al., 2017, p. 113). This issue is most prevalent upon release from prison, because participants in that situation had lost contact with family and friends and could not find a job. All respondents state that follow-up after treatment is crucial but that they rarely experienced it, particularly after incarceration.

Concerning alternative treatment methods, five participants had travelled to Turkey to get clean in a family environment or during their compulsory military service (De Kock et al., 2017, p. 109). However, these participants continued their use after returning to Belgium, because of a perceived lack of external support for their abstinence. Lastly, as mentioned in the previous section, five participants turned to an imam or hoja for help.

Meso: frames among mental health providers

Rondelez and colleagues (2018) studied the frames applied by 31 mental health professionals in their contact with Muslim clients. They identified recurring statements related to three overlapping frames: a biomedical, re-socialisation or culturalising frame.

Firstly, a biomedical frame was reflected in the recurring statement that Muslims have more psychosomatic complaints because they seem less aware of mental health problems. According to these participants, this results in Muslim clients presenting more often to general practitioners. Nevertheless, it should be noted that in European literature, the reason for presenting more often to general practitioners is related to access and knowledge rather than culture (Cuadra, 2012; Dauvrin and Lorant, 2014). The biomedical frame among Rondelez's participants is exemplified by professionals stating, for example, that 'their [Muslim] reasoning often takes the form of "the doctor will give me a pill so that my complaints will pass"' (Rondelez et al., 2018, p. 406). It could be argued that these professionals frame clients based on what they perceive of as characteristic (cultural) traits as opposed to their own views on good treatment, overlooking issues related to access and knowledge.

Secondly, a predominant re-socialisation frame was identified among providers that interpret mental health symptoms as clients' intention to avoid personal responsibility, and providers seeing personal responsibility for re-socialisation as the main aim of treatment. Similar to the moralising 'dangerous classes' discourse, Muslim clients are often portrayed as unwilling or rationally 'incapable' of taking responsibility (Silver, 1996) for their own re-socialisation. This is exemplified in statements such as 'they [Muslim clients] expect that they will change by taking a pill, without doing anything themselves' (Rondelez et al., 2018, p. 407). Considering that respondents consistently refer to 'Muslim client' characteristics in these re-socialisation and biomedical frames, these frames can be considered as 'other-ing' strategies among the participating providers.

Third, some providers appeared to construct cultural difference as an indicator of a progressive and independent 'we', as opposed to a religious and dependent 'they' (Rondelez et al., 2018). One respondent, for instance, argues that the Qu'ran is more important than a doctor among 'these clients' (Rondelez et al., 2018, p. 409). This frame does not reflect the diverse views on Islam reported by the Turkish participants, elaborated on earlier. Another participant in Rondelez's study notes that 'they [Muslim clients] try to solve these problems within the family as long as possible, until it is no longer sustainable' (Rondelez et al., 2018, p. 409). Once again, similar to the framing of American underclasses, it could be argued that these participants unwittingly attest of an idea of alleged 'cultural' reproduction (solving within the family) within a certain population as the evidence of rejecting mainstream values of society (in this case 'good treatment') (Murray 1984 in Morris, 1996, p. 162) instead of enquiring into the root causes of relying only on family members instead of mainstream services (i.e. because of low knowledge and/or access).

Rondelez concludes by noting that some professionals do recognise that they might excessively focus on their own normative framework, and that this might be a barrier in treatment. She further stresses that, across the identified frames, the agency of Muslim clients is strikingly absent. This reproduction of cultural stereotypes, assumptions and biases was also documented by Olcón and Gulbas (2018) and Madeira and colleagues (2018) (see introduction). It can be harmful to the quality and success of drug treatment considering that a relationship of trust between client and service provider is at the core of the clinical encounter.

Macro: the cultural competence frame

A similar unexplored notion of 'culture' was identified in a review of cultural competence (CC in what follows) in drug treatment (De Kock, 2019a) that was based on the 'What's the problem represented to be?' approach (Bacchi, 2012). I studied (1) the origin and nature of CC and derivatives in substance use treatment (SUT) (2007–2017), (2) the presuppositions as well as (3) how CC and derivatives in SUT are questioned and (4) what is left unquestioned.

Strikingly, only 8 of 41 studies about cultural competence included a clear definition of culture. In the majority of papers, culture was staged as a seemingly agency-free concept, although authors implicitly referred to clients' cultural background. The included papers referred to a much lesser extent to issues at the level of the health system (macro) or among professionals (meso) that could also well be defined in terms of underlying (treatment) cultures.

It is striking that most of the identified arguments in favour of CC and derivatives in SUT are located at the macro-level, including predominantly poorer (mental) health, lower disability adjusted life years (DALYs) and institutional racism, but that in practice CC is consistently more often aimed at client micro-level characteristics. This is reflected in the fact that only a small number of studies use macro outcome indicators that represent the influence of cultural competence on treatment disparities (i.e. access, satisfaction rates, adherence).

It remains unclear why culture is the point of departure in reducing drug treatment disparities amongst MEM. By overemphasising the individual service user 'culture' in treatment, CC proponents might unwittingly add to the isolation of and static views on MEM, which in turn diverts attention from systemic issues that are causing greater problems among MEM (Shaw and Armin, 2011) such as generalist services not meeting the responsibility to fulfil the right to mental health for all (Fountain and Hicks, 2010) and social correlates contributing to harmful substance use.

Discussion

Although the concept of 'dangerous classes' is fundamentally rooted in the US- and UK-based literature and has permeated the European debate on migration and ethnicity to a much lesser extent, the question posed by scholars such as Wacquant in the denomination of 'underclasses' as well as identifying 'risk factors' in the psy-disciplines (Castel, 1986) is pertinent to framing European migrants and ethnic minorities, especially in the drug treatment context.

While among professionals in Rondelez's study and in the review of cultural competence, 'culture' in treatment indeed often refers to client habits or customs in a static and 'othering' (Said, 1979) perspective and as 'risk factors', fleshing out what ethnicity means for problem users with a Turkish migration background paints a different picture. A remarkable similarity among these participants is that all agree that a Turkish community exists in Ghent and all but three identify as Muslims. Nevertheless, comparing recreational and recovered users to problem users and users in recovery reveals the complexity of these statements. Recreational and, to a lesser extent, recovered users link being 'Belgian', 'Turkish' and 'Muslim' explicitly to positive feelings of belonging. They also address the blurred delineation of 'being Muslim' and 'belonging to a community' by stating, for instance, that drinking alcohol or not praying does not mean that one is not Muslim.

Contrarily, problem users and users in recovery tend to link being 'Belgian', 'Turkish' and 'Muslim' to negative feelings of exclusion. They stress internalised shame and stigma towards what they perceive as the boundaries of these identities. They also appear to have less flexible ideas on what a 'good Muslim' should be and consider themselves 'bad Muslims'. They experience mutually conflicting and dependent conditions: they feel more Turkish partly because of a feeling of exclusion from general society, they have most contact with Turkish people (De Kock and Decorte, 2017), but they also feel excluded from the Turkish community. This double (Gary, 2005) or even triple stigma leads to label avoidance behaviour by withdrawing from what is conceived of as the Turkish and religious community and consequently losing the associated social support.

Van Kerckem and colleagues define part of this dynamic in this same community as 'ethnic conformity pressure'. It is a mechanism that could be considered as 'self-framing', exerted by group members, reinforced and strengthened by societal exclusion and expressed in direct discourse (gossip, ridicule) and indirectly through social control (Van Kerckem et al., 2014, p. 286). They identify three individual negotiation strategies to deal with this social pressure: conformation, creativity and disregard. In this study, only recreational and, to a lesser extent, recovered users demonstrate creativity and disregard in blurring these perceived ethnic boundaries.

Similar to Wacquant's study of French banlieu 'underclasses', we see that what for outsiders appears to be a monolithic ensemble (the Turkish community) is in fact very diverse. Moreover, the consciousness of stigmatisation in general society stimulates practices of internal social differentiation which in turn decreases interpersonal trust and undercuts solidarity (Wacquant, 1996, p. 244). Respondents overstress their moral worth as individuals and join dominant discourse that could contrarily work to confirm essentialist categories of 'the Turkish'. This is exemplified by recreational users stressing that they are different compared to other Turkish because they are higher educated, come from a city instead of a village or because they are less conservative. They deploy distancing strategies and thereby validate negative outsider perceptions.

Concerning religion, whereas some research suggests that being religious may be protective for the initiation of use and increased problem use, this study demonstrates that this is often not the case for continued problem use and studies among the same group demonstrate it is not protective for delinquency (Duchateau et al., 2006). A minority of the respondents find strength in their beliefs and only a few find support in a religious community. This is in line with studies that point out that when the religious community is perceived as too critical or demanding, distress may occur and in turn well-being may diminish (Schieman et al., 2013).

On the subject of help-seeking, it appears, as demonstrated in previous research in this population (Vardar et al., 2012), that the participants have sufficient knowledge of and make use of a broad array of treatment services. A small minority also consulted an imam or hoja, or went to Turkey to start their recovery. From a 'health bricolage' perspective, one could argue that those struggling with mental health issues – including problem drug use – will often draw upon a variety of perspectives on mental health and healing, depending on what is available to them (Phillimore et al., 2017). In the same line, attributing the widespread consultation of general practitioners for mental health problems to cultural understanding of mental health (see Rondelez et al., 2018) does not reflect the complexity of Turkish (potential) clients help-seeking behaviour.

A study among imams in Flanders (Loobuyck and Meier, 2014) confirms that imams feel that providing psychological support is one of their core tasks. Furthermore, the recent establishment of a 'Muslim advice point' in Ghent illustrates that imams can play a role in giving information, counselling or referring to other services. However, while some suggest that including imams and hojas in mental health care could increase access to and the relevance of care (Lim et al., 2015) (e.g. because they understand spiritual perspectives on mental health issues), the current study nuances this statement.

The inclusion of imams and hojas in treatment might in some cases lead to the enforcement of ethnic conformity pressure, not only out of fear that personal information might be passed in the community but also because of the possible imposition of a normative framework that is not helpful or even harmful to the client. Additionally, the majority of the participants in this study state that imams and hojas are not best placed and are insufficiently trained to deal with problem use.

Concerning treatment, whereas the presented provider and CC perspectives mainly focus on client–provider differences presented in biomedical, resocialisation, culturalising (habits, customs) and 'othering' frames, problem users themselves report other issues in treatment. They refer to exclusion (from the community, from general society, from treatment), waiting lists (and blacklists), treatment-mismatch and a lack of follow-up after treatment, all issues that are unrelated to their own 'culture'. These user narratives reveal aspects of what could be considered a treatment culture: the habit of having waiting lists and offering insufficient follow-up as well as the unspoken norm of referring clients to blacklists if their profile is considered 'too hard to handle' (or dangerous). In this sense, culture and exclusion as barriers to and in treatment should be perceived as barriers not only at the micro-level (client/substance user) but also at the meso-level (service provision) and macro-level (theoretical discourse as well as macro disparities).

Concluding remarks

A feeling of exclusion echoes throughout most of the problem user narratives in this research. Recreational and recovered users in turn argue that the Turkish community and being Muslim are layered and have different meanings to different individuals. These narratives demonstrate that the continuous construction and embodiment of what is perceived of as Turkish, Muslim and Belgian is far more significant in the lives of the participants than 'the cultural stuff' that is enclosed within the perceived boundaries of these concepts.

Taking into account that social isolation and a lack of social bounds have been identified as significant contributors to substance dependence (Alexander et al., 1980), it is vital to focus in treatment on problem users' social relations and clients' own feelings of exclusion in their perceived ethnic community, treatment and general society.

Furthermore, Rondelez et al. (2016; Rondelez et al., 2018) pointed out that 'othering' mechanisms rely on the failure to recognise the agency of 'the other'. Consequently, 'culture' is often presented as an agency-free concept. Rather than overrelying on 'the culture of clients' as risk factors, providers should focus on building a relation of trust to help clients disentangle what ethnic boundaries mean to them, what determines the construction of these boundaries and which other issues, in other life domains, are hindering their personal recovery. They should also be given the organisational support to self-reflect about culture and to consider the structural barriers that impact the lives of their clients.

Based on this critical reflection, one can question to what degree the cultural competence movement can reach its goals of equal access and quality treatment for MEM when it focuses its arguments predominantly on culture, thereby adhering to the discourse that fosters inequality in the first place. It seems as if the CC movement conflates a critique to dominant individualistic and biomedical discourse on 'good treatment' with the need for respect for cultural understandings and ways of dealing with it. Instead of pointing out what is going wrong in treatment for all, the debate gets focused on one fraction of the client population, setting this critique aside from other critiques (i.e. social recovery movement) to dominant treatment perspectives.

This in turn, results in the fact that the socio-economic causes that contribute to problem use in these populations are downscaled, and that providers are inclined not to counter the dominant treatment paradigms but rather locate the 'problem' in the culture of the client as risk factors. Instead of identifying, analysing and deconstructing certain perceived characteristics as co-causing mental problems, 'cultural traits' are often used to constitute a specific group of 'others'. When identifying complex underlying causes of mental health problems and substance use as constituting static characteristics of a population, these clients become 'others among others': a population designated as difficult to treat because they are other than the other – already 'othered' – clients.

Examining ethnic boundary-making processes and taking agency as well as societal constraints as a point of departure might be a useful way to 'work with and against' (Lather, 2007) categories of difference in research and to understand how problem users 'talk through and back' to these categories (Nordgren, 2017) in treatment and in broader society. Lastly, it is essential to identify and offer alternatives to the limitations inherent to the health system, such as waiting lists and blacklists, mismatches between preferred treatment and available treatment, the lack of treatment follow-up and also treatment accessibility issues for diverse MEM populations.

Notes

1 Epidemiological findings that frame substance use and treatment in an ethnic versus non-ethnic dichotomy have given rise to a growing research interest in differential patterns of use and treatment outcomes among MEM across continents. The emphasis on these ethnicity-based differences has been criticised for focusing too much on the strength of the relationship between two variables (substance use and ethnicity and culture) and too little on their nature (Hunt et al., 2004) and the underlying intersecting mechanisms at the micro-, meso- and macro-levels (De Kock et al., 2017; Meloni, 2014).

2 In 2012, the nationality proxy was removed from the European Treatment Demand Indicator protocol (CocoTDI report 23/11/2012). Although nationality is indeed a flawed proxy for studying ethnicity in substance use treatment, this choice leaves researchers and policy makers with little to no indicators for studying the situation of this target group in treatment.

3 About 10.5% of the Ghent population has a Turkish migration background (parent or grandparents migrated). The presence of this population is largely traced back to the labour agreements concluded between Belgium and Turkey and 1.7% has the Turkish nationality

(Laban, 2015). The remainder of inhabitants with a Turkish migration background possesses both the Belgian and Turkish nationality or only the Belgian nationality.

4 We excluded seven medicinal users (as opposed to De Kock and Decorte, 2017, 55 respondents) because they cannot strictly be subdivided into the fourfold categorisation.

5 Considering that the community researchers were free to select respondents and that respondents self-describing 'problem use', I also included a 'problem gambler' selected by the community researchers.

6 A study on the frames applied by mental health providers working with Muslim clients, as analysed by Rondelez and colleagues (2016, 2018) among 31 providers in Ghent.

7 Zolberg and Woon (1999) consider three types of ethnic boundary change: 'boundary blurring', 'boundary shifting' and 'boundary crossing'. Boundary crossing refers to the individual-level process of moving from one group to another, without any real change to the boundary itself. Boundary blurring implies a process in which the social profile of a boundary becomes less distinct, where 'the clarity of the social distinction involved has become clouded, and individuals' location with respect to the boundary may appear indeterminate' (2005). Boundary shifting, finally, involves 'the relocation of a boundary so that populations once situated on one side are now included on the other' (Van Kerckem et al., 2014, p. 282; Wimmer, 2013).

8 An imam is a person who leads prayers in a mosque in Sunni Islam. Further, the imam can be seen as a community leader and a person who provides religious guidance. In Shia Islam, imams have a more weighty position because they are believed to be appointed by God himself. Hodja's in turn are harder to define. Some say that they have performed the 'hajj' (pilgrimage to Mecca) but in popular speech and in the interviews, we hear that hodjas are wise people in some way or another (i.e. by having studied Qu'ran or having enjoyed higher education) and are called upon for religious and other guidance. In some studies, hodjas are called faith healers (Edirne et al., 2010).

References

Alegria, M., Carson, N., Goncalves, M., and Keefe, K. 2011. Disparities in treatment for substance use disorders and co-occurring disorders for ethnic/racial minority youth. *Journal of the American Academy of Child & Adolescent Psychiatry* 50 (1), pp. 22–31.

Alexander, B., Hadaway, P., and Coambs, R. 1980. Rat park chronicle. *British Columbia Medical Journal* 22 (2), pp. 32–45.

Andrade, L.H., Alonso, J., Mneimneh, Z., Wells, J.E., et al. 2014. Barriers to mental health treatment: Results from the WHO world mental health surveys. *Psychological Medicine* 44 (6), pp. 1303–17.

Bacchi, C. 2012. Introducing the "What's the problem represented to be?" Approach. In: Bletsas, A., and Beasly, C. (Eds.), *Engaging with Carol Bacchi: Strategic Interventions and Exchanges*. Adelaide: University of Adelaide Press, pp. 21–4.

Balibar, E. 1992. Inégalités, fractionnement social, exclusion: Nouvelles formes de l'antagonisme de classe? In: Affichard, J., and de Foucald, J.-B. (Eds.), Paris: Editions Esprit, pp. 141–61.

Barth, F. 1969/1998. *Ethnic Groups and Boundaries: The Social Organization of Culture Difference*. Long Grove: Waveland Press.

Berger, P.L., and Luckmann, T. 1966. *The Social Construction of Reality: A Treatise in the Sociology of Knowledge*. New York: Garden City, First Anchor.

Best, D., Albertson, K., Irving, J., Lightowlers, C., et al. 2016. *UK Life in Recovery Survey 2015*. Sheffield Hallam University. Available at: http://shura.shu.ac.uk/12200/1/FINAL%20UK%20Life%20in%20Recovery%20Survey%202015%20report.pdf

Blackman, L.M. 1996. The dangerous classes: Retelling the psychiatric story. *Feminism & Psychology* 6 (3), pp. 361–79.

Bourgois, P. 1996. *In Search of Respect: Selling Crack in El Barrio.* Cambridge: University Press.

Bourgois, P. 1996. In search of masculinity: violence, respect and sexuality among Puerto Rican crack dealers in East Harlem. *The British Journal of Criminology,* 36 (3), pp. 412–27.

Bucerius, S. 2014. *Unwanted: Muslim Immigrants, Dignity, and Drug Dealing.* Oxford: Oxford University Press.

Castel, R. 1986. From dangerousness to risk. In: Burchell, G., Gordon, C., and Miller, P. (Eds.), *The Foucault Effect,* pp. 119–27. Chicago: The University of Chicago Press.

Cuadra, C.B. 2012. Right of access to health care for undocumented migrants in EU: A comparative study of national policies. *European Journal of Public Health* 22 (2), pp. 267–71. doi:10.1093/eurpub/ckr049.

Dauvrin, M., Derluyn, I., Coune, I., Verrept, H., and Lorant, V. 2012. Towards fair health policies for migrants and ethnic minorities: The case-study of ETHEALTH in Belgium. *BMC Public Health* 12 (1), p. 726.

Dauvrin, M., and Lorant, V. 2014. Adaptation of health care for migrants: Whose responsibility? *BMC Health Services Research* 14 (1), p. 294.

De Kock, C. 2019a. Cultural competence and derivatives in substance use treatment for migrants and ethnic minorities: What's the problem represented to be? *Social Theory & Health* (advance online publication). Available at: https://link.springer.com/article/10.1057/s41285-019-00113-0.

De Kock, C. 2019b. Migration and ethnicity related indicators in European drug treatment demand (TDI) registries. *Journal of Ethnicity in Substance Abuse* (advance online publication). Available at: https://www.tandfonline.com/doi/abs/10.1080/15332640.2019.1664962

De Kock, C., and Decorte, T. 2017. Exploring problem use, discrimination, ethnic identity and social networks. *Drugs and Alcohol Today* 17 (4), pp. 269–79.

De Kock, C., Decorte, T., Schamp, J., Vanderplasschen, W., et al. 2017. *Substance Use Among People with a Migration Background: A Community-Based Participatory Research Study.* Antwerpen: Garant.

De Kock, C., Decorte, T., Vanderplasschen, W., Derluyn, I., and Sacco, M. 2017. Studying ethnicity, problem substance use and treatment: From epidemiology to social change. *Drugs: Education, Prevention and Policy* 24 (3), pp. 230–39.

Duchateau, K., Van Pouck, B., and Hebberecht, P. 2006. *Het levensverhaal van jongeren van Turkse en Marokkaanse origine met een instellingsverleden.* Gent: Onderzoeksgroep Criminologie & Rechtssociologie UGent.

Edirne, T., Arica, S.G., Gucuk, S., Yildizhan, R., et al. 2010. Use of complementary and alternative medicines by a sample of Turkish women for infertility enhancement: A descriptive study. *BMC Complementary and Alternative Medicine* 10 (1), p. 11.

Farkas, L. 2017. Analysis and comparative review of equality data collection practices in the European Union. Data collection in the field of ethnicity. *Report commissioned by the European Commission, Directorate-General for Justice and Consumers.*

Fountain, J., and Hicks, J. 2010. *Delivering Race Equality in Mental Health Care: Report on the Findings and Outcomes of the Community Engagement Programme 2005–2008.* Central Lancashire: University of Central Lancashire.

Gary, F.A. 2005. Stigma: Barrier to mental health care among ethnic minorities. *Issues in Mental Health Nursing* 26 (10), pp. 979–99.

Hordijk, R., Hendrickx, K., Lanting, K., MacFarlane, et al. 2018. Defining a framework for medical teachers' competencies to teach ethnic and cultural diversity: Results of a European Delphi study. *Medical Teacher,* pp. 1–7.

Horvat, L., Horey, D., Romios, P., and Kis-Rigo, J. 2014. Cultural competence education for health professionals. *Cochrane Database of Systematic Reviews* (5).

Horyniak, D., Melo, J.S., Farrell, R.M., Ojeda, V.D., and Strathdee, S.A. 2016. Epidemiology of substance use among forced migrants: A global systematic review. *PLoS One* 11 (7). doi:10.1371/journal.pone.0159134.

Hunt, L.M., Schneider, S., and Comer, B. 2004. Should "acculturation" be a variable in health research? A critical review of research on US Hispanics. *Social Science & Medicine* 59 (5), pp. 973–86. doi:10.1016/j.socscimed.2003.12.009.

Karl-Trummer, U., Novak-Zezula, S., and Metzler, B. 2010. Access to health care for undocumented migrants in the EU. *Eurohealth* 16 (1), pp. 13–16.

Krieger, N. 2012. Methods for the scientific study of discrimination and health: An ecosocial approach. *American Journal of Public Health* 102 (5), pp. 936–44.

Laban, C.J. 2015. *Lokale inburgerings- en integratiemonitor*. Editie.

Lalander, P. (2017). Staging "Chileanness": Ethnicity, illegal drug economy and social structures. *Drugs: Education, Prevention and Policy*, 24 (3), pp. 240–47.

Lather, P. 2007. *Getting Lost*. New York: SUNY Press.

Lemmens, P., Dupont, H., and Roosen, I. 2017. Migrants, asylum seekers and refugees: An overview of the literature relating to drug use and access to services. *Background Paper Commissioned by the EMCDDA*. Lisbon: EMCDDA.

Lim, A., Hoek, H.W., and Blom, J.D. 2015. The attribution of psychotic symptoms to jinn in Islamic patients. *Transcultural Psychiatry* 52 (1), pp. 18–32.

Loobuyck, P., and Meier, P. 2014. Imams in Flanders: A research note. *Islam and Christian–Muslim Relations* 25 (4), pp. 471–87.

Madeira, A.F., Pereira, C.R., Gama, A., and Dias, S. 2018. Justifying treatment bias: The legitimizing role of threat perception and immigrant – provider contact in healthcare. *Cultural Diversity and Ethnic Minority Psychology* 24 (2), pp. 294–301.

Martiniello, M. 2013. *Penser l'ethnicité. Identité, Culture et Relations Sociales*. Liège: Presses Universitaires de Liège.

Meloni, M. 2014. How biology became social, and what it means for social theory. *The Sociological Review* 62 (3), pp. 593–614. doi:10.1111/1467-954X.12151.

Mingione, E. 1996. *Urban Poverty and the Underclass: A Reader*. Cambridge and Oxford: Blackwell Publishers.

Missinne, S., and Bracke, P. 2012. Depressive symptoms among immigrants and ethnic minorities: A population based study in 23 European countries. *Social Psychiatry and Psychiatric Epidemiology* 47 (1), pp. 97–109. doi:10.1007/s00127-010-0321-0.

Moore, R. 1989. Ethnic divisions and class in Western Europe. In: Scase, R. (Ed.), *Industrial Societies (Routledge Revivals): Crisis and Division in Western Capitalism*. London: Routledge, p. 146.

Moore, R. 2015. Ethnic divisions and class in Western Europe. In: Scase, R. (Ed.), *Industrial Societies (Routledge Revivals): Crisis and Division in Western Capitalism*. London: Routledge, p. 146.

Morris, L. 1996. Dangerous classes: Neglected aspects of the underclass debate. In: Mingione, E. (Ed.), *Urban Poverty and the Underclass: A Reader*. Oxford: Blackwell publishers, pp. 160–75.

Napier, A., Arcano, C., Butler, B., Calabrese, J., et al. 2014. Culture and health. *The Lancet* 384 (9954), pp. 1607–39. doi:10.1080/01459740.2015.1030644.

Nordgren, J. 2017. Making up the "Drug-Abusing Immigrant" knowledge production in Swedish social work and drug treatment contexts, 1960s – 2011. *Contemporary Drug Problems* 44 (1), pp. 49–68.

Olcoń, K., and Gulbas, L.E. 2018. "Because That's the Culture": Providers' perspectives on the mental health of Latino immigrant youth. *Qualitative Health Research* 28 (12), pp. 1944–54.

Phillimore, J., Bradby, H., Knecht, M., Padilla, B., and Pemberton, S. 2017. Bricolage as conceptual tool for understanding access to healthcare in superdiverse populations. *Social Theory & Health*, pp. 1–22. Available at: https://doi.org/10.1057/s41285-018-0075-4.

Rechel, B., Mladovsky, P., Ingleby, D., Mackenbach, J.P., and McKee, M. 2013. Migration and health in an increasingly diverse Europe. *The Lancet* 381 (9873), pp. 1235–45.

Rein, M., and Schön, D. 1996. Frame-critical policy analysis and frame-reflective policy practice. *Knowledge and Policy* 9 (1), pp. 85–104.

Rondelez, E., Bracke, S., Roets, G., and Bracke, P. 2016. Racism, migration, and mental health. Theoretical reflections from Belgium. *Subjectivity* 9 (3), pp. 313–32.

Rondelez, E., Bracke, S., Roets, G., Vandekinderen, C., and Bracke, P. 2018. Revisiting Goffman: Frames of mental health in the interactions of mental healthcare professionals with diasporic Muslims. *Social Theory & Health* 1–18.

Said, E. 1979. *Orientalism*. New York: Vintage.

Scheppers, E., van Dongen, E., Dekker, J., Geertzen, J., and Dekker, J. 2006. Potential barriers to the use of health services among ethnic minorities: A review. *Family Practice* 23 (3), pp. 325–48.

Schieman, S., Bierman, A., and Ellison, C.G. 2013. Religion and mental health. In: *Handbook of the Sociology of Mental Health*. New York: Springer, pp. 457–78.

Shaw, S.J., and Armin, J. 2011. The ethical self-fashioning of physicians and health care systems in culturally appropriate health care. *Culture, Medicine, and Psychiatry* 35 (2), pp. 236–61.

Silver, H. 1996. Culture, politics and national discourses of the new urban poverty. In: Mingione, E. (Ed.), *Urban Poverty and the Underclass: A Reader*. Oxford: Blackwell Publishers, pp. 105–38.

Sorensen, J., Smith Jervelund, S., Norredam, M., Kristiansen, M., and Krasnik, A. 2017. Cultural competence in medical education: A questionnaire study of Danish medical teachers' perceptions of and preparedness to teach cultural competence. *Scandinavian Journal of Public Health* 45 (2), pp. 153–60.

Van Kerckem, K., Van de Putte, B., and Stevens, P.A.J. 2014. Pushing the boundaries: Responses to ethnic conformity pressure in two Turkish communities in Belgium. *Qualitative Sociology* 37 (3), pp. 277–300. doi:10.1007/s11133-014-9283-y.

Vardar, A., Kluge, U., and Penka, S. 2012. How to express mental health problems: Turkish immigrants in Berlin compared to native Germans in Berlin and Turks in Istanbul. *European Psychiatry* 27, pp. S50–S55.

Wacquant, L.J. 1996. Red belt, black belt: Racial division, class inequality and the state in the French urban periphery and the American ghetto. In: Mingione, E. (Ed.), *Urban Poverty and the Underclass: A Reader*. Oxford: Blackwell Publishers, pp. 234–74.

Wimmer, A. 2013. *Ethnic Boundary Making: Institutions, Power, Networks*. Oxford: Oxford University Press.

Zolberg, A.R., and Woon, L.L. 1999. Why Islam is like Spanish: Cultural incorporation in Europe and the United States. *Politics and Society* 27 (1), pp. 5–38.

8 The contemporary complexities of Irish Traveller navigation of drug risk environments

Marie Claire Van Hout

Introduction

The human rights of Travellers and Gypsies in Europe have long been violated throughout history in their experiences of persecutions, enforced assimilation through coerced settlement and cultural genocide by fostering of Traveller children through social care systems (Cemlyn and Briskman, 2002). Levels of contemporary human rights denial range from socio-political exclusions to the denial of their status as an ethnic minority group (Cemlyn, 2008). Despite persecution, Travellers and Gypsies strive to maintain a strong sense of ethnic identity, attachment and affiliation to their culture (McVeigh, 1997; Vanderbeck, 2005). The Traveller community known in Ireland as 'pikeys' and 'tinkers' are identified 'as an ethnic minority people with a shared history, language, culture and traditions including, historically, a nomadic way of life and value system on the island of Ireland' (NiShuinear, 1994) and are recorded in Irish history since the twelfth century (Joyce, 2002). They are a distinct ethnic group with a history of nomadism and, despite having a common Irish origin, are socially isolated from the surrounding, 'settled' Irish people (Gilbert et al., 2017). Irish Travellers exist as a marginalised group, which exacerbates their visibility as a social problem and yet, also, their invisibility within public discourse as an ethnic minority (Cemlyn and Briskman, 2002). The scale of ethnic homogeneity in Ireland is such that the Irish census did not include a general question on race/ethnicity until 2006. (It included a question on membership of the Traveller community in the 2002 census.) The most recent Irish census (CSO, 2011) recorded 29,573 Travellers in Ireland, representing 0.6 per cent of the total Irish population. As of March 1, 2017, Travellers are recognised by the Irish government as a distinct ethnic group within the fabric of Irish society (Radio Telifis Eireann, RTE, 2017). Despite this recognition, in March 2018, the Monitoring Report by Pavee Point in Ireland revealed continued high rates of racism and prejudice, poverty and social exclusion of Travellers in Ireland.

Social situation of Irish Travellers on the fringe

> Although Travellers resent being separated from non-Travellers, many I knew valued the separation, providing they could cross the border on their own terms, when they chose.
>
> (Griffin, 2002, p. 69)

Historically, Irish Traveller existence as a 'dangerous class' within Irish society has been fraught with a multiplicity of socio-economic disadvantage, public discriminatory attitudes and hostility. Traveller communities traditionally reinforce their identity as an ethnic nomadic group in Ireland by choice of separateness from the settled Irish population. Gmelch (1996, p. 177) emphasised: 'Travellers do not work or live in a vacuum, their identity and lifestyle is unquestionably influenced by their connexion to the larger society'. He asserted that the Traveller claim for ethnic separateness was grounded in Traveller culture and identity, supported by their close-knit social bonds and inner social capital rather than by the historical basis. Helleiner (2000, p. 101) quoted as follows: 'I argue that Traveller culture and identity have been and continue to be produced out of sets of unequal social relations . . . [that are] deeply structured by class, gender, and generation'. The limited interaction historically with settled Irish people and the marked inner community boundaries have contributed to public prejudice of the 'itinerant way of life' and the labelling of Travellers as criminals. The Irish Travellers have epitomised the problem of 'mobility' for decades as represented by other groups such as illegal immigrants, criminal networks and other disreputable individuals and groups (Weber and Bowling, 2008; Shubin and Swanson, 2010; Mulcahy, 2012). In 1963, following the publication of the Report of the Commission on Itinerancy, the Irish Government implemented the national programme for the 'settlement', 'assimilation' and 'rehabilitation' of Irish Travellers. This has ultimately led to the demise of Traveller control over their own culture. The Report stated that among settled people, Travellers evoked feelings of 'bitter hostility often accompanied by fear', and it observed that 'in nearly all areas, itinerants are despised as inferior beings and are regarded as the dregs of society' (1963, p. 102). Mass level public attitudes towards Travellers are characterised by anti-Traveller racism (MacGréil, 1977, 1996, 2010, 2011; Helleiner, 2000; Crowley and Kitchin, 2015; Fetzer, 2016). Public hysteria around Travellers appears to stem from concerns around 'feud fighting', extreme violence and low trust in the Irish police, or Gardai, in resolving ongoing disputes (Okley, 2005). Travellers are equally negatively referred to by the criminal justice system (Walsh, 2000; Bhreatnach, 2007; Fanning, 2009; Hourigan, 2011; MacGabhann, 2011; Mulcahy, 2012).

Since the 1950s, Traveller assimilationist policy by the Irish government ('boulder' policies,[1] oppressive housing policies) and social changes in Ireland have contributed to Traveller displacement into urban areas, with loss of traditional forms of income generation (trade and craftwork) and the nomadic way of life (Van Hout, 2011a). This has contributed to their marginal status and relegation to the fringes of Irish society. The very reinforcement of Traveller rights, values and cultural traditions as distinction between their culture and 'way of life' and that of the settled Irish population have resulted in a lack of tolerance and inclusion within individual, public and political discourse (Blighe, 2001; Pavee Point, 2005). Sadly, the Traveller appeared to be drifting within contemporary Ireland, amidst coercive attempts by local authorities to house Traveller families and remove them from social visibility. Reports of residential harassment are high, with many Traveller families intimidated on the estates where they lived. Culture shocks are similar to those reported in the UK and include 'isolation' and 'dislocation' from the extended Traveller family as most 'settled' housing is restricted to accommodating the nuclear family, whereas the extended Traveller family is a central focus of Traveller culture (Cemlyn, 2000; Parry et al., 2004; Cemlyn, 2008). Essentially, this fragmentation of Traveller culture through oppressive housing policies and restrictions on mobility has contributed to Travellers not only being dubbed a 'dangerous class' but also equally their situation in societal spaces in halting sites, group housing schemes and social housing areas as 'dangerous spaces'. This forms the basis for discussion in this chapter as it relates to the Traveller connection and engagement in illegal drug activity and the resultant social and health consequences for this ethnic group. Despite governmental efforts to provide culturally specific housing and other culturally mediated social supports, Irish Travellers continue to experience multiple socio-economic disadvantages in contemporary Irish society (Walsh, 2010; Staniewicz and Van Hout, 2012; Van Hout and Staniewicz, 2012; MacGabhann, 2013; Nolan, 2014), all of which heighten their vulnerability to drug abuse and addiction (Van Hout, 2011a, 2010c, 2010d; Van Hout and Hearne, 2016; Claffey et al., 2017).

Drug use and the Irish Traveller community

> Originally their cultural norms protected them from drug use, but as they become increasingly settled and involved in the settled community . . . their drug use is increasing.
>
> (Agency Worker, Van Hout, 2009c, p. 20)

Traditionally, the Traveller community, both young and old, was protected from illicit drug use by strong family bonds and traditional anti-drug norms reinforced by elders within their marked inner boundaries from the 'settled' community (Pavee Point, 2005; Van Hout and Connor, 2008; Van Hout, 2009a, 2009b, 2010a, 2010b, 2010c, 2010d, 2011a, 2011b; Van Hout and Hearne, 2016; Claffey et al., 2017). In 1995, the Report of Task Force on the Travelling Community made no reference to illicit drug use within the Traveller community. By virtue of their contested social and physical space and separation from settled society, illicit drug use and addiction was not an issue within Traveller communities in Ireland. Their religious and patriarchal cultural values traditionally protected Travellers from self-medication or intoxication behaviours and sanctioned those who crossed the line (Van Hout and Connor, 2008; Van Hout, 2009a, 2009b, 2009c, 2010c). However, since the early 2000s, social and cultural upheaval through enforced dislocation of Traveller families, breaking up of Traveller networks via dispersal and severe poverty and social exclusion have heightened Traveller vulnerability to psycho-social distress, poor mental and physical health outcomes, and consequently a steep rise in substance abuse and addiction amongst Travellers has been observed (Van Hout, 2010a, 2010c, 2010d, 2011a, 2011b; Van Hout and Hearne, 2016; Claffey et al., 2017).

The National Drug Treatment System (NDTRS) commenced recording of the ethnicity of those accessing drug treatment and rehabilitation services in 2007. By 2010, 66 per cent of Travellers surveyed in the All Ireland Traveller Health Study (AITHS, 2010) said that illicit drugs were a recent and concerning problem in their community. Increases in alcohol and drug abuse among Irish Travellers since 2009 are attributed to the gradual erosion of traditional Traveller cultural values placed on religiosity and patriarchal family systems, high rates of Traveller male incarceration, loss of traditional forms of (nomadic) income, drug availability and use where Travellers are housed and development of normative and reciprocal relationships in drug activities with the settled community (Pavee Point, 2005; Van Hout and Connor, 2008; AITHS, 2010; Costello, 2014; Van Hout, 2010a, 2010b, 2011a; Walsh, 2010; MacGabhann, 2013; Van Hout and Hearne, 2016). As drug abuse is occurring within the Traveller family and extended groups of Travellers, it will become increasingly difficult for this not to have a serious impact on young Travellers, most particularly when confronted with this type of behaviour at close proximity, whether in the halting site, in caravans or among close relatives (Van Hout and Connor, 2008; Van Hout, 2009c, 2010d).

Rising concerns in 2016 and 2017 are evident around the impact of addiction and associated health and social impacts affecting Traveller families and their communities (Van Hout, 2011a, 2011b; Nolan, 2014; Van Hout and Hearne, 2016). Treatment and prison treatment indicators remain the only real indicator of the extent of Traveller substance abuse (AITHS, 2010; MacGabhann, 2011; Carew et al., 2013; Costello, 2014). Risky drinking of alcohol remains a significant problem among Travellers, particularly due to social acceptability of use among Traveller men and unmarried Traveller women and due to the lack of understanding of alcohol dependency and the downplaying of problematic use patterns (Fountain, 2006; Van Hout, 2009b; AITHS, 2010; Pavee Point, 2011; Nolan, 2014). Gender differences are illustrated in both qualitative studies and treatment data with Traveller men predominantly using cocaine, amphetamine, natural and synthetic cannabis and ecstasy, and Traveller women reporting prescription medication abuse (i.e. combination opioid analgesics, benzodiazepine and Z-hypnotics) (Fountain, 2006; Van Hout, 2009a, 2009b; Walsh, 2010; Pavee Point, 2011; Carew et al., 2013; Van Hout and Hearne, 2016,). Opiate use is less common, but with high risk of heroin use and anabolic steroids during incarceration, especially for Traveller men (Fountain, 2006; Van Hout, 2009a, 2009b; MacGabhann, 2013; Costello, 2014; Van Hout and Hearne, 2016). Difficulties with drug dependence in Traveller men and women, including heroin and prescription opioids, are observed (Van Hout and Hearne, 2016; Claffey et al., 2017) along with high rates of poor mental health including suicides among both genders of Travellers (AITHS, 2010).

Dangerous spaces and navigation of drug-related risk

> Traveller substance use is more than a coping mechanism. It is a set of circumstances.
>
> (Van Hout, 2009c, p. 25)

'Dangerous spaces' encountered by Travellers in contemporary Ireland now consist of drug (availability, use and dealing) risk environments, as their families, communities and networks are exposed to illicit drug availability and contact with drug trafficking gangs, increasingly disenfranchised and/or incarcerated male youth and with their own members seeking alternative routes for income generation in drug dealing and drug-related crimes. Drug use itself can create 'parallel lives' to counteract day-to-day uncertainty (Moore and Miles, 2004), in this instance spanning the impacts of social exclusion, bereavement, frustration, depression and incarceration. The Traveller drugs risk environment within Irish society can therefore be viewed as a 'social space' whereby a multiplicity of social, ethnic and cultural factors interact to discourage, facilitate and mediate forms of drug activity (Van Hout, 2010c). Individual and group risk negotiation and harm formations are imbibed in 'socially constructed discourses of risk and morality' (Rhodes, 2002, p. 86) and constructed as linear and non-linear complexities between individuals and their immediate environments (Galea et al., 2009). The contextual constraints of contemporary 'risk society' necessitate understanding within consideration of the presence of power resources between individual and situational agency within their risk environment (Rhodes, 1997a, 1997b). This is particularly salient with regard to Traveller identity and situation within modernist settled Irish society. Lupton (1995, p. 35) has argued that risk is, 'inevitably mediated through . . . social processes and can never be known in isolation from these processes'. Thus, the processes of drug risk neutralisation or denial for Irish Travellers over time can be better understood when distinctive cultural, individual, social and ethnic variables within lay associational life are considered in understanding drug behaviours. Emerging drug trends point to an increased filtering of so-called legitimate drug use between mainstream and Traveller groups, whereby one must recognise that within social navigation of drug risk, changes in attitude and drug consumptive intent may be reflected by shifts in normative beliefs about a certain drug, perceived prevalence and acceptability of drug consumption. Travellers are now housed in areas where drugs are commonplace.

Travellers are persistently constructed as a criminogenic community (Dillon, 2006; Drummond, 2006; Kabachnik, 2009). Diversification of Traveller criminal networks into drug trafficking has occurred as a natural market response. Drug dealing within the Traveller communities is reportedly increasing and represents the potential acquisition of resources, social space, agency and status during the assimilation process (Van Hout, 2011a; Van Hout and Hearne, 2016). Whilst Travellers are increasingly entrepreneurial and able to navigate 'dangerous spaces' in the context of crime, they remain ill-equipped to deal with the profound harms caused by drug abuse, often confounded by their life and social circumstances.

> The fighting comes from them settled thugs . . . we never had it like this before . . . stabbings and shootings is part of Traveller life now.
>
> (Traveller, Van Hout, 2011a, p. 209)

Traveller habitus and drugs

> I'll always be a Traveller . . . they won't ever take that away from me . . . I want my kids to understand the life.
>
> (Van Hout, 2011a, p. 209)

Social shifts caused by social housing policies which destroy Traveller networks remain a threat in terms of potential for drug abuse, as drug-using members of Travellers families will inadvertently influence members of their own family over time, even in the context of previous fear of drug use within the halting site. Traveller communities have experienced the influx of drug activity and through inexperience and stigma surrounding drug use, as well as low engagement with school-based drug prevention, and poor literacy levels were not as apt to respond. The continued prejudices against Travellers by the settled Irish community exacerbate the invisibility of problematic drug use and heightened drug activity within the Traveller networks and families, making it increasingly difficult to control, quantify and address (Van Hout, 2011a; Claffey et al., 2017). The traditional Traveller way of dealing with a problem was 'to pack up and leave', which is now compromised by governmental restraint on Traveller nomadism in contemporary Ireland and resulting in Traveller communities 'closing shop' and attempting to resolve issues within themselves. The Traveller community in their day-to-day experiences with contemporary discriminatory Ireland present with low levels of institutional trust, which creates a problem in terms of increasing problematic substance use and reluctance to access services, due to frequent discrimination and lack of cultural acceptance. Hence, the impacts of drug addiction within Traveller families continue to be observed and are compounded. The National Traveller Centre Pavee Point has underscored how Travellers and their family members struggle to reveal addiction due to issues of shame and generally attempt to deal with the issue themselves (Pavee Point, 2005, 2011; Nolan, 2014). Home detoxification attempts and religious faith healing are common attempts within Traveller families (Van Hout, 2010b). Efforts to deal with addiction remain firmly within the closed networks of Traveller families, where stigma of addiction remains high (Van Hout and Hearne, 2016; Claffey et al., 2017).

> The problem and the solution come from within the Traveller community itself. . . . [T]hey will dictate how they deal with it . . . whether with closed doors or with us.
>
> (Van Hout, 2011b, p. 56)

> It's the likes of the older generation of Travellers that's stopping the younger ones from coming to centres.
>
> (Claffey et al., 2017, p. 8)

The fragile sense of contemporary Traveller community identity has contributed to increased dissipation of traditional Traveller culture within greater social structures.

The potent sense of familialism within inner Traveller networks once provided by older Travellers with history of living in large community networks, thereby offering support, solidarity and connectiveness in Traveller community life, is weakened. Hence, the concept of habitus (Bourdieu, 1990) may offer some added illustration and comprehension into the repercussions of forced assimilation of Travellers over time in Ireland and their negotiation of new and existing drug-risk environments both around them and within their families and networks (Ryder, 2017).

As Irish Traveller culture is dissipating in its strength and also adapting somewhat to 'settled' values and norms, this may result in distinct habitus evolving for younger generations of Travellers. Similar changing Traveller identities and cultures have been observed by Ryder (2017). Bourdieu (1977) describes the influence of habitus as limiting the options, which individuals possess through their culture and precedents set by generations of their ethnic group before them. The Traveller environment as it meets and navigates the 'new' sedentarist risk environment has yielded an entirely new set of action schemas over time, with prevalence of addiction and drug-related criminal activity occurring in response to heightened contact with illicit drugs in day-to-day life. Previous and traditionally held views and values continue to be enforced by elders (Claffey et al., 2017) in countering the rise in youth and Traveller women's engagement in adoption of new stocks of knowledge around drug practices and consumption. Bourdieu (1984) described distinct consumption practices in social groups in terms of meaning and expression and reflected in perceived risk, strategic decision-making and sanctioned or condoned forms of behaviour within certain cultural norms. Consumption patterns and modes of drug use are part of the habitus which become unconscious reflexes over time. As habitus is deemed to limit certain responses to risk situations, the question remains: whether inherent Traveller abuse of alcohol and now in recent times of drugs is a reflexive action or partially reflexive in the assimilation, yet socially excluded process, characterised by the undercurrent of frustration, tension and discrimination in Traveller lives. Drug activity whether use or dealing within the Traveller community may be seen, therefore, as attempts to seek recognition or status within groups by the so-called illicit means, the creation of new space or new cultural capital spanning the settled society. When applied to the older Traveller generations, resilience to drug and alcohol use may be viewed as an attempt to counteract dominant values. Drug use by male Travellers has become a medium not only in its capacity for group membership and support but also as a mechanism for raising one's profile or status based on reciprocity and trust within society, however underground this may operate.

> If you have no education and no skills, you more than likely have no job, then kids that have no opportunities, they seek an opportunity and an easy way out. Some kids take the drugs for their own use and they take extra and are selling it to their friends, and it's like a skill, like a job.
>
> (Van Hout, 2009a, p. 44)

Traveller women despite high levels of partner incarceration exist as 'passive objects of power' (Neale, 2002, p. 45) in their world. The Traveller woman's consumption of drugs appears limited to prescription medications, heroin and alcohol and deeply rooted in a lack of empowerment and coping skills (Claffey et al., 2017). Traveller women, in particular, present to services with much higher levels of depression than the general population (Barry, 1996; Smart et al., 2003).

Conclusion

The restricted 'sense of Traveller belonging' in dominant Irish discourse is the crux of the problem for Irish Travellers and yet appears reinforced both by Travellers themselves and the sedentarist population. Lack of Traveller institutional trust remains strong as a consequence of aggressive sedentarisation in Ireland, where attempts to coerce Travellers to behave like non-Travellers continue and policies ignore their individual values, beliefs and concerns. The process of assimilation whether by choice or enforced, therefore, contributes to a relinquishing of Traveller social capital. One must note that for Travellers, integration does not infer assimilation and 'social inclusion and social integration should not be equated with the homogenisation of minority ethnic groups' (Pavee Point, 2005).

The uncritical settled perspective where Traveller cultural identities are perceived to be criminal, pathological and deviant continues (see 'othering', Cemlyn, 2008). Irish Travellers experience a myriad of identified risk factors for substance use and in the relative absence of resilience. This weakened resilience occurs within the context of enforced assimilation, reorganisation of Traveller habitus and the identified clash between older Travellers resisting 'settled' values and Traveller youth integrating within sedentarist communities. Thus, drug exposure and activity, whether consumption or dealing, represent an interesting paradigm for Traveller integration, selective assimilation or simply 'just contact' within settled Irish society. Eroded Traveller community characteristics in terms of disorder, stress, poor mental health, lowered social cohesion, trust, safety and bonding are linked to drug use. Complexities in dealing with the impact of drug-related crime and addiction within Traveller families are underpinned by shame, stigma and attempts to self-manage (home detoxification, faith healing, sanctioning with domestic violence and outcasting of users and addicts) from within. This contributes to the renewed framing of the Traveller community as a 'dangerous class' operating within contemporary criminal environments as 'dangerous spaces'. One cannot underestimate the importance of the lay 'voices' in the exploration of the concept of risk and drug use and the power relations in decision-making and drug use, in terms of social environments, peer crowds and cliques, the balance of being 'in' or being 'different' and consequences relating to risk-taking behaviours. Targeted and successful drug prevention must be increasingly driven by the science of risk and vulnerability within the complex and competitive social environment of changing social encounters with drugs. Contemporary drug policies must consider the contextual constraints of the 'Traveller risk society', which impact on inherent individual 'power resources', whereby individual agency and drug taking are better understood within situational agency of 'localised' social, gender, ethnic and cultural capital.

Note

1 Council policy whereby traditional roadside campsites have been blocked with huge obstacles once families have been moved on.

References

All Ireland Traveller Health Study (AITHS). 2010. *All Ireland Traveller Health Study; Summary of Findings*. Dublin: School of Public Health, UCD. Available at: www.paveepoint.ie/resources/our-geels-allireland-traveller-health-study.

Barry, J.M.G. 1996. *Maternal and Infant Health of Irish Travellers*. Dublin, MD, Trinity College, University of Dublin.

Bhreatnach, A. 2007. Policing the community: Homicide and violence in traveller and settled society. *Irish Economic and Social History* 34, pp. 47–64.

Blighe, P. 2001. *Report on Travellers Needs in the Roscommon Area*. Roscommon: Roscommon County Development Board.

Bourdieu, P. 1977. *Outline of a Theory of Practice*. London: Cambridge University Press.

Bourdieu, P. 1984. *Distinction: A Social Critique of the Judgement of Taste*. Cambridge, MA: Harvard University Press.

Bourdieu, P. 1990. *The Logic of Practice*. Cambridge: Polity Press.

Carew, A.M., Cafferty, S., Long, J., Bellerose, D., and Lyons, S. 2013. Travellers accessing addiction services in Ireland (2007 to 2010): Analysis of routine surveillance data. *Journal of Ethnicity in Substance Abuse* 12 pp. 339–55. doi:10.1080/15332640.2013.830943.

Cemlyn, S. 2000. Assimilation, control, mediation or advocacy? Social work dilemmas in providing anti-oppressive services for traveller children and families. *Child and Family Social Work* 5 (4), pp. 327–41.

Cemlyn, S. 2008. Human rights and gypsies and travellers: An exploration of the application of a human rights perspective to social work with a minority community in Britain. *British Journal of Social Work* 38 (1), pp. 153–73.

Cemlyn, S., and Briskman, L. 2002. Social (dys) welfare within a hostile state. *Social Work Education* 21 (1), pp. 49–69.

Claffey, C., MacLachlan, M., Crowley, D., and Van Hout, M.C. 2017. Exploring Irish Travellers' experiences of opioid substitute treatment: A phenomenological study. *Heroin Addiction and Related Clinical Problems* 19 (6), pp. 73–80.

Commission on Itinerancy. 1963. *Report of the Commission on Itinerancy*. Dublin: Stationery Office.

Costello, L. 2014. *Travellers in the Irish Prison System: A Qualitative Study*. Dublin: Irish Penal Reform Trust.

Crowley, U., and Kitchin, R. 2015. Academic 'truth' and the perpetuation of negative attitudes and intolerance toward Irish Travellers in contemporary Ireland. In: Honohan, I., and Rougier, N. (Eds.), *Tolerance and Diversity in Ireland, North and South*. Manchester: Manchester University Press, pp. 153–70.

CSO. 2011. *Irish Census*. Cork: CSO Publishing. Available at: www.cso.ie/en/census/census2011reports/.

Dillon, E. 2006. *The Outsiders: Exposing the Secretive World of Ireland's Travellers*. Dublin: Merlin.

Drummond, A. 2006. Cultural denigration: Media representation of Irish Travellers as criminal. In: Hayes, M., and Acton, T. (Eds.), *Counterhegemony and the Postcolonial 'Other'*. Newcastle: Cambridge Scholars Press, pp. 75–85.

Fanning, B. 2009. *New Guests of the Irish Nation*. Dublin: Irish Academic Press.

Fetzer, J.S. 2016. Opposition to Irish travellers' halting sites in the republic of Ireland: Realistic group conflict or symbolic politics? *Irish Journal of Sociology* 25 (2), pp. 195–206.

Fountain, J. 2006. *An Exploratory Study of an Overview of the Nature and Extent of Illicit Drug Use Amongst the Traveller Community*. Dublin: National Advisory Committee on Drugs. Available at: www.drugs.ie/resourcesfiles/research/2006/NACDTraveller ReportFinal.pdf.

Galea, S., Hall, C., and Kaplan, G.A. 2009. Social epidemiology and complex system dynamic modelling as applied to health behaviour and drug use research. *International Journal of Drug Policy* 20, pp. 209–16.

Gilbert, E., Carmi, S., Ennis, S., Wilson, J.F., and Cavalleri, G.L. 2017. Genomic insights into the population structure and history of the Irish travellers. *Scientific Reports* 7 (42187). doi:10.1038/srep42187.

Gmelch, G. 1996. Irish travellers: Culture and ethnicity. *Journal of the Royal Anthropological Institute* 2 (1), p. 176.

Griffin, C.C.M. 2002. The religion and social organisation of Irish travellers on a London caravan site (part I). *Nomadic Peoples* 6 (1), pp. 45–69.

Helleiner, J. 2000. *Irish Travellers: Racism and the Politics of Culture*. Toronto: University of Toronto Press.

Hourigan, N. 2011. The sociology of feuding: Limerick gangland and Travellers' feuds compared. In: Hourigan, N. (Ed.), *Understanding Limerick*. Cork: Cork University Press.

Joyce, D. 2002. *Charting a Future Strategy for Traveller Accommodation*. Dublin: Irish Traveller Movement.

Kabachnik, P. 2009. The culture of crime: Examining representations of Irish Travellers, in Traveller and the Riches. *Romani Studies* 19, pp. 49–63.

Lupton, D. 1995. *Risk*. London: Routledge.

MacGabhann, C. 2011. *Voices Unheard. A Study of Irish Travellers in Prison*. Irish Chaplaincy in Britain, London.

MacGabhann, C. 2013. Irish travellers in prison – The unknown prisoners. *Prison Service Journal* 206, pp. 19–26.

MacGréil, M. 1977. *Prejudice and Tolerance in Ireland*. Dublin, OH: College of Industrial Relations.

MacGréil, M. 1996. *Prejudice in Ireland Revisited*. Maynooth: St. Patrick's College.

MacGréil, M. 2010. *Emancipation of the Travelling People: A Report on the Attitudes and Prejudices of the Irish People Towards the Travellers Based on a National Social Survey 2007 – '08. Research Report*. Maynooth: National University of Ireland Maynooth.

MacGréil, M. 2011. *Pluralism and Diversity in Ireland*. New York: Columbia University Press.

McVeigh, R. 1997. Theorising sedentarism: The roots of anti-nomadism. In: Acton, T. (Ed.), *Gypsy Politics and Traveller Identity*. Hatfield: University of Hertfordshire Press, pp. 7–25.

Moore, K., and Miles, S. 2004. Young people, dance and the sub-cultural consumption of drugs. *Addiction Research and Theory* 12 (6), pp. 507–23.

Mulcahy, A. 2012. 'Alright in their own place': Policing and the spatial regulation of Irish Travellers. *Criminology & Criminal Justice* 12 (3), pp. 307–27.

Neale, J. 2002. *Drug Users in Society*. London: Macmillan.

NiShuinear, S. 1994. Irish Travellers, ethnicity and the origins question. In: McCann, M.O., Siochain, S., and Ruane, J. (Eds.), *Irish Travellers Culture and Ethnicity*. Belfast: Institute of Irish Studies, pp. 54–77.

Nolan, S. 2014. *The Needs Assessment on the Problematic Use of Drugs and Alcohol within the Traveller Community in the ECRDTF Area*. Wicklow: Wicklow Travellers Group.

Okley, J. 2005. Gypsy justice versus Gorgio law: Interrelations of difference. *Sociological Review* 53 (4), pp. 691–709.

Parry, G., van Cleemput, P., Peters, J., Walters, S., Thomas, K., and Cooper, C. 2004. *The Health Status of Gypsies and Travellers in England. A Report for the Department of Health*. The School of Health and Related Research (ScHARR). Sheffield: University of Sheffield.

Pavee Point. 2005. Moving forward: Exploring responses to drug issues in the traveller community. *Conference Proceedings*, May 2005. Dublin: Pavee Point Travellers Centre.

Pavee Point. 2011. *The Use of Benzodiazepines within the Traveller Community: An Overview of the Extent of the Problem with Recommended Actions for Change*. Dublin: Pavee Point Travellers Centre. Available at: www.paveepoint.ie/resources/drugs/.

Radio Telifis Eireann. 2017. *Taoiseach: Travellers 'a People within Our People' as Ethnicity Recognised*. Available at: www.rte.ie/news/2017/0301/856293-travellers-etnic-status/.

Rhodes, T. 1997a. Risk theory in epidemic times: Sex, drugs and the social organisation of "risk behaviour". *Sociology of Health and Illness* 19, pp. 737–48.

Rhodes, T. 1997b. Risk theory in epidemic times. *Sociology of Health and Illness* 19, pp. 208–27.

Rhodes, T. 2002. The 'risk environment': A framework for understanding and reducing drug-related harm. *International Journal of Drug Policy* 13, pp. 85–94.

Ryder, A. 2017. *Sites of Resistance: Gypsies, Roma and Travellers in School, Community and the Academy*. London: Trentham Press.

Shubin, S., and Swanson, K. 2010. 'I'm an Imaginary Figure': Unravelling the mobility and marginalisation of Scottish gypsy travellers. *Geoforum* 41 (6), pp. 919–29.

Smart, H., Titterton, M., and Clark, C. 2003. A literature review of the health of Gypsy/ Traveller families in Scotland. *Health Education* 103, pp. 156–65.

Staniewicz, T., and Van Hout, M.C. 2012. 'The Lost Road': Traveller housing in contemporary Ireland, and its interplay with cultural erosion and health. In: Lewis, C. (Ed.), *Ireland: Economic, Political and Social Issues*. Hauppauge, NY: Nova Science, pp. 1–10.

Van Hout, M.C. 2009a. Irish travellers and drug use- An exploratory study. *Ethnicity and Inequalities in Health and Social Care* 2 (1), pp. 42–9.

Van Hout, M.C. 2009b. Alcohol use and the traveller community in the West of Ireland. *Drug and Alcohol Review* 29, pp. 59–63.

Van Hout, M.C. 2009c. *Substance Misuse in the Traveller Community: A Regional Needs Assessment*. Galway: Western Region Drugs Task Force.

Van Hout, M.C. 2010a. Travellers and substance use – Implications for service provision. *International Journal of Health Promotion and Education* 48 (2), pp. 36–41.

Van Hout, M.C. 2010b. Traveller health and primary health care – A stakeholders perspective. *Community Practitioner* 85 (5), pp. 25–8.

Van Hout, M.C. 2010c. The Irish traveller community, social capital and drug use – An exploratory study. *Journal of Ethnicity in Substance Abuse* 9 (3), pp. 186–205.

Van Hout, M.C. 2010d. Traveller drug use and the school setting: Friend or Foe? *Journal of Alcohol and Drug Education* 54 (2), pp. 7–16.

Van Hout, M.C. 2011a. Assimilation, habitus and drug use among Irish travellers. *Critical Public Health* 21 (2), pp. 203–21.

Van Hout, M.C. 2011b. Travellers and substance use in Ireland-recommendations for drug and alcohol policy. *Drugs Education, Prevention and Policy* 18 (1), pp. 53–9.

Van Hout, M.C., and Connor, S. 2008. The normalisation of substance abuse among young travellers in Ireland- implications for practice. *Journal of Ethnicity of Substance Abuse* 7 (1), pp. 5–23.

Van Hout, M.C., and Hearne, E. 2016. The changing landscape of Irish traveller alcohol and drug use. *Drugs Education Prevention and Policy* 24 (2), pp. 220–30.

Van Hout, M.C., and Staniewicz, T. 2012. Roma and traveller housing and health disparity – A public health concern. *Critical Public Health* 22 (2), pp. 193–207.

Vanderbeck, R. 2005. Anti-nomadism, institutions and the geographies of childhood. *Environment and Planning D: Society and Space* 23 (1), pp. 71–94.

Walsh, B. 2010. *Cultural Dislocation and Consequences: An Exploratory Study of Illicit Drug Activity Among a Traveller Community in North Dublin*. Dublin: Blanchardstown Local Drugs Task Force.

Walsh, D. 2000. Policing pluralism. In: MacLachlan, M., and O'Connell, M. (Eds.), *Cultivating Pluralism*. Dublin: Oak Tree Press, pp. 152–74.

Weber, L., and Bowling, B. 2008. Valiant beggars and global vagabonds: Select, eject, immobilise. *Theoretical Criminology* 12 (3), pp. 355–75.

9 Drink, drugs and the 'dangerous poor'

Fear and loathing in contemporary cities

Susanne MacGregor and Aileen O'Gorman

Introduction

In this chapter, we utilise framing and reframing theories and apply them to perceptions and policies on drugs, drink and the poor. Our general approach rests on social constructionism, which is a set of theories that draw attention to the social construction of target populations, defining images and stereotypes and attributing value (deserving or undeserving, clean or dirty) to objects, people and events (Stone, 1989).

We pay particular attention to ideas deriving from Schön and Rein (1994). The value of their approach is that they focus on intractable policy controversies. Both consumption of drink and drugs and poverty are characterised by divergent, intractable, opposing viewpoints and policies. Disputes are highly resistant to resolution by appeal to evidence, research or reasoned argument. Schön and Rein tell us that the parties to policy controversies see issues, policies and policy situations in different and conflicting ways that embody different systems of belief and related prescriptions for action, often crystallised in generative metaphors: 'these frames determine what counts as a fact and how one makes the normative leap from facts to prescriptions for action' (Schön and Rein, 1994, p. xviii).

They also draw attention to the role of underlying assumptions and the use of metaphors, narratives and storylines. Each story conveys a very different view of reality and represents a special way of seeing (Schön and Rein, 1994, p. 26). They describe what is wrong in such a way as to set the direction for future transformation. Schön and Rein point to a process which involves both framing and reframing. 'Policy positions rest on underlying structures of belief, perception and appreciation which we call frames' (Schön and Rein, 1994, p. 23). Generative metaphors play a key role as 'the taken for granted assumptional structures' that influence both policy and research (Schön and Rein, 1994, p. viii).

We also build on insights deriving from Bacchi's 'What's the problem represented to be?' (WPR) approach to policy analysis: 'that what we say we want to do about something indicates what we think needs to change and hence how we constitute the "problem"' (Bacchi, 2012, p. 5). Starting from this position, we offer a critical review of key policy themes relating to drugs, drink and the poor.

We will identify the key assumptions in discourses and assess the socially harmful impacts of policy framing.

Over time, a variety of representations of 'the poor' and 'drug and alcohol users' can be seen with some being more prominent at different times or in different places. For example, at one time, certain diseases, described as 'social diseases', were seen as principally of the poor – such as tuberculosis, venereal diseases and alcoholism (Bryder, 1988) – to which drugs (along with smoking and obesity) have now been added. Faced with these diseases, the goal of spreading new values, habits and lifestyles has often justified authoritarian intervention strategies – either mainly compassionate (paternalism) or primarily punitive (excessive coercion). Fears about the 'dangerous classes' have tended to emerge at times of economic and social upheaval (Gordon, 1994). In periods of crisis, it seems there is less tolerance of difference, and fear and loathing of 'deviants' increase. Fear arises when routine measures of control seem not to be working, threatening the reproduction of power relations. Equally, certain spaces (inner cities, ghettos, schemes/social housing estates) have been defined as 'dangerous', explained as being to do with the types of people who gather there – often immigrant communities, 'drug addicts' or homeless people. Whole neighbourhoods have been stigmatised, with these areas and their residents constructed as aggressive and violent. Insecurity seems to heighten the perception of danger.

Perceptions of danger are social constructions which depend on social categorisations and social context. Our argument in this chapter is that it is the social status of the person using drugs or alcohol which determines how much that person is demonised rather than the substance itself or the pattern of use – important though those factors are. Another key argument of this chapter is that ideas matter. Words are actions and actions have consequences. Powerful images construct social perceptions of problems and shape policy responses.

We have noted over recent years an increasingly ideological presentation of social issues, that is, a more emphatic and intransigent discourse. This, we argue, is linked to the rise of populist politics, a polarisation of opinion and the decay of the middle ground and any willingness to compromise. There has been an increasingly punitive response to some groups of people, a hardening of attitudes and a decline in sympathy. What happens to groups like people who use drugs and alcohol or poor people depends on how these are portrayed – which groups are seen as 'one of us' and which are seen as 'enemies of the people'. Powerful images of dangerous groups have been manufactured to justify authoritarian and despotic populism: reflecting the link between ideas and interests. While these are commonly presented as outsiders or immigrants, links have also been made to the poor and to people who use drugs and alcohol. The outstanding example of this is in the Philippines where Duterte's War on Drug Users has led to the deaths of 5,000 officially and perhaps between 12,000 and over 20,000 mainly poor people according to human rights groups.[1] Similar processes appear to be at work in other countries, such as Hungary where homelessness has been criminalised and Opiate Substitution Treatment and Needle Syringe Programmes curtailed. However, populism does not inevitably lead to harsher drug and alcohol policies. In the

United States, currently, more health-oriented policies are being developed for some people who use drugs.[2]

To explain these differences, we need to look in closer detail at the links between images/frames and the networks that link interest groups, politicians and the media. The right-wing press have played a key role in demonising the welfare poor in some countries – especially we have observed this trend in the UK. There the argument has been made that those who are receiving welfare benefits are irresponsible and undeserving, spending too much of their income on drink and drugs. In a similar way, certain areas associated with low-income groups have been stigmatised, especially social housing estates and tower blocks. As we shall demonstrate in this chapter, the reality of course differs markedly from the inaccurate and prejudiced images found in political rhetoric, the media and some policy statements.

Underlying these frames is the trend to explain poverty not as a result of low income but as a result of behavioural choices. Policies built on these assumptions have borne down on poor people. On occasions, however, the people affected have resisted these images and through community action have constructed alternative images and offered alternative policy solutions.

In approaching this analysis, we draw on work which has pointed to the capacity of actors to influence others' normative and cognitive beliefs through the use of ideational elements such as discourse, practices and symbols. For example, the types of ideational power Carstensen and Schmidt (2016) identified: power *through* ideas – the capacity of actors to persuade others to accept and adopt their views through the use of ideational elements; power *over* ideas – the imposition of ideas and the power to resist the inclusion of alternative ideas into the policy-making arena. This perspective illustrates how ideas matter and are important for understanding relations and structures of power. Sets of ideas provide interpretive frameworks that give definition to values and preferences and make political and economic interests actionable.

Paradigms of social policy: problematisations and policies

Drawing on literature reviews and observation of policy trends over a more than 30-year period, we outline three types of social policy paradigm or types of ideational power (welfare state, neoliberal and populist) to trace the trajectory of the problematisation policy response nexus with regard to people who are poor and/or use drink or drugs (see Table 9.1). These paradigms are presented as analytic ideal types to help explain trends.

In the welfare state period (1945–1979), the stress was on shared norms and values and people who misused drugs and alcohol were seen largely as sick or deviant. In the 1960s, drug use became associated with rebellious or counter-cultural behaviour, especially among students and hippies. The working class had little contact with people who used drugs apart from occasional family members. Later, rising use of drink and drugs was linked to generational change along with increased affluence and availability. HIV/AIDs appeared towards the end of this

Table 9.1 Paradigms of social policy: perceptions and policy responses

Overarching paradigms	Welfare state (1945–1979)	Neoliberalism (1979–2008)	Populism (2008–the present)
Perception of the poor	Contempt Inadequate Small and residual group	Poor choices Lack of education Under-socialised Criminalisation of the poor/poverty	The poor as a whole associated with drugs, drink, obesity, disability, mental illness
Perception of people who use drugs and alcohol	Deviant Sick	Irresponsible Unhealthy lifestyles Risky behaviour Acquisitive crime Public nuisance	Outsiders Welfare dependent or criminal Sub-human Racist or xenophobic categories Dangerous
Policy response	Medicine Social work Social security and social assistance Habitual drinkers and vagrants – prisons, police and reception centres	Multi-agency partnerships, including criminal justice Selectivist/residual benefits	Conditionality Sanctions Exclusion
Perceived links between drug use or drinking and working class and poor	Drug scenes belong to bohemians, artists or eccentrics Respectable working class abstemious; rough working class more likely to drink Increase in prevalence of drinking linked to affluence Alcoholics move down social scale	Heroin and opioid epidemics in deprived former manufacturing places/rust belt Collapse of community among de-industrialised working class – social problems linked to drink and drugs	Stereotypes of the poor justify cuts in public expenditure Wasteful expenditure on drink and drugs Opposition presented between hard-working ordinary people and lazy drug or drink users
Key terms	Need Inequality	Lifestyles Harm Risk Concentrated risk	Danger Threat Dependence Recovery Abstinence
Economy and politics	Economic growth Tripartism Trade Unions Social Democratic or Labour parties	Prosperity Consumer capitalism Globalisation Market dominance Decline of trade unions	Recession Austerity Protectionism Collapse of centre parties

period and in some countries harm reduction became a new frame for policy – a development from the former medical or social work models aiming at treatment and rehabilitation.

In the period of neoliberalism (1979–2008), policies veered between malign and benign. The malign neglect of the early years of neoliberalism led to riots and rising crime. In the United States, use of harsh drug laws led to mass incarceration of African Americans as a form of social control, the new Jim Crow (Alexander, 2012). In the UK, following restructuring to create a new enterprise state under Thatcher, 'third way' policies accepted the market as the economic policy driver but incorporated forms of social policy aimed at tackling social exclusion and disadvantage. New Labour shared many Thatcherite assumptions: what used to be seen as matters of social justice were presented as the consequences of personal behaviour, individual defects and lifestyle choices and translated into policies for welfare reform, criminal justice and addiction policies. Drug problems were framed as a working-class issue, either because of lack of treatment for family members or because of acquisitive crime or discarded syringes causing public nuisance. Drug policies were given attention and increased expenditure, and some achievements can be seen (MacGregor, 2017). By contrast, alcohol use was encouraged as part of the night-time economy and urban regeneration programmes but concentrations of problems, for example, in city centres, led to targeted interventions.

Following the financial crisis of 2008, state expenditures were cut and justified by the construction of a new image of users of public services – one which largely blamed them for their own misfortune: hostile policy and practice environments were deliberately developed.

Underpinning these latter paradigms, a process of 'criminalisation of the poor' can be identified: the poor were constructed as a dangerous class, beginning in the 1980s with the arrival of Thatcherism/Reaganism and neoliberalism. The process got underway when the concept of 'the underclass' came into social policy debates as part of a radical Right/neoliberal critique of the 'welfare state' (Lemann, 1986; Murray, 1984). With the American reconstruction of the poor as an underclass (Auletta, 1982), hustlers, traumatised drunks and 'the passive poor' (long-term welfare dependents) were portrayed as the dominant image of poverty. A particularly noteworthy aspect of current contemporary constructions is the use of the term 'dependence' – stressing passivity and lack of control with regard to use of drugs, drink and welfare. This image is counterposed to concepts of independence, strength and individualism. Poor people were blamed for an array of social problems, constructed as unemployable and seen as dependent on welfare and drugs. Rhetoric and dominant images focused on the pathologies of the 'welfare poor'. It was also at this time in the UK that social security or social assistance began to be talked about as 'welfare' – another American import to discourse – heralding a shift from a universalist to a selectivist/residual policy paradigm. Where public services are provided selectively rather than universally, a central question is always who are entitled to benefits or services? Policies are then delivered in ways based on degrees of deservingness, assessing who is most in need and who will benefit, involving often complex calculations and assignment of people to administrative categories. The administration of services on the ground impacts on both those delivering and those receiving them. The experience of being on the end of these labels and assessments can be demeaning, and likely to involve feelings of rejection, exclusion and insult and lowered self-esteem – commonly referred to today as 'stigma'. Degradation and surveillance are constant features of policies towards the poor as they have been towards 'addicts' and 'alcoholics'.

In the following two sections, examples from the UK, the United States and elsewhere illustrate this link between framing and policy.

Poverty, drugs and alcohol: examples from the UK

In a characteristic counter-propaganda strategy, the term social justice (central to social democracy but avoided by the UK New Labour government (1997–2010) who replaced it with social exclusion) was appropriated by the Right-wing, who then used it against the very social groups for whom it is most relevant.

A prime mover in this policy shift, the Conservative politician Ian Duncan Smith was one of the main architects of the punitive policy turn as the founder of the influential think tank the Centre for Social Justice (CSJ) and also as Secretary of State for Work and Pensions in the Coalition and later Conservative governments (after 2010).

The CSJ's vigorous criticism of harm reduction and expansion of methadone treatment under the Labour administration (in their report *Addicted Britain*, 2007) heavily influenced the Coalition government's drugs policy shift towards abstinence-based recovery. CSJ also promoted the image of the 'welfare scrounger' dependent on both drugs and welfare, which served to justify enhanced levels of conditionality before poor people could access state support (Wincup and Monaghan, 2016).

During his tenure, IDS – as he is known – sought to redefine poverty in terms of behaviour, emphasising drugs, alcohol, worklessness, family stability and parenting skills. These images became embedded in policy in the document *Social Justice: Transforming Lives* (DWP, 2012), a report which 'completely reframed a concern for social justice with a focus on very troubled families' (Shildrick, 2018, p. 32). In this policy, the problematised groups were households identified as being involved in crime and antisocial behaviour, having children not in school, having an adult on benefits and causing high costs to the public purse. A health criterion included emotional and mental health problems, drug and alcohol misuse, long-term health conditions, health problems caused by domestic abuse and under 18 conceptions. Drugs and alcohol were part of a complex of conditions where individual failure and inadequacy was the defining feature.

The Troubled Families Programme was introduced after the extensive 2011 urban riots, which were framed as caused by a hard core of rioters coming from 'a feral underclass' who were seen as having a twisted moral code and an absence of self-restraint (Crossley, 2018, p. 1). At the launch of the new Troubled Families Programme in December 2011, Prime Minister Cameron stated:

> [W]hatever you call them, we've known for years that a relatively small number of families are the source of a large proportion of the problems in society. Drug addiction, alcohol abuse, crime, a culture of disruption and irresponsibility cascades through generations.[3]

A similar distorted view was presented by IDS who, introducing the Troubled Families programme, referred to a photograph of children in a room with their drug-addicted parents, implying that this was a key explanation of the situation.

The Troubled Families programme operated in England through local authorities who would receive funding on a payment by results basis. JobCentre Plus (the UK government-funded employment agency and social security office) was expected to devise approaches to support people dependent on drugs and alcohol back into employment. However, implementation proved difficult. There was some resistance at the local level. Crossley noted that 'workers do not always agree with all aspects of the policy they are asked to implement' (Crossley, 2018, p. 119). Local authorities resisted some of the shaming aspects of the programme: 'almost all local authorities called their local troubled families work by another name in an attempt to soften the stigmatising tone of the programme' (Crossley, 2018, p. 173). Crossley's assessment is damning: 'the programme from start to finish and from top to bottom has relied on dirty data, deceitful practices and dubious claims throughout' (Crossley, 2018, p. 180). An evaluation report found 93 per cent of the so-called troubled families had no adults clinically diagnosed as being dependent on alcohol and a similar 93 per cent of families had no adults clinically diagnosed as being dependent on non-prescription drugs (Crossley, 2018, p. 153). However, the hostile rhetoric was maintained with vignettes of extreme and atypical families being presented as case studies (Crossley, 2018, p. 160).

Indeed, the evidence shows only a small proportion of poverty is associated with problem substance misuse and low-income people drink less than others (ONS, 2018). Researchers for the Joseph Rowntree Foundation reviewed the data and concluded that 'the problem of addiction, while severe for those affected, is not common among those that are in poverty – only a small fraction are affected' (Harkness et al., 2012, p. 32). While 'one-in-four working age adults living in a couple with children are poor . . . fewer than three percent are alcohol dependent and less than one per cent drug dependent' (Harkness et al., 2012, p. 32; HBAI, 2011; Gould, 2006). In spite of this, they add, 'the public perception appears to be that these problems are a common cause of poverty. . . . [D]ata from the British Social Attitudes Survey (2011) found the factor most commonly cited as a reason for child poverty was drug and alcohol addiction, 75 per cent thinking it was a reason for children living in poverty while drug and alcohol addiction has been cited as an argument against increasing the incomes of people in poverty'.[4] (Harkness et al., 2012, pp. 32–3).

In the last ten years, since the financial crash, poverty and inequality have gained a new public presence in the UK. Korte and Zipp note that at a time of social expenditure cuts and new austerity measures, 'a rhetoric about "Broken Britain" poverty is present in the public imagination and it is visible on the streets of British cities' (Korte and Zipp, 2014, p. 1). The poor have been treated as cultural others and associated with 'brutality, crime, alcoholism and neglect' (Korte and Zipp, 2014, p. 17). Images such as those in the television programmes *Little Britain* and *Benefits Street* exude class contempt. They conclude that 'the council estate in particular has emerged as the equivalent of the Victorian slum. Poor people thus appear as marginalised not only in social but also spatial terms' (Korte and Zipp, 2014, p. 125). The tower block is particularly maligned. Shildrick sums up this perspective well:

> poverty and other associated disadvantages are increasingly explained (away) by individual behaviours and problematic drug and alcohol use has a central place in these ever more animated and vitriolic debates. Problematic drug and alcohol use is not only identified as one of the key causes of poverty but increasingly drug and alcohol use by those in poverty is understood as being problematic. The regular deployment of extreme and sometimes downright fantastical examples are drawn upon by those in political power (aided by a right wing media) to depict life for those at the bottom as riven by prolific and problematic drug consumption (and drug selling) behaviours.
>
> (Shildrick, 2018, p. 266)

The linking of the use of drink and drugs to low-income people served to produce fear in others and led to distancing, avoiding the places where they live. People who have little contact with each other do not know that the image is incorrect. So the image presented in the media dominates – until a crisis event, like that of the tragic and devastating fire at Grenfell Tower in London 2017, breaks through to show the reality of the lives of the hard-working, articulate and responsible people living there.

The political advantage of such discussions of poverty (whether intentional or not), which emphasise problematic drug and alcohol use or focus on 'troubled families', is to stoke anger at the welfare state and justify austerity policies and cuts in welfare provision and in public services generally, including in drug and alcohol treatment and care (Shildrick, 2018, p. 133). The main function of this construction is to delegitimise state expenditure on welfare/social security and on health and social services, a development that coincided with reductions in public expenditure under the name of 'austerity' policies following the 2008 financial crisis.

Tracy Shildrick has discussed this situation at length in her work arguing that 'poverty propaganda – deliberately and often very carefully crafted myths and misrepresentations about poverty and those who experience the conditions – has the biggest influence on how poverty is understood in the contemporary context' (Shildrick, 2018, p. 2). She notes that poverty has been 'demonised to such a degree that its real causes and consequences are barely discussed . . . [allowing] punitive and sometimes downright cruel policies' (Shildrick, 2018, p. 2). She adds, 'in popular and political debates poverty is presented as a personal failure that can be resolved by individual determination and hard work' (Shildrick, 2018, p. 6). What she terms 'poverty propaganda' is characterised by the way it manufactures the unusual into the usual. Propaganda is 'used to justify policy developments that amount to little more than punitive and aggressive assaults on the conditions of life for those with the least' (Shildrick, 2018, p. 20). As an example, she cites *ITV News, December 18, 2012* where a Yorkshire MP called for a ban on 'state handouts from being spent on booze'.

Another illustration of poverty propaganda was the attempt to denigrate and cut income support for people with disabilities: an online newspaper reported '£435 million in sickness benefit handed out to drunks and junkies with 75,000 signed off work for their addictions given up to £108 a week'.[5] Similarly, poverty was presented as a result of bad habits by a Conservative city councillor who said that there was no need for food banks – donating to them allowed recipients to spend more money on alcohol and cigarettes (quoted in Shildrick, 2018, p. 62).

From welfare to workfare

Welfare policy in Britain in recent years has moved to a system of workfare characterised by increased conditionality – linking welfare rights to 'responsible' behaviour. The origins of this shift may be traced to the Thatcher government's policy change from 'unemployment benefit' to 'jobseekers allowance', expanded under New Labour and then escalated under the Coalition government. These trends were further developed under the current Conservative administration whose rejoinder to all criticisms of their policies is to say that 'work is the best answer to poverty', despite the fact that poverty among working people is rising with growing low-paid, insecure employment.

This policy focus on welfare conditionality is evident in the government's establishment of the Black Inquiry in 2015 – another initiative which backfired. Its terms of reference were to conduct an independent review into the challenges faced by individuals seeking, returning to and remaining in work when they are addicted to alcohol or drugs or are obese (the three contemporary hate figures framing the poor). The review was to consider how best to support benefit claimants with these potentially treatable conditions back into work – including considering the case for linking benefit entitlements to take up of appropriate treatment or support. The issue was problematised in by now familiar terms. In the call for evidence under a section headed 'Why change is needed', the DWP stated:

> Long-term conditions such as drug addiction and alcohol dependence, or obesity, can seriously affect people's chances of taking up and remaining in

rewarding employment. In England alone, research from 2008 and 2010 indicated that:

- 1 in 15 working-age benefit claimants is dependent on drugs such as heroin and crack cocaine[6]
- 1 in 25 working-age benefit claimants are suffering from alcohol dependency.[7] Assuming these ratios have remained broadly constant since the research was conducted, this analysis suggests that around 280,000 working-age benefit claimants are suffering from addiction to opiates, and 170,000 from alcohol dependency (as of August 2014).

(DWP, 2015, p. 6)

A moment's reflection tells us that this means that 14 out of 15 working-age claimants are not dependent on drugs and 24 out of 25 are not suffering from alcohol dependency. At first, we may react with shock and horror. But what is the sense of these numbers? Are they huge or not? Without relevant comparators, the numbers (the facts) alone are meaningless. Harmful alcohol consumption was estimated to cost around £3.5 billion per year to the NHS, £11 billion in crime and over £7 billion to the economy in lost productivity and the societal costs of drug addiction were estimated to be £15.4 billion. Again, it is pertinent to point out that without putting such bald figures into context, it is difficult to interpret them. And are poor people alone responsible for these costs?

After careful review of the available evidence, the Black Inquiry concluded, however, that most obese people were in work and it was not possible to use the welfare system to encourage drug- and alcohol-dependent people into work (Black, 2016). Introducing her report, Prof. Dame Carol Black said: 'After a searching inquiry we are clear that a fresh approach is needed, one that brings together health, social, and employment agencies in new collaborative ways, personalised to the circumstances of each individual'.[8]

The examples in this section show how the UK Conservative governments were able to build on developments under the previous New Labour administrations to bring about a harsh turn in policy. Under New Labour, dangerous drugs became associated with deprived communities and heavy drinking with public nuisance as well as domestic violence and other problematic behaviours. The Conservative governments saw these behaviours as concentrated among a distinctive group of 'troubled families', and welfare claimants were presented as a burden on social services and a troubling cost to the state (MacGregor, 2017). Drug-taking was portrayed as one small part of a complex of problems concentrated in one strata of society, a facet of intergenerational poverty and explained in moralistic terms. As a result of this framing, this group are condemned as a burden on society.

In the following section, we examine similar examples from the United States and Australia.

Poverty, drugs and alcohol: examples from the United States and Australia

The radical right ideas which dominate in discussions of poverty and addiction in England had their origins in the underclass discourse developed in the United States. These ideas were taken up by the Democrat administration through Clinton's *Personal Responsibility and Work Opportunities Act 1996* that focused on the pathologies of the welfare poor and signalled a rightwards shift for the Democratic Party. These changes served to revamp assistance treating 'the dependent poor as a troublesome population to be subdued and "corrected" through stern behavioural controls and paternalistic sanctions' (Wacquant, 2009, p. 79). What was specific about the US discourse was its explicit racialisation of poverty. 'In the debate leading to the 1996 "reform" four racialised figures coalesced into a new controlling image of the issue by offering vivid incarnations of "dependency" and its corrosive consequences' (Wacquant, 2009, p. 84). These four images were 'the "welfare queen" a wily and fecund black matriarch who shirks employment, cheats the public aid bureaucracy and spends her assistance check high on drugs and liquor, leaving her many children in appalling neglect' (Wacquant, 2009, p. 84). The other three were the teenage mother, the lower-class deadbeat dad and the elderly immigrant.

Clinton's reforms to the 'cash benefit programme' instituted a work requirement along with a time limit in the Temporary Assistance for Needy Families programme. Subsequently, the number of claimants fell, though some attributed this to improvements in the economy. More recently in 2018, Kentucky considered becoming the first state to require some Medicaid recipients to work; other states with Republican governors, including Indiana and Arkansas, aimed to follow. Able-bodied adults enrolled in Medicaid risk losing their insurance if they do not fulfil a community engagement requirement of 20 hours of work, job seeking or volunteering each week. While activity requirements regarding receipt of social security/welfare payments are now well established as part of activation policies in many Western countries (for example, in England, those in receipt of unemployment benefits have to apply via the Internet for about 30 jobs per week), what is new here is a work requirement to access health care. The rationale for these changes appears to be more to do with morality than money: the aim is to weed out malingerers.[9] A consequence also is that such framing acts to stigmatise all Medicaid recipients as malingerers. Stigma acts as a deterrent to claiming and accessing services. Early estimates suggest that as many as 6.3 million people could lose access to health care if these reforms were to be carried through (O'Hara, 2018).

Under discussion in Australia was a Federal plan put forward in the budget proposals for 2017 to drug test welfare recipients. Under the plan, 5,000 new welfare recipients on Newstart and Youth Allowance would be tested in a trial programme. Saliva, hair follicle and urine testing would be used to detect drugs including ecstasy, marijuana and ice. The project would be administered by a private contractor and conducted during appointments at the Department of Human

Services. Under the trial, those who failed a drug test would be placed on income management and 80 per cent of their welfare would be quarantined to a Basics card – a cashless welfare card with funds available to spend only on approved items (not alcohol). A second failed test would prompt a referral to treatment and the government would establish a treatment fund to help access to services.

Malcolm Turnbull, the then Prime Minister, said the plan would be doing people a huge favour because substance abuse has a very high correlation with unemployment.[10] Again, we see the slippage where unemployment is blamed on the behaviour of the unemployed rather than on structural conditions to be responded to by different policies.

These proposals, however, met with concerns from across the sectors – doctors, drug and alcohol researchers, infectious disease experts, local government, charities and community representatives – and eventually were dropped. A 2018 Senate enquiry into the Bill noted the concerns from these sectors: that the drug testing proposals were overly punitive and would perpetuate issues of marginalisation for the most vulnerable; that they would drive people away from support services and the social security system forcing them to find other ways to support their addiction. Furthermore, other people would be caught up in the net who have no issue with substance abuse but are being targeted because they need to make use of the social security system.

Nationally and locally in Australia, there is a shortage of rehabilitation services, leading Lisa Maher, an expert researcher, to comment that the proposals would have risked increasing rates of HIV and hepatitis C. She said that

> this is clearly a very vulnerable population and attempts to penalise this group by attempting to reduce their access to benefits could have potentially significant public health implications: one of the ways in which this could happen is by displacing or driving this group underground and further away from health services.

Another eminent researcher, Alison Ritter, said the tests did nothing to identify addiction – they merely identified drug use – and they risked pushing people onto riskier synthetic drugs which would not be identified by the tests (both quoted in Knaus, 2018).

Thus, we have seen from these examples that over the years, and at a time of rising populism, certain dominant ideas have been translated into policy proposals but have also met with resistance.

Policy shifts: the US opioid crisis

In 2017, more than 70,200 Americans died from drug overdoses, including illicit drugs and prescription opioids.[11] More than 382,000 Americans have overdosed on opioids since 2000 – greater than the number of American combat deaths in World War II, the Korean, and the Vietnam wars combined.[12] The response to the opioid crisis in the United States offers, in contrast to the preceding sections, an interesting illustration of what happens when problematic drug use is framed as a problem of ordinary people not of the poor – suddenly different policy and public responses emerge.

Alexander has persuasively argued that the War on Drugs has operated as a new Jim Crow regime, targeting African American men (Alexander, 2012). As a result, the American criminal justice system has functioned as a system of racial control, relegating millions to permanent second class status. However, a policy shift can be seen to have occurred when it was white people who seemed to be most affected by the opioid crisis. A surprising about-turn has occurred under Trump's populist regime with an unusual cross-party consensus to tackle the opioid crisis. Civil action is being taken to challenge the pharmaceutical companies for irresponsible marketing.

In late 2018, President Trump signed legislation aimed at helping people overcome addiction and preventing addictions before they start, saying 'Together we are going to end the scourge of drug addiction in America'.[13] Trump framed the opioid crisis as a public health emergency. A package of measures focused on improving access to treatment services by lifting certain restrictions on Medicaid and Medicare coverage, as well as backing the creation of comprehensive opioid recovery centres and attempting to address over-prescription of opioids. Government research into non-addictive drugs that could be used for pain management was authorised.

What happened was that partly as a result of measures to curtail the availability of prescription medication, some people then turned to heroin accessed through the black market. As a result of policy and practice changes, such as the use of naloxone by first responders, a flattening or reduction in the rate of increase in opioid deaths occurred. Support has also grown for medication-based treatment using methadone, for the availability of drug-testing kits and provision of safe injection sites. What is not known at present is whether the policy change will impact differently on different racial groups – with, for example, white people being diverted into treatment and black people continuing to be sent to jail. (Trump's suggestion that the death penalty be used for drug dealers does not bode well for those who come into contact with the criminal justice system.)

Major social changes are seen to lie beneath this shift in perspective. Case and Deaton have documented a marked increase in all-cause mortality of middle-aged, white, non-Hispanic men and women in the United States between 1999 and 2013 (Case and Deaton, 2015). Mobilising this new evidence helped to reframe the issue. The increase in mortality for whites was largely accounted for by increasing death rates from drug and alcohol poisoning, suicide and chronic liver diseases and cirrhosis. Those with less education saw the most marked increases. These rising midlife mortality rates were paralleled by increases in midlife morbidity. There were self-reported declines in health, mental health and ability to conduct activities of daily living and increases in chronic pain and inability to work, as well as clinically measured deteriorations in liver function. Case and Deaton describe a process of cumulative disadvantage for generations over time, triggered by progressively worsening labour market opportunities at the time of entry, for whites with low levels of education. They predict that those in midlife now are likely to do much worse in old age than those currently older than 65 (Case and Deaton, 2015). What they are pointing to is the importance of life course experiences and especially the influence of context and the opportunities available at the crucial point of entry to the labour market. This bleak long-term social and economic outlook underpins the 'diseases of despair' and 'deaths of despair' explanations for drug-related deaths.

The shift in the policy response in the United States has come out of a reframing of the issue, by a broad range of actors, including the pharmaceutical industry. For example, Shaun Thaxter, Chief Executive of Indivior, facilitated this reframing in his (re)construction of opioid users: 'this is not the stereotyped image of an inject-ing heroin user living on the street – we are talking about people from all levels of society' (Kollewe, 2017). Stupplebeen has shown how media accounts switched to health-oriented rather than crime-oriented themes (Stupplebeen, 2018). This shift from a criminal justice to a public health response in the United States, along with the radical changes there in marijuana policies, shows that the movement for change can go in either direction – progressive or reactionary. Who, or which, groups, or places, are identified as being mainly involved decides whether we are talking simply about 'risk' or the more alarming 'danger'.

Dangerous places: resistance from affected communities

Resistance to recent neoliberal and populist constructions of poverty as caused by drink and drug excesses has come from experts and practitioners, as in the aforementioned examples in the UK and Australia, but also from those affected – those below. The construction of certain spaces (inner cities, projects. ghettos, schemes) as dangerous has led to whole neighbourhoods being stigmatised and their residents represented as aggressive and violent. However, there is a striking difference between internal and external views of neighbourhoods deemed poor and dangerous. Research from the community studies tradition depicts a more complex and nuanced picture than the dominant view espoused by politicians and the media or via crime and deprivation statistics. Residents from maligned areas report many positive aspects to life in their neighbourhoods: the friendli-ness, the greetings in the street, the informal support networks especially among women and migrant communities in the area and the sense of solidarity (Batty et al., 2011).

This is not to suggest that danger, violence, drug use and drug-related harms are not part of the lived experience in poor areas. However, the experience from the communities' perspective is somewhat different. For example, residents express frustration that drug use is portrayed predominantly as a problem in and for their communities when it is actually a society-wide phenomenon (O'Gorman et al., 2016). This inequity has been explored in community studies by O'Gorman (2016) and Shildrick (2016) who found that the normalisation of drug use is dif-ferentiated by the social status of the person using the drugs in that their drug use and drug-using behaviour are differentially accommodated and accepted by mainstream society.

Other evidence-based analyses of the drug-related harms faced by communities challenge the populist view of drug-related violence as an individualistic and pharma-centric phenomenon – a construction that elicits support for punitive law enforcement and welfare policies. For example, the role of the drugs economy and local drug markets in disadvantaged neighbourhoods, seen in the context of the increased demand for drugs in the general population and the extent of joblessness and cuts in welfare support in an area, suggests the need for a more benign social policy response. In this reading, marginalised young people with aspirations for status and financial success, but with little opportunity to achieve these through the formal economy, are drawn to working in the drugs economy (Bourgois, 1996; Nightingale, 1993). Physically as well as socially marginalised housing estates provide the space and the supply of labour for the organisation of the drugs economy to bag, store and distribute drugs and money (O'Gorman, 2014). Also, systemic violence accompanies the organisation of the drugs economy as a means to regulate its illicit business with disputes over sales territory, drug debts, suspected informants and stolen or seized consignments of drugs liable to be resolved by violent means (Goldstein, 1985; Hammersley, 2008; Reuter, 2009). Young people participating in the drugs economy who are portrayed as demons and monsters turn out often to be just young offenders, as described by one participant in the local drugs economy:

> The young fellas are really just full of fear running around, it's sad. Like on the outside its 'scumbag coke dealers' but they're just afraid scared little boys out there trying to make a name for themselves fuelled up by fear.
>
> (O'Gorman et al., 2016, p. 28)

From the residents' perspective, the experience of structural violence by the state – defined as the avoidable impairment of fundamental human needs (Farmer, 2004; Galtung, 1990) – is the source of their most constant fear, that of not having sufficient finances for themselves and their families' basic needs such as food, rent, and utilities (Batty et al., 2011). This perspective, and the disproportionate extent of policy-induced harms experienced by the poor and vulnerable, is rarely given voice.

The community development sector in the UK and in Ireland has a strong tradition of voicing these views and advocating for social justice. Under the benign phase of neoliberalism, the sector was allocated space in multi-agency partnerships to participate in policy-making processes. As Mayo notes, there have been extraordinary examples of community solidarity and resistance with community activists resisting being 'othered' and persisting to 'tell it as it is' and offer alternative policy solutions (Mayo, 2016, p. 18). However, under populism, the multi-agency partnership approach has all but disappeared: although policy rhetoric maintains the language of partnership, this no longer translates into experience on the ground (O'Gorman et al., 2016).

Conclusion – from risk to danger

In this account, we have tried to show how dominant paradigms or sets of ideas affect the details of specific policies for the poor and for those affected by drug or alcohol use and dependency. As different paradigms come to prominence, some interests benefit and others lose out. So ideas and interests are interconnected, perhaps not explicitly with intention but certainly in their effects. Often what appear as harsh and punitive policies are presented in moralistic tones as being for the public good or to improve the moral fibre and well-being of those impacted.

In recent years, social and addiction policies have increasingly drawn a stark distinction between the deserving and the undeserving, the motivated and the unmotivated. Extreme examples have been deployed to create scapegoats based on stereotypes of dangerous people, who are portrayed as irresponsible and a burden on the hard-working moral majority. Poverty and other associated disadvantages have been increasingly constructed as individual behaviours reflecting personal choices rather than the result of structural conditions. Any drug or alcohol use by those in poverty is understood as being problematic and as one of the key causes of poverty.

Scapegoating and stigmatising, by linking the poor to drink and drugs, are part of a process of dehumanising, which justifies extreme measures and exclusionary practices. The undeserving poor (Matza, 1961) are presented as unable to exercise self-control, volatile, violent and disorderly. A central aspect of this process is amplification: the use of drink or drugs and the threat posed by these are distorted and exaggerated. The issue is given disproportionate attention relative to other hazards and harms which may be equally or more dangerous to health and stability, such as air pollution, bad housing, or other social and structural determinants of health. As the poor are blamed for social ills, the policies that follow become more punitive, designed to catch people out and deny them access to services.

These problematisations and use of ideas to frame perceptions and policies are set in wider overarching paradigms of social, economic and political arrangements. In the UK, and arguably in other countries, there has been a shift over time from welfare state to malign or benign neoliberalism to the current situation of populism. While these three phases can be associated with specific time periods, as outlined earlier, elements of each can be seen at any one time in any one of the case study countries. There is not a sudden shift between periods but continuity along with change.

A key argument here is that the seeds of populism were present in the neoliberal period. The excessive individualisation of problems and the epidemiological focus on risky behaviours, and thence on the concentration of unhealthy and high-risk behaviours in certain groups, laid the foundations for the identification of the very poor as addicts and drunkards. The poor were constructed as an underclass and associated with drugs, crime and single mothers: when funds were available, policies were strict and controlling but not harsh and brutal. With austerity, drug treatment and other services were cut back and need neglected. Arbitrary treatment in the welfare system became common. Although Ireland has not shown the same signs of populism as other countries, remaining within the neoliberal paradigm, it is interesting to note that there the terminology and discourse of partnership have continued as a policy motif while in practice a new set of policy responses were developing – ones which were more harsh and exclusionary (O'Gorman et al., 2016).

It is the social status of the person using drugs or alcohol which influences the extent to which they are demonised and portrayed as dangerous, rather than merely being an 'at risk group'. Right-wing rhetoric, neoliberal and populist, has attacked both the poor and those with addiction problems. When those who are suffering are seen to be 'one of us' – to belong to the same community – then more compassionate policies follow. Although we have focused mainly on top-down framings as they shape political and public opinion and policy responses, framings are always challenged sooner or later on the basis of experience from below. What happens next depends on the balance of power.

The key role played by the media in shifting frames has been noted. Whether changes in constructions then lead to changes in policy depends on the presence and effectiveness of links between networks of image makers and decision takers. However, the contradictions and paradoxes within frames and policies provide spaces and opportunities within which resistance and change may develop. Spaces may be filled by alliances of actors, some involving experts and practitioners and some linking community activists to decision takers. What happens is not predetermined but relies on the organised actions of concerned people acting either in progressive or reactionary ways. The outcome depends on who wins in this battle of ideas and interests.

Notes

1 Ellis-Petersen, H. 2018. Duterte's Philippines drug war death toll rises above 5,000. *The Guardian*, 19 December. Available at: www.theguardian.com/world/2018/dec/19/dutertes-philippines-drug-war-death-toll-rises-above-5000.
2 White House Fact Sheets. 2018. President Donald J. Trump Is Combatting the Opioid Crisis. 1 March. Available at: www.whitehouse.gov/briefings-statements/president-donald-j-trump-combatting-opioid-crisis/.
3 Cameron, D. 2011. Troubled Families Speech. *Gov.UK,* 15 December. Available at: htps://www.gov.uk/government/speeches/troubled-families-speech.
4 See, for example, Iain Duncan Smith's Speech to the London School of Economics, December 1, 2011. Available at: http://www2.lse.ac.uk/assets/richmedia/channels/publicLecturesAndEvents/transcripts/20111201_1830_familiesAndYoungPeople_tr.pdf.
5 Beckford, M. 2015. £435MILLION in sickness benefit handed to drunks and junkies, with 75,000 signed off work for their addictions given up to £108 a week. *Daily Mail,* 1 February. Available at: https://www.dailymail.co.uk/news/article-2934798/435MILLION-sickness-benefit-handed-drunks-junkies-75-000-signed-work-addictions-given-108-week.html.
6 Hay, G., and Bauld, L. (2008) Population Estimates of Problematic Drug Users in England Who Access DWP Benefits: A Feasibility Study, *DWP Working Paper No. 46.* London: Department for Work and Pensions.

7 Hay, G. and Bauld, L. (2011) Population Estimates of Alcohol Misusers Who Access DWP Benefits, *DWP Working Paper No. 94* [online]. Department for Work and Pensions. Available at: www.gov.uk/government/uploads/system/uploads/attachment_data/file/214391/WP94.pdf (Accessed June 3rd, 2015).
8 Gov.UK. 2016. Dame Carol Black publishes review on links between work and addiction. *Press Release,* 5 December. Available at: www.gov.uk/government/news/dame-carol-black-publishes-review-on-links-between-work-and-addiction.
9 *The Economist,* January 20th, 2018, pp. 37–38.
10 Knaus, C. 2017. Drug-testing will demonise Australians on welfare, experts say. *The Guardian,* 10 May. Available at: www.theguardian.com/australia-news/2017/may/10/budget-2017-drug-testing-will-demonise-australians-on-welfare-experts-say.
11 National Institute on Drug Abuse. 2019. Overdose Death Rates. Revised January. Available at: www.drugabuse.gov/related-topics/trends-statistics/overdose-death-rates.
12 *The Economist,* June 2, 2018, p. 42.
13 NPR Politics Newsletter. 2018. Signing Opioid Law, Trump Pledges to End 'Scourge' of Drug Addiction. 24 October. Available at: www.npr.org/2018/10/24/660205718/signing-opioid-law-trump-pledges-to-end-scourge-of-drug-addiction.

References

Alexander, M. 2012. *The New Jim Crow*. New York: The New Press.
Auletta, K. 1982. *The Underclass*. New York: Random House.
Bacchi, C. 2012. Why study problematizations? Making politics visible. *Open Journal of Political Science* 2 (1), pp. 1–8.
Batty, E., Cole, I., and Green, S. 2011. *Low-Income Neighbourhoods in Britain. The Gap Between Policy Ideas and Residents' Realities*. York: Joseph Rowntree Foundation.
Black, Dame C. 2016. *An Independent Review into the Impact on Employment Outcomes of Drug or Alcohol Addiction, and Obesity*. London: HMSO, Cm 9336.
Bourgois, P. 1996. *In Search of Respect: Selling Crack in El Barrio*. Cambridge: University Press.
British Social Attitudes Survey. 2011. *British Social Attitudes 28*. London: National Centre for Social Research/Sage Publications.
Bryder, L. 1988. *Below the Magic Mountain: A Social History of Tuberculosis in Twentieth Century Britain*. Oxford: Clarendon Press.
Carstensen, M.B., and Schmidt, V.A. 2016. Power through, over and in ideas: Conceptualizing ideational power in discursive institutionalism. *Journal of European Public Policy* 23 (3), pp. 318–37.
Case, A., and Deaton, A. 2015. Rising morbidity and mortality in midlife among white non-hispanic Americans in the 21st century. *PNAS* 112 (49), pp. 15078–83.
Crossley, S. 2018. *Troublemakers: The Construction of 'Troubled Families' as a Social Problem*. Bristol: Policy Press.
DWP (Department of Work and Pensions). 2012. *Social Justice: Transforming Lives*. London: HMSO.
DWP. 2015. *An Independent Review into the Impact on Employment Outcomes of Drug or Alcohol Addiction, and Obesity: Call for Evidence*. July. London: DWP.
Farmer, P. 2004. An anthropology of structural violence. *Current Anthropology* 45 (3), pp. 305–25.
Galtung, J. 1990. Cultural violence. *Journal of Peace Research* 27 (3), pp. 291–305.
Goldstein, P.J. 1985. The drugs/violence nexus: A tripartite conceptual framework. *Journal of Drug Issues* 15 (4), pp. 493–508.

Gordon, D. 1994. *The Return of the Dangerous Classes – Drug Prohibition and Policy Politics*. New York: W.W. Norton.

Gould, N. 2006. *Mental Health and Child Poverty*. York: Joseph Rowntree Foundation.

Hammersley, R. 2008. *Drugs and Crime: Theories and Practices*. Cambridge: Polity Press.

Harkness, S., Gregg, P., and MacMillan, L. 2012. *Poverty: The Role of Institutions, Behaviours and Culture*. JRF Programme Paper Poverty (June) JRF.

HBAI. 2011. *Households Below Average Income 1994/5 to 2009/10*. London: Department for Work and Pensions.

Knaus, C. 2018. Drug testing welfare recipients could lead to more crime, Mayor says. *The Guardian*, 23 April. Available at: www.theguardian.com/australia-news/2018/apr/23/drug-testing-welfare-recipients-could-lead-to-more-mayor-says.

Kollewe, J. 2017. Drugs firms join fight against painkiller deaths epidemic. *Observer*, 2 December. Available at: www.theguardian.com/business/2017/dec/02/drugs-firms-join-fight-against-opioid-painkiller-deaths-epidemic.

Korte, B., and Zipp, G. 2014. *Poverty in Contemporary Literature*. Basingstoke: Palgrave Macmillan.

Lemann, N. 1986. The origins of the underclass. *The Atlantic* 257 (6), pp. 31–55.

MacGregor, S. 2017. *The Politics of Drugs: Perceptions, Power and Policies*. Basingstoke: Palgrave Macmillan.

Matza, D. 1961. Poverty and disrepute. In: Merton, R.K., and Nisbet, R.A. (Eds.), *Contemporary Social Problems*. New York: Harcourt Brace Jovanavich.

Mayo, M. 2016. CDJ 50 years anniversary conference presentation: Looking backwards, looking forwards – from the present. *Community Development Journal* 51 (1), pp. 8–22.

Murray, C. 1984. *Losing Ground: American Social Policy, 1950–1980*. New York: Basic Books.

Nightingale, C.H. 1993. *On the Edge: A History of Poor Black Children and Their American Dreams*. New York: Basic Books.

O'Gorman, A. 2014. Drug use, drug markets and area-based responses. In: Norris, M. (Ed.), *Social Housing and Liveability: Ten Years of Change in Social Housing Neighbourhoods*. New York: Routledge.

O'Gorman, A. 2016. Chillin, buzzin, getting mangled, and coming down: Doing differentiated normalisation in risk environments. *Drugs: Education, Prevention and Policy* 23 (3), pp. 247–54.

O'Gorman, A., Driscoll, A., Moore, K., and Roantree, D. 2016. *Outcomes: Drug Harms, Policy Harms, Poverty and Inequality*. Dublin: Clondalkin Drug and Alcohol Task Force.

O'Hara, M. 2018. Lesson from America. *The Guardian*, 21 February, p. 35.

ONS [Office for National Statistics]. 2018. *Adult Drinking Habits in Great Britain: 2017, Statistical Bulletin*, 1 May. Available at: www.ons.gov.uk/.

Reuter, P. 2009. Systemic violence in drug markets. *Crime, Law and Social Change* 52 (3), pp. 275–84.

Schön, D.A., and Rein, M. 1994. *Frame Reflection: Toward the Resolution of Intractable Policy Controversies*. New York: Basic Books.

Shildrick, T. 2016. Normalisation, youth transitions and austerity. *Drugs: Education, Prevention and Policy* 23 (3), pp. 264–6.

Shildrick, T. 2018. *Poverty Propaganda – Exploring the Myths*. Bristol: Policy Press.

Stone, D. 1989. Causal stories and the formation of policy agendas. *Political Science Quarterly* 104, pp. 281–300.

Stupplebeen, D.A. 2018. People who inject drugs and HIV crisis in Pence's Indiana: A media analysis using two policymaking theories. *International Journal of Drugs Policy* 57, pp. 79–85.

Wacquant, L. 2009. *Punishing the Poor: The Neoliberal Government of Social Insecurity*. Durham, NC: Duke University Press.

Wincup, E., and Monaghan, M.P. 2016. Scrounger narratives and dependent drug users: Welfare, workfare and warfare. *Journal of Poverty and Social Justice* 24 (3), pp. 261–75.

10 Framing and reframing drug 'problems' in prison spaces and populations

Karen Duke and Torsten Kolind

Introduction

During the last 20–30 years, drug use and dealing have emerged as prioritised 'problems' within many prison contexts around the world. Most Western prison systems have responded with dual policies consisting of offering drug treatment and rehabilitation and imposing increasing control and disciplinary sanctioning for drug use and involvement in drug supply. The drug issue is simultaneously framed as both a 'problem' of crime and control and a 'problem' of well-being and health and these frames often compete, conflict, converge and overlap with one another. MacGregor (2017, p. 133) argues that the drugs debate is framed in terms of oppositions: zero tolerance versus harm reduction; prohibition versus legalisation; abstinence versus maintenance; care versus control; public health versus law and order and so on. Different institutions and stakeholders are associated with the different sides of the debate. When we transfer the drugs debate into the prison space, these oppositions or conflicts become even more pronounced and explicit (Duke, 2003). Due to their histories of offending and sometimes violent behaviour, prison populations can be perceived to be 'dangerous', 'threatening' and 'risky' and in need of surveillance and control. The prison environment itself constitutes a 'dangerous space' by exacerbating and often creating problems of violence, harmful drug use, drug dependence, physical and mental illness and transmission of infectious disease (EMCDDA, 2012; WHO, 2014; Sturop-Toft et al., 2018). Within prison settings, an inmate culture characterised by drug sales, drug debt, threats, violence and a range of 'pains of imprisonment' can work as drivers towards initiation, continuation or increasing of prisoner's drug use (Crewe, 2005, 2006; Tompkins, 2016).

People in prison often come from marginalised and under-served groups and experience significant health inequalities. Compared to the general population, they experience a higher burden of communicable and non-communicable disease and mental health and substance use problems (Sturop-Toft et al., 2018). World Health Organisation (WHO) figures from Europe (2014) indicate that there are high rates of lifetime prevalence of illicit drug use and injecting drug use among prison populations and many people enter prison with severe drug problems. A high proportion of people use drugs in prisons and those who inject drugs often share needles. There is a high rate of relapse and overdose on release from prison. There are also high rates of smoking, alcohol use and dependence in prison populations. Mental health problems and co-morbidity (dual diagnosis) of mental health and alcohol/drug problems are common in prison populations. Rates of TB, HIV and Hep C are much higher for people in prison than in the community. People in prison are more likely to self-harm and die by suicide than in the general population. The context of prisons with overcrowding, unsanitary conditions and lack of staffing exacerbates these conditions and practices. As WHO (2014, p. xi) states, 'prisons are not healthy places'. A high-risk population is therefore imported into a high-risk environment and eventually released into the community. People who use drugs in prisons can be framed and categorised as 'vulnerable' and 'at risk' and in need of care, treatment and rehabilitation. Given their increased risk of infectious disease, they can be framed as a threat to public health and in need of monitoring and surveillance. Those involved in drugs in prisons can also be framed and categorised as 'dangerous', a threat to 'order, security and control' and in need of discipline and punishment, particularly participants in the drug trade. Prisoners can thus be framed as offenders and criminals and/or as patients and clients.

The crime and health framings are present in the prison drug policies in many Western countries, but the emphasis on the individual frames fluctuates across space and time (Garland, 2001). Different countries vary in their placement on this continuum of control and treatment (Duke and Kolind, 2017). Political, social and economic factors shape and influence these frames at national levels. In this chapter, we will analyse how the drug 'problem' is framed within prison spaces and populations at the international and national levels of policy, what influences these frames, as well as how prisoners respond to and at times resist these frames. In this view, framing takes place from above and to some extent from below and these different levels of framing can interact and shape each other. We argue that framing is a constant power struggle. Frames can be established at policy level and become embedded over time, but reframing can occur as these frames are contested, circumvented or resisted by different actors in the penal system.

Conceptual framework

According to Rein and Schon (1993), policy actors construct and make sense of problematic policy issues through a process of 'framing' which is defined as 'a way of selecting, organising, interpreting, and making sense of a complex reality to provide guideposts for knowing, analyzing, persuading, and acting' (Rein and Schon, 1993, p. 146). Within this framework, the complementary processes of naming and framing define what is problematic about the issue and suggest what courses of action and policies would be appropriate to tackle the 'problem'. In this sense, policy representations direct how social services act upon certain kinds of issues and social problems (Jöhncke, 2009). In prison drugs policy, framing could highlight issues around prevention, treatment, harm reduction, release and throughcare, drug testing, security, control and punishment. Each framing of the issue is likely to select out and name different features of the 'problem' and ignore or exclude others. For example, in the case of the 'problem' of drugs in prisons, health issues connected with drug use, such as withdrawal, relapse or overdose, could be selected out for attention or alternatively security issues connected with the drugs trade, such as supply reduction or violence, could be highlighted. Once certain features of a situation are named and selected, attempts are made to bind these elements together into a coherent and comprehensible pattern or story. In this way, framing results in different views of the world and creates multiple social realities which often results in tensions between different frames and the corresponding policy actors regarding what constitutes the 'problem'. Within the prison space, the crime and control framing of the drugs 'problem' can conflict, but it can also converge with the health and treatment framing.

Van Hulst and Yanow (2016) have elaborated on Rein and Schon's original work and suggest firstly that framing as an analytical concept should also include a focus on sense-making. That is, policy actors draw on their own knowledge, values and experience to define and frame the 'problem' which results in different solutions and responses. Secondly, 'categorising' helps to draw distinctions and highlights some aspects of a problematic situation or a population while occluding or silencing other aspects. Practitioners select certain features of their client populations in order to categorise their clients for different interventions, and in this way they assist in creating 'institutional selves' in organisational settings (Gubrium and Holstein, 2001). In this sense, they transform the 'problems' of clients into 'more or less distinct troubled identities that match the working logic of the treatment system' (Järvinen and Andersen, 2009, p. 865). Policy-makers also categorise populations or the targets of policy whereby distinctions are drawn between populations who are perceived to be deserving versus undeserving, legitimate versus illegitimate, worthy versus unworthy and sympathetic versus threatening (Rochefort and Cobb, 1993; Presser, 2004). Characteristics such as race, gender, class and age are also considered. Often, 'deviants' and other excluded groups do not receive equivalent considerations; for example, people in prison who use drugs are often categorised as 'criminals' and 'addicts' and therefore framed as undeserving, illegitimate, unworthy and threatening. Historically, the discourse of 'less eligibility' has infiltrated the development of Western penal policy and ensured that the conditions and services available to prisoners are not superior to those available to the working classes or they will not be deterred from committing crime (Melossi and Pavarini, 1981). However, people in prison who use drugs can also be categorised as 'vulnerable', 'deserving' and in need of help, treatment and rehabilitation. As Donahue and Moore (2009) have argued from a Canadian context, the institutional identity of the 'offender' increasingly coexists with that of the 'client' in need of therapeutic attention. This development is also seen in other parts of the world, for example, in the United States, parts of Europe and Australia (see also Fox, 2001; Nielsen and Kolind, 2016; Walker et al., 2018). Moreover, with the growth of prison-based drug treatment programmes, drug users in prisons are also represented as people with the right to be treated and served in many Western countries. The way in which affected populations are perceived and categorised by different policy actors and the public are therefore crucial in terms of determining the balance between care and control in policy design (Rochefort and Cobb., 1993; Kolind et al., 2013).

The ways in which the drug issue in prison is framed and debated and the setting out of policy options are influenced by wider forces or a 'nested context' (Rein and Schon, 1993, p. 154). In this view, policy issues emerge in connection with governmental programmes, which exist within a wider policy environment, which is part of a broader political, social and economic setting, which is situated within a historical era. Features of this context shift and impact on each other, often resulting in the reframing of a policy issue. In this chapter, we are interested in examining the framing of the drug 'problem' in prison at the international level through the work of the INCB, UNODC and WHO and the documents and guidance they produce and how these frames attempt to set the framework for the development of policies and practices at the national level of drugs policy in prisons. Our focus drills down from a consideration of policies at the level of international institutions to the European institutional level and then down to certain national examples where there have been analyses of the development of prison drugs policy. It is not our intention to compare national policies.

The framings taking place in policy development and subsequently informing practice naturally have consequences for the prisoners being 'framed'. That is, the prisoner's troubles or issues are turned into 'problems' and then acted upon. However, it is also important to note that even though prison policies and services construct subject positions and typifications (e.g. criminal, drug user, sick, empowered, etc.), the connection between prisoners' personal selves and troubled identities needs to be negotiated and formed (Gubrium and Holstein, 2001). Naturally, individuals cannot transform discourses or frames at will, particularly inmates whose every movement is surveilled and monitored, but they can relate themselves and their actions to them, thereby resisting, rejecting, reproducing or surrendering to the discourses and policies that frame them (Hacking, 1986). This makes room for what we would call reframing or everyday forms of prison resistance (Ugelvik, 2011) by the 'objects' of policy and practice or those who are subjected to the framing, but also for adaptations to the policy and practice (Crewe, 2009) or even acceptance of the power of the prison if it is experienced as legitimate (Sparks and Bottoms, 1995). After having identified the main framings of drug 'problems' in prisons in the first part of this chapter, we will, in the second, offer examples of such reframing.

Framing from above: framing the drug 'problem' in prison at international and national levels

International level

Historically, the two pillars of the international drug control system have been supply reduction and demand reduction (Babor et al., 2010), with harm reduction emerging during the HIV epidemic in the 1980s. Aligned to these policy goals, the drugs issue has been primarily framed as a 'problem' of crime and/or a 'problem' of health. The UN Conventions 1961, 1971 and 1988 form the basis of international drugs control and prohibit the production and use of narcotic and synthetic pharmaceutical drugs (except for medical and scientific purposes), increase controls around drug trafficking and money laundering and require Member States to criminalise the production, manufacture, sale, possession or purchase of any narcotic drug or psychotropic substance for non-medical and non-scientific purposes, which effectively criminalises people who use drugs. The treaties are overseen by the Commission on Narcotic Drugs (CND), the United Nations Office on Drugs and Crime (UNODC) and the International Narcotics Control Board (INCB). Through the INCB, the crime and control framings are exemplified in its hardline, punitive approach and its emphasis on supply reduction, while the health framing manifests itself mainly through the work of the World Health Organisation which provides medical and scientific expertise on the scheduling of substances and guidance on health responses. As Ritter et al. (2017) argue, although historically the treaties and structure afforded little room to manoeuvre within this punitive, prohibitionist framework, this has changed in recent years with a greater emphasis on public health and human rights approaches to drug policy and movement away from criminalisation and penalisation. For example, there have been moves towards developing more public health-oriented drug strategies, greater recognition of the place of harm reduction services within treatment and increasing support for depenalisation and decriminalisation by the UNODC and WHO (UNODC, 2013; WHO, 2014). It is important to note that statements from these international institutions represent the views of a particular set of advocates who have engaged in battles of ideas within these institutions to ensure their perspectives around harm reduction, human rights, depenalisation and decriminalisation are instituted. These approaches are embedded in Western values and opposition to these ideas and reforms continues to come from prohibitionist countries like China, Russia and the Philippines (MacGregor, 2017).

Following UNGASS 2016, the movement away from penalisation can be seen in the guidance of UNODC and WHO on providing treatment as an alternative to conviction or punishment for those people with drug use disorders who are in contact with the criminal justice system. The UNODC (2018, p. 22) argues that 'drug use disorders' should be treated in the health care system and that providing drug treatment as an alternative in this way is an effective public health and public safety strategy. Such alternatives have the potential to reduce the prison population, overcrowding and the detrimental effects of a prison sentence. However, this drive from the UNODC to facilitate treatment interventions as alternatives or additions to conviction or punishment has not been universally applied within individual countries. The UNODC has also put forward a number of principles enshrined in the international legal framework which relate to the treatment of people with drug use disorders in contact with the criminal justice system. Two of these apply directly to those who are in prison settings and aim to frame prison drugs policies at the national levels. The first principle is that 'prisoners with drug use disorders may not be deprived of their right to health and are entitled to the same level of treatment as the general population' and the second principle is that 'drug use disorders are a public health concern requiring responses that are health-centred. Individuals with drug use disorders should not be punished for their drug use disorder but provided with appropriate treatment' (UNODC, 2018, p. 20).

In international law, the right to health is universal and non-discriminatory in application and therefore applies to people who have been deprived of liberty. The UN Standard Minimum Rules for the Treatment of Prisoners (SMR) (i.e. Mandela Rules) emphasise the *principle of equivalence* or the idea that people in prison must 'have access to the health services available in the country without discrimination on the grounds of their legal situation'. The HIV/AIDS crisis prompted further emphasis on access to HIV treatment and services as a human right for people inside and outside custody and on the principle of equivalence for HIV provision and harm reduction initiatives (Csete et al., 2018). This 'human rights framing' has been developed into policy and practice guidance by UNODC, UNAIDS and WHO around the treatment of drug dependence. Along with the principle of equivalence, the UN promotes the following treatment principles: treatment must be voluntary; treatment approaches should be chosen and implemented with meaningful involvement of the patient; treatment must be scientifically sound, humane and low-threshold and be overseen by qualified health professionals; people with drug dependence should have access to several kinds of treatment; treatment programmes must not exclude people because of criminal records; women, especially pregnant women, and people with psychiatric co-morbidities should be given priority in treatment; and treatment as an alternative to imprisonment or other penal sanctions should be made available to drug-dependent offenders (UNODC, 2009).

Despite the work of WHO and UNODC on promoting the health of prisoners through effective drug treatment policy, many Member States do not meet their responsibility to protect the health of prison populations and implement the principle of equivalence. Csete et al. (2018, p. 179) argue that the human rights protections for people in prison (particularly for those who use drugs) in both international and national law and guidelines are often flouted:

> Although the right to health of prisoners is broadly protected under human rights norms, ensuring these guarantees in practice is rare. In reality, the rights of people who use drugs – and of prisoners more broadly – are flagrantly violated in prisons in many countries with no opportunity for complaint or redress.

In practice, research illustrates the complexities surrounding the interpretations and applications of the principle of equivalence in prison settings, particularly within the context of increasing prison populations and their complex health needs, austerity measures and the prevailing focus on enforcement, security and control (Ismail and deViaggani, 2018b). Prisoners are often denied evidence-based treatment options that might be available in the community such as opioid substitution therapy (OST) which reduces the risk of HIV and hepatitis C transmission and overdose (Stover et al., 2004; Degenhardt et al., 2014). In 2016, an estimated 52 countries provided OST in prison – much lower than the number of countries which provide OST in the community (Stone, 2016). However, in practice, even where OST and other proven treatments are offered in prisons, the treatment may only be offered in some prisons and may not be available to all prisoners depending on screening procedures (Larney and Dolan, 2009). Similarly, needle and syringe exchange schemes are available in the community in some countries, but this is not usually part of service provision in prison environments with only eight countries providing this service in at least one prison (Stöver and Hariga, 2016; Stone, 2016). Despite the shifting landscape of drug policy at national and local levels, harm reduction still remains highly controversial politically, particularly for prison populations (de Andrade, 2018; Zurhold and Stöver, 2016). In many countries, harm reduction initiatives are seen to conflict with criminal justice goals of enforcement, zero tolerance and abstinence.

Mold (2018) argues that the public health framing of drug use has started to gain momentum, although this can be defined in multiple ways and exists alongside and sometimes converges with other frames such as the medical/psychiatric and penal/criminological approaches. In line with a public health framing, WHO (2014, p. xi) argues that 'prison health is part of public health and prisons are part of our society'. Good health and well-being in prison populations is seen to be in the interests of the wider society and cost-effective because it improves the health of the whole community, reduces public health expenditure, improves reintegration into society and reduces reoffending, and reduces health inequalities (WHO, 2015). With prison populations, there is not only an emphasis on public health but also a preoccupation with public safety. The Doha Declaration, which was adopted at the 13th UN Congress on Crime Prevention and Criminal Justice, focuses on rehabilitation and social integration of prisoners into the community (UNODC, 2017a). UNODC provides Member States with technical guidance on how to initiate and enhance rehabilitation based on the UN Standard Minimum Rules for the Treatment of Prisoners and such rehabilitation programmes are viewed as 'one of the best and cost-effective ways of preventing their reoffending, with significant benefits for not only the individuals concerned, but also for public safety more broadly' (UNODC, 2017b, p. 1). A New Chance programme has been proposed for future development in order to increase skills, income, employability and self-esteem of prisoners. These types of initiatives frame people in prison as needing transformation and change through rehabilitation and treatment in order for them to make contributions to society, as well as to protect the public. The emphasis is on converting an 'unproductive population' into productive, active and contributing citizens, who do not pose a threat or risk to the wider public.

In 1995, the WHO introduced the Healthy Prisons Agenda in order to protect and improve the health of people in prisons. The UNODC (2018, p. 64) views the criminal justice system as a 'gateway to treatment' and important setting for drug interventions. Although the limits of prison settings in terms of delivering health care are recognised and WHO (2014, p. 91) argues that 'prisons are not therapeutic institutions', prison sentences are framed as 'opportunities' for improving health and reducing health inequalities through drug treatment. How-ever, when we examine what is occurring with health in prisons at the national level, it is evident that the Healthy Prisons Agenda has not been implemented in many jurisdictions. For example, research conducted in England uncovered vari-ous challenges to the implementation of the Healthy Prisons Agenda linked to sec-toral, institutional and occupational barriers, including constraints on resources and staffing, lack of training around health issues, conflicts between professional groups in prisons and the subordination of the health agenda to that of immediate security and control priorities. Ismail and deViggiani (2018a, p. 94) concluded that within English prisons there is 'widespread prevalence of a command-and-control ethos . . . underpinned by a prevailing security culture that dismisses prison-based health-promoting activities. Health in prisons is portrayed as an uto-pian oxymoron, inferior to the punitive aims of the prison'. Similarly, a recent study of the level of infectious risk in prisons in five European countries measured to what extent the prison system adheres to WHO/UNODC recommendations and found low availability of preventive measures. As a result, infectious risk remains extremely high in prisons (Michel et al., 2015).

National level

At the national level, the health and crime framings manifest themselves in vari-ous prison drug policy and practice initiatives around the world. For example, in British prisons, there is an emphasis on providing treatment and rehabilitation for those with drug use problems as well as on various security and control meas-ures that have been implemented to control the supply and use of drugs in pris-ons, including searching procedures and equipment, sniffer dogs, drone/mobile phone blocking technology, CCTV, mandatory drug testing and the introduction of a range of sanctions for those who contravene the rules surrounding use and supply. The intensification of security and control measures, such as mandatory drug testing and increased searching and surveillance, has resulted in prisoners engaging in risky behaviours such as holding drugs and other contraband inter-nally and switching to less detectable substances through testing (e.g. opiates and synthetic cannabinoids) (Boys et al., 2002; HM Inspectorate of Prisons, 2015; User Voice, 2016; Ralphs et al., 2017). Although harm reduction was successfully implemented in the community during the HIV crisis in the late 1980s, this was extremely difficult to extend into prisons as it was viewed as politically unten-able (Duke, 2003, 2011). The lack of effective harm reduction in prisons has also resulted in risky practices, including needle sharing (Swann and James, 1998). Within the prison context and particularly during periods of 'crisis', the security and control frames often take precedence over the treatment and health frames in pursuit of the goal to eradicate the drug 'problem' and achieve a drug-free prison, leaving drug treatment provision under-resourced and low priority. In times of austerity, drug treatment and rehabilitation programmes have suffered major cuts to funding (ACMD, 2017). The crime and health framings conflict with each other as prisoners are offered treatment and care for their drug use problems, while simultaneously punished with a range of sanctions (Duke, 2003). They also converge and overlap; for example, mandatory drug testing is a multifunctional initiative in the prison setting. It is employed as a method to identify and assess those in need of treatment and encourage them to access it, a way to measure the drug 'problem' in prisons by providing quantifiable indicators of use, a measure to deter prisoners from using drugs and as a punitive practice to administer sanctions for drug use.

These framings around care and control are also found in prison drugs policies of other countries. In Australia, Walker et al. (2018) reveal the multiple representations of the drugs 'problem' in prison drug policy in Victoria and how the merging of a tough, control-focused approach with a focus on health, welfare and treatment leads to plurality and diversity in the modes of governing those who are involved in drugs use and supply. They show how the Identified Drug User Programme is underpinned by the dividing practices of care and control and how the conflicting discourses constitute young men as 'criminal', 'untrustworthy' and 'deserving of punishment', but simultaneously constitute them as 'rational', 'self-governing' and 'deserving of treatment'. These dividing practices and conflicting discourses produce harmful effects (e.g. closed visits) which cause distress and pain to people in prison and their families and limit the way the drug 'problem' can be conceptualised in policy and practice. In a similar vein, Watson (2016) argues that the Correctional Service of Canada's pursuit of 'drug-free' prisons and the adoption of enhanced enforcement and zero tolerance policies have produced a number of adverse effects, including continued efforts to smuggle drugs into prison, increased tension and violence, prisoners switching drugs, health-related harms, deterrence of visitors and staff involvement in the drug trade. In the Nordic countries, drug treatment programmes have increased over the last 15 years. Such development might be considered in line with the 'exceptional' prisons of the Nordic countries, characterised by more humane living conditions and low prison populations (Pratt, 2008). However, despite this attempt to offer the prison population adequate drug treatment, the 'treatment' framing is still competing with the 'zero tolerance' and 'tough on drugs' framings with these latter frames dominating (Kolind et al., 2013), and prison drug treatment programmes do not meet the same standards as community treatment (Kolind, 2017).

It is clear that two organising frames of drug policy – health and crime – are present at the international level through the work of INCB, WHO and UNODC and impact on the guidance produced for prisons and their populations. However, there appears to be a clear disjuncture between the international level which has placed more stress on harm reduction, health and depenalisation in recent years and what is happening on the ground in terms of implementation of drugs policy initiatives in prisons at the national level. Many interventions available in the community such as OST, naloxone distribution, needle exchange and other harm reduction techniques are difficult to extend to the prison environment (Michel et al., 2015; Stone, 2016; Stöver and Hariga, 2016). As has been argued in relation to the implementation of health initiatives in some prison systems, this is due to political resistance, austerity, lack of resources and the dominance of the law and order ethos (Duke, 2003; Kolind et al., 2013; Ismail and deViggiani, 2018a). The conflicts between the health and crime framings intensify within the prison space and have implications for the ways in which the people in prison who use drugs themselves are framed by policy-makers and for the drug interventions available within this environment, but also for ways in which prisoners themselves respond to, adapt and resist these framings. The next section will explore the framing and reframing actions and practices of those imprisoned around drugs issues.

Framing and reframing from below

In prisons, those who use drugs frame and also reframe several different subjectivities. As argued so far, framing drug using prisoners as either 'criminal' or 'in need of treatment' (sick/diseased) are the two most dominant frames in present political discourse at both global and national levels. These framings inform practice, practices that both restrict and enable the ways prisoners can act, and together framings and practices are important for the ways prisoners understand and identify themselves. However, it is also important to understand that some reframing or even resistance by prisoners also takes place. That is, prisoners challenge, exploit or avoid the more global framings and the practices that follow from these framings. In the following section, we will explore how prisoners reframe the drug using prisoner as 'criminal' and 'in need of treatment', respectively.

We would like to stress that overarching policy frames are not translated directly into practice. The discretionary practices (i.e. blending personal and professional judgements) of street-level bureaucrats (Lipsky, 1980) – such as prison officers, prison health personnel and counsellors – change, adjust and modify the policy frames to suit concrete situations. Hence, a difference exists between policy frames and policy in practice (Shore and Wright, 1997). For instance, when drug treatment programmes are implemented in a prison setting, they are often regarded as being of secondary importance to the discipline and order involved in running the prison (Craig, 2004; McIntosh and Saville, 2006). As a result, such programmes often face restrictions limiting the services provided (Kolind et al., 2013). But pragmatic adjustment of prison policy may also reverse control as when prison officers turn a blind eye to inmates' use of cannabis, as too rigid a deployment of control measures could generate conflict (Kolind, 2015a). In this chapter, we do not have the space to elaborate on the consequences of such a 'policy in practice' perspective for the framing and reframing of policy representations. However, it is important to be aware that prisoners' reframings are cast within the policy translations of prison staff.

Reframing the drug-involved prisoner as 'criminal'

As already argued, a 'tough on drugs' policy prevails in many prisons worldwide. In practice, such policy consists of, for example, mandatory drug testing, intensive cell searches and different kinds of punishments (e.g. fines, restrictions on leave, additional days, etc.). The goal of this policy is to stop prisoners from using or selling drugs and, at times, it is also argued as being part of a strategy to moti-vate/force prisoners into entering drug treatment programmes. While this policy may work at times, it often also has unintended consequences.

Firstly, it can be argued that the strict security and control measures imple-mented in prisons as a part of framing drug use as a crime 'problem' foster the development of low trust and highly controlled environments. In this way, they exacerbate the 'pains of imprisonment' (Sykes, 1958) experienced by prisoners, including loss of privacy, deprivation of personal autonomy, denial of social rela-tionships, boredom and violence. As research has documented, a commonly used strategy by many prisoners to cope with such 'pains' is to engage in drug use as a form of self-medication. At times, prisoners start to use drugs in prison while oth-ers continue or enlarge their repertoire of drug use after being imprisoned (Strang et al., 2006; Stover and Weilandt, 2007; Indig et al., 2010). Prisoners prefer using heroin or cannabis due to their sedative and calming effects in order to relieve stress, to facilitate sleep and ultimately to relieve the pains of imprisonment (Boys et al., 2002; Ritter et al., 2013; Kolind, 2015a). Interestingly, studies also show that officers sometimes tolerate or turn a blind eye to inmates' cannabis use as this tends to help keep inmates calm and quiet and make their work in keeping order on the wings easier, but also because officers recognise that cannabis use helps inmates cope with prison life (see also Duke, 2003; Carlin, 2005; Kolind, 2015b).

Another unintended consequence of the framing of drug 'problems' as crime in prisons relates to the prison drug economy. While a strict controlling and sanc-tioning prison drug policy does not in itself create the drug markets in prisons, it seems reasonable to suggest that prisoners react strategically to and exploit such policy initiatives for their own benefit. For instance, some prisoners gain economically in engaging with drug selling and smuggling in a highly controlled environment. Moreover, not only do they profit economically, they also reframe or reinterpret the intentions of the policy and exploit it in order to create prestig-ious social identities. There are limited studies of drug supply and drug dealing in prisons (however, see Munson et al., 1973; Crewe, 2005, 2006; Mjåland, 2014a; Tompkins, 2016). Crewe's long-term fieldwork on drug dealing in a British prison shows that although the financial power of drugs is important, drug dealing in prisons must be understood as more than simply an economic activity. Drug sell-ing is also strongly bound up with masculinity, self-identity, emotions and internal hierarchies. Drug dealing can enhance the dealers' status and symbolic capital, for instance, by being able to bring drugs into prisons, making connections to outside drug and criminal networks and displaying courage. Moreover, engaging in the prison drug economy can add to the feeling among inmates that they are part of a larger social group (Crewe, 2005, 2006). In addition, drug trafficking can also carry subversive meanings for prisoners in a highly controlled and stigmatised environment. As Mjåland shows from a Norwegian prison, diversion of medi-cine (buprenorphine) is an example of a relatively small and seemingly trivial, rule-violating behaviour but adds to a feeling of collective resistance among pris-oners. Moreover, only rarely did Mjåland encounter more confrontational pro-tests among the prisoners (Mjåland, 2015). Furthermore, drug use and selling in prisons and also drug treatment appear to be linked to ethnic identifications. That is, although ethnic stereotypes are imported into prisons, they become highly intensified in this space because of how drug dealing and selling are organised and articulated inside. For instance, in our study we found that Danish prisoners spending time in a treatment wing were often viewed as 'soft' and' weak' by prisoners with ethnic minority backgrounds in regular wings, whereas these prisoners in regular wings were in turn perceived as troublemakers and chaotic by the ethnic Danish prisoners in drug treatment (Haller and Kolind, 2018). In short, the display of, for instance, a prestigious masculinity, street capital (Sandberg, 2008) and an entrepreneurial approach related to drug selling in prisons is on a daily basis negotiated along ethnic lines (Haller and Kolind, 2018). In sum, drug dealing and drug taking play central roles in the forming of important social and personal identities in the prison. However, the illegal prison drug economy is not always violent and focused on individual gain. As Mjåland (2014a) has demonstrated from a Norwegian prison, a culture of drug sharing may also be central among prisoners. However, even in such instances, we see how prisoners reframe or reinterpret the framing of them as 'criminal'. In this way, policy framings are never neutral; rather, they have consequences for the way people understand themselves and the way they act in order to counter or reframe the social identities inherent in the wider policy frames in which they are subjected.

Reframing the drug-using prisoner as in need of treatment

The framing in contemporary prison drug policy of prisoners as not only criminal but also as legitimate recipients of health services also has consequences for the prisoners in their daily lives. As part of the public health framing, we find prison-based drug treatment programmes – both medically assisted (substitutes, e.g. methadone or buprenorphine) and/or social pedagogical/psychosocial drug treatment services. In this section, such programmes will serve as the case for understanding processes of reframing of health services as seen from the perspectives of the prisoners.

Although drug treatment programmes have increased in many prisons and are recommended by the WHO (2014) and European Monitoring Centre on Drugs and Drug Addiction (2012), they are still lacking in many countries (EMCDDA, 2012, pp. 20–6). Moreover, prison-based drug treatment programmes have to adapt to what is still seen as the prisons' primary goal: control and security (see, for example Walker et al., 2018). In this way, the programmes become subjected to the framing of prisoners as criminal. Nevertheless, with the introduction of prison drug treatment programmes over the last 30 years, a 'new' framing of prisoners has developed. As Donohue and Moore (2009) argue, with the growth in prison drug treatment programmes, the traditional 'inmate' or the 'offender' now increasingly coexists with the 'client': a consumer of welfare services who requires therapeutic attention. In this view, prisoners are not only to be punished and controlled, they also increasingly have individual rights and should be seen as the recipients of health services in line with other citizens. This shift in framing is particular to Western liberal progressive societies and coincides with the growing narratives of consumerism and managerialism in recent Western political thought and practice (see also Moore, 2007). For prisoners, this alternative framing, focusing on them not only as criminals but also as 'consumers', offers new opportunities. However, this framing also makes new demands on the prisoner. The 'client' that has emerged in prison drug policy and practice has to be motivated to take responsibility for his/her own treatment and recovery. Clients are seen as rational individuals who actively choose and self-reflectively engage with their own recovery. This also means that those who cannot honour these demands (for instance, the most severely affected and marginalised prisoners who often are more in need of care than treatment) are often left to themselves or left to an intensified criminalisation (Kolind, 2017; see also Bjerge and Nielsen, 2014). This is because prisons often operate a dual policy: either prisoners are categorised as a motivated and responsibilised prisoner in treatment or categorised as a criminal, irredeemable and face intensified sanctions (Haller, 2015). Moreover, as Donahue and Moore (2009, p. 329) argue:

> The notion that people in conflict with the law have choice or empowerment or agency afforded to them by the State is perhaps one of the greatest (if not most effective) mythologies of contemporary punishment. Framing people in conflict with the law thusly, however, is an extremely effective governing strategy that all but erases the potential for resistance or alternate thinking on the part of so-called clients.

However, it could be argued that this is an exaggeration and 'alternate' thinking or practices can exist. A study of prisoners' experiences with drug treatment programmes in Denmark (Frank et al., 2015) shows that even though some prisoners do buy into the ideology of the programmes (i.e. seeing themselves as active clients who with the help of the counsellors (re)discover their real selves and recover), alternative strategies and reframing also exist. For some of the clients, the treatment programmes were actively used in order to try to reduce or overcome their drug misuse, but also to better individuals' lives both inside and outside the prisons. In short, these prisoners at times actively embraced the framing of them as 'clients' in need of treatment to take on a new direction in life. At the same time however, most prisoners also had a somewhat pragmatic stance to the programmes. For instance, as positive urine tests resulted in fines and deprivation of weekend leaves, some prisoners engaged positively with the treatment ideology of (re)discovering their authentic inner core and they did stay drug free for a period of time. However, several prisoners also admitted that within two to three weeks before their release, they would go back to using drugs, as the prison sanction (i.e. deprivation of weekend leaves) would not matter much because the prisoners would be so close to their release dates. The framing of them as 'recovering clients', in this way, was useful for a time.

For other prisoners, neither abstinence nor the wish to recover was their key motive for entering the drug treatment programme. Some prisoners started in treatment and displayed overt positive motivation because this would make it easier for them to obtain favourable reports and, consequently, be transferred to an open prison: a strategy that in many ways interfaces well with the Danish national drug action plan and its principle of 'something-for-something' (Regeringen, 2003) or if you behave well, you are rewarded. For other prisoners, it was the brutal side of prison life that motivated them to start drug treatment. A good part of prison life is characterised by violence, threats, fights and drug debts (Crewe, 2005). By moving to a safer dedicated treatment wing and engaging in treatment, some prisoners tried to escape the more violent regular wings. This is not to say that they did not in time become positively involved in the treatment programme, but it is an example of how the framing of the client and the practices that follow are also used strategically by prisoners.

At this point, one might consider Carr's (2011) analysis of script flipping among female drug users in a drug treatment programme in the United States. It is a practice characterised by borrowing the language of the powerful (for instance, by acting like a recovering and motivated 'client') and then skilfully redirecting its political force. That is, by skilfully performing prescribed ways of speaking, the women could, for instance, obtain shelter, food or even regain/maintain custody of their children (Carr, 2011, p. 222). In sum, it appears that prisoners' motives for entering prison drug treatment programmes are related to both the prisoners' actual drug problems *and* factors related to serving prison sentences (see Williams et al., 2008; Kaskela and Tourunen, 2018). One can argue that starting in drug treatment programmes for some prisoners is a 'survival strategy' alleviating the pains of imprisonment (Kolind et al., 2013); prisoners 'play the game' (Schwaebe, 2003) or 'tell them [treatment staff] what they want to hear' (Patenaude, 2005).

This section has provided examples of how prisoners reframe the institutional identities and categorisations to which they are subjected as a consequence of the framings in policy and practice. At times, they resist these framings. Often, however, they redirect, deflect, strategically 'play the game' or 'flip the script' and pragmatically adjust to the framings in order to better survive imprisonment. More to the point, prisoners' reframing practices are complex. It is not that they either submit to the policy frames and just play out the identities which these frames outline or that they resist and develop alternative and more authentic identifications. Rather, as we have already demonstrated, prisoners alternate between the different frames available depending on what is most opportune and feasible. In addition, they at times resist, adjust or pragmatically exploit the frames within the constraints of the prison space.

The section focuses mainly on individual adaptations to the environment. According to Crewe (2009), the lack of collective resistance among prisoners in contemporary prisons is largely due to the ways in which sentencing is increasingly individualised: incentive schemes, progression in sentencing and individualised discretionary arrangements (see also Mjåland, 2015, p. 782). However, it should be noted that resistance also comes from organised user groups in the form of more coherent policy consultations, proposals and critiques. The UK NGO User Voice is an example of this collective resistance. They conduct consultations and research led by former service users. For example, in a recent report, they found that young people in secure settings and youth custody in Britain used drugs mainly in order to deal with grief and anger. Moreover, they found that a majority of the young people had no trust in the professionals involved in their care. These results have been used by User Voice to call for action and improvements to service provision for young people (User Voice, 2018).

Conclusion

We have illustrated some of the intricate interplay between policy framings and prisoners' reframing. We have argued that prisoners pragmatically adjust to, exploit, resist but also subvert the policy frames. In this way, prisoners should not be seen as passive recipients of policy framings and completely subjected to the powers of prison policy and practice. Rather, they are active agents reflecting on and acting within the circumstances they are placed in. Naturally, prisoners cannot resist the formidable powers of the prison and the robust policy framings at will. Prison drug policies set the agenda and parameters for the life prisoners can live, but counter-strategies, everyday pragmatics and ingenious evasions are also put into play. There is limited space to manoeuvre, but the room to manoeuvre and resist these framings are still present. On the other hand, we do not want to romanticise prisoners' counter-strategies. As we also argue in the following, the rigid policy framings may well contribute to creating prisons as dangerous places. Therefore, in order to analytically conceptualise prisoner's reframing, we suggest viewing prisoners' counter-practices in line with what de Certeau (1988) calls 'tactics'. Whereas 'strategies' refer to the institutional logic of the powerful, tactics are employed by those in weak positions. Tactics are subjected to the agenda and actions of the powerful and to the institutional and political logic on which such strategies draw (Desjarlais, 1997; see also Carr, 2011). But tactics are also often defensive and opportunistic. In other words, prisoners do practice some degree of reframing, but they do this from institutionally assigned positions set by the policy framings. To what extent such tactics have the potential to actually reframe and challenge the powerful policy framings is debatable. Nevertheless, tactics can work for prisoners as a way to 'survive' everyday prison life, adapt to rigid policy framings and to construct alternative identifications for prisoners in their daily prison life that might generate feelings of empowerment.

As Christie (1981) reminded us some decades ago, the intention of prisons is to inflict pain. Framing prisoners as 'criminals' legitimises practices that are intended to remind prisoners and the general population that people in prisons are secondary and deserve punishment. However, prison populations are also framed as in need of treatment, but only those prisoners who are seen as and can present themselves as in need and also willing to change. However, as demonstrated in this chapter, prisoners often pragmatically play or reframe the framing of them as either criminal *or* in need of treatment. Prisoners often move tactically or pragmatically between the different framings available depending on the situation. In our view, this is a predicament of the everyday life in total institutions – rules and framings are (re)worked (Goffman, 1961). As a consequence, if the framings from policy levels set too rigid an agenda, those prisoners who cannot comply with and display appropriate behaviour and positions (e.g. the framing of them as sick and in need of treatment), or those who cannot find their pragmatic way in the 'cracks' of the framings, they are only left with the framing of them as 'criminals' to adhere to. For instance, long-term drug-dependent prisoners who are severely affected socially and psychologically and not sufficiently skilled in 'playing the game' most often face disciplinary punishments. Often, they do not manage to stay in drug treatment (as they are discharged for using drugs) and often they are harassed and exploited by more powerful prisoners in the drug market (Crewe, 2005; Kolind et al., 2013). Prisons therefore may unintentionally become dangerous spaces or 'risk environments' (Rhodes, 2009) or spaces where a range of factors interact to increase the chances of drug-related harm occurring. As shown, prisoners often constitute a risk population with multiple problems: drug and alcohol problems, health problems, social problems, criminality and psychological problems. When this group of people are 'imported' into a prison setting with a detrimental inmate culture, an everyday existence characterised by a range of pains of imprisonment and rigid policy framings that favour the stronger and less affected population, then prisoners' problems may be amplified and we can talk about 'dangerous places': dangerous places that host, produce and reproduce problems. In line with this, Rein and Schon called for policy actors to consider how their own frames contribute to policy problems: 'if actors were willing and able to reflect on their frames, frame shifts – reframing – might occur, and problems that had seemed irresolvable might be resolved after all' (Van Hulst and Yanow, 2016, p. 96). In the case of prison drugs policy, there is a need for policy actors to consider and reflect on the predominant framings and their unintended consequences in further exacerbating existing problems and producing new problems.

References

Advisory Council on the Misuse of Drugs (ACMD). 2017. *Commissioning Impact on Drug Treatment: The Extent to Which Commissioning Structures, the Financial Environment and Wider Changes to Health and Social Welfare Impact on Drug Misuse Treatment and Recovery*. London: ACMD.

Babor, T., Caulkins, J., Edwards, G., Fischer, B., Foxcroft, D., Humphreys, K., Obot, I., Rehm, J., Reuter, P., Room, R., Rossow, I., and Strang, J. 2010. *Drug Policy and the Public Good*. Oxford: Oxford University Press.

Bjerge, B., and Nielsen, B. 2014. Empowered and self-managing users in methadone treatment? *European Journal of Social Work* 17 (1), pp. 74–87.

Boys, A., Farrell, M., Bebbington, P., Brugha, T., Coid, Jenkins, R., Lewis, G., Marsden, J., Meltzer, H., Singleton, N., and Taylor, C. 2002. Drug use and initiation in prison: Results from a national prison survey in England and Wales. *Addiction* 97, 1551–60.

Carlin, T. 2005. An exploration of prisoners' and prison staff's perception of the methadone maintenance programme in Mountjoy male prison, Dublin. *Drugs: Education, Prevention and Policy* 12, pp. 405–16.

Carr, E.S. 2011. *Scripting Addiction: The Politics of Therapeutic Talk and American Sobriety*. Princeton and Oxford: Princeton University Press.

Christie, N. 1981. *Pinens Begrensning (Limits to Pain)*. Oslo: Universitetsforlaget.

Craig, S.C. 2004. Rehabilitation versus control: An organizational theory of prison management. *The Prison Journal* 84 (4), pp. 92–114.

Crewe, B. 2005. Prisoner society in the era of hard drugs. *Punishment & Society* 7 (4), pp. 457–81.

Crewe, B. 2006. Prison drug dealing and the ethnographic lens. *The Howard Journal of Criminal Justice* 45 (4), pp. 347–68.

Crewe, B. 2009. *The Prisoner Society. Power, Adaptation, and Social Life in an English Prison*. Oxford: Oxford University Press.

Csete, J., Lines, R., and Jurgens, R. 2018. Drug use and prison: The challenge of making human rights protections a reality. In: Kinner, S.A., and Rich, J.D. (Eds.), *Drug Use in Prisoners: Epidemiology, Implications, and Policy Responses*. Oxford: Oxford University Press, pp. 175–84.

De Andrade, D. 2018. The drugs-crime nexus. In: Kinner, S.A., and Rich, J.D. (Eds.), *Drug Use in Prisoners: Epidemiology, Implications, and Policy Responses*. Oxford: Oxford University Press, pp. 1–16.

de Certeau, M. 1988. *The Practice of Everyday Life*. Berkeley: University of California Press.

Degenhardt, L., et al. 2014. The impact of opioid substitution therapy on mortality post-release from prison: Retrospective data linkage study. *Addiction* 109 (8), pp. 1306–17.

Desjarlais, R. 1997. *Shelter Blues: Sanity and Selfhood Among the Homeless*. Philadelphia: University of Pennsylvania Press.

Donahue, E., and Moore, D. 2009. When is an offender not an offender? Power, the client and shifting penal subjectivities. *Punishment & Society* 11 (3), pp. 319–36.

Duke, K. 2003. *Drugs, Prisons and Policy Making*. London: Palgrave Macmillan.

Duke, K. 2011. Reconceptualising harm reduction in prisons. In: Fraser, S., and Moore, D. (Eds.), *The Drug Effect: Health, Crime and Society*. Cambridge: Cambridge University Press, pp. 209–24.

Duke, K., and Kolind, T. 2017. The prison population and illegal drug use. In: Kolind, T., Thom, B., and Hunt, G. (Eds.), *The Sage Handbook of Drug and Alcohol Studies*. London: Sage.

EMCDDA. 2012. *Prisons and Drug Use in Europe: The Problem and Responses*. Luxembourg, European Monitoring Centre for Drugs and Drug Addiction.

Fox, K.J. 2001. Self-change and resistance in prison. In: Gubrium, J.F., and Holstein, J.A. (Eds.), *Institutional Selves*. New York: Oxford University Press, pp. 176–91.

Frank, V.A., et al. 2015. Inmates' perspectives on prison drug treatment: A qualitative study from three prisons in Denmark. *Probation Journal* 62 (2), pp. 156–71.

Garland, D. 2001. *The Culture of Control: Crime and Social Order in Contemporary Society*. Oxford: Oxford University Press.

Goffman, E. 1961. *Asylums. Essays on the Social Situation of Mental Patients and Other Inmates*. New York: Anchor Books.

Gubrium, J.F., and Holstein, J. 2001. *Institutional Selves – Troubled Identities in a Postmodern World*. Oxford: Oxford University Press.

Hacking, I. 1986. Making up people. In: Heller, T., Sosna, M., and Wellbery, D.E. (Eds.), *Reconstructing Individualism*. Stanford: Stanford University Press, pp. 222–36.

Haller, M.B. 2015. *Spaces of Possibility. The Contrasting Meanings of Regular and Treatment Wings in a Danish Prison.* PhD. Department of Psychology and Behavioral Sciences. Aarhus, Aarhus University, p. 260.

Haller, M.B., and Kolind, T. 2018. Space and ethnic identification in a Danish prison. *Punishment & Society* 20 (5), pp. 580–98.

HM Inspectorate of Prisons. 2015. *Changing Patterns of Substance Misuse in Adult Prisons and Service Responses: A Thematic Review by HM Inspectorate of Prisons.* London: HMIP.

Indig, D., Topp, L., Ross, B., Mamoon, H., Border, B., Kumar, S., and McNamara, M. 2010. *2009 NSW Inmate Health Survey: Key Findings Report.* Sydney: Justice Health.

Ismail, N., and deViggiani, N. 2018a. Challenges for prison governors and staff in implementing the healthy prisons agenda in English prisons. *Public Health* 162, pp. 91–7.

Ismail, N., and deViggiani, N. 2018b. How do policymakers interpret and implement the principle of equivalence with regard to prison health? A qualitative study among key policymakers in England. *Journal of Medical Ethics*, early online.

Järvinen, M., and Andersen, D. 2009. The making of the chronic addict. *Substance Use & Misuse* 44, pp. 865–85.

Jöhncke, S. 2009. Treatmentality and the governing of drug use. *Drugs and Alcohol Today* 9 (4), pp. 14–17.

Kaskela, T., and Tourunen, J. 2018. Facing drug problems and advancing sentence plan: Prisoners' perspectives on drug treatment programmes in Finland. *International Journal of Comparative and Applied Criminal Justice* 42 (2–3), pp. 195–213.

Kolind, T. 2015. Drugs and discretionary power in prisons: The officer's perspective. *International Journal of Drug Policy* 26 (9), pp. 799–807.

Kolind, T. 2017. Is prison drug treatment a welfare service? In: Smith, P.S., and Ugelvik, T. (Eds.), *Scandinavian Penal History, Culture and Prison Practice.* London: Palgrave Macmillan, pp. 205–24.

Kolind, T., et al. 2013. Prison-based drug treatment in Nordic political discourse: An elastic discursive construct. *European Journal of Criminology* 10 (6), pp. 659–74.

Kolind, T., et al. 2015. Officers and drug counsellors: New occupational identities in Nordic prisons. *British Journal of Criminology* 55 (2), pp. 303–20.

Larney, S., and Dolan, K. 2009. A literature review of international implementation of opioid substitution treatment in prisons: Equivalence of care? *European Addiction Research* 15 (2), pp. 107–12.

Lipsky, M. 1980. *Street-Level Bureaucracy. Dilemmas of the Individual in Public Services.* New York: Russell Sage Foundation.

MacGregor, S. 2017. *The Politics of Drugs: Perceptions, Power and Policies.* London: Palgrave Macmillan.

McIntosh, J., and Saville, E. 2006. The challenges associated with drug treatment in prison. *Probation Journal* 53 (3), pp. 230–47.

Melossi, D., and Pavarini, M. 1981. *The Prison and the Factory: The Origins of the Penitentiary System.* London: Palgrave Macmillan.

Michel, L., et al. 2015. Insufficient access to harm reduction measures in prisons in 5 countries (PRIDE Europe): A shared European public health concern. *BMC Public Health* 15 (1), p. 1093.

Mjåland, K. 2014a. 'A culture of sharing': Drug exchange in a Norwegian prison. *Punishment & Society* 16 (3), pp. 336–52.

Mjåland, K. 2015. The paradox of control: An ethnographic analysis of opiate maintenance treatment in a Norwegian prison. *International Journal of Drug Policy* 26, pp. 781–9.

Mold, A. 2018. Framing drug and alcohol use as a public health problem in Britain: Past and present. *Nordic Studies on Alcohol and Drugs* 35 (2), pp. 93–9.

Moore, D. 2007. *Criminal Artefacts: Governing Drugs and Drug Users*. Vancouver: UBC Press.

Munson, N., Rexed, I., Packard, R., and Blum, R. 1973. Prisons. In: Blum, R. (Ed.), *Drug Dealers: Taking Action*. San Francisco: Jossey-Bass, pp. 171–200.

Nielsen, B., and Kolind, T. 2016. Offender and/or client? Fuzzy institutional identities in prison-based drug treatment in Denmark. *Punishment & Society* 18 (2), pp. 131–50.

Patenaude, A. 2005. A qualitative exploration into a prison substance abuse treatment program: "I tell them what they want to hear". In: Sims, B. (Eds.), *Substance Abuse Treatment with Correctional Clients: Practical Implications for Institutional and Community Settings*. Binghamton, NY: Haworth Publishing, ch. 5, pp. 73–93.

Pratt, J. 2008. Scandinavian exceptionalism in an era of penal excess. Part I: The nature and roots of Scandinavian exceptionalism. *British Journal of Criminology* 48, pp. 119–37.

Presser, L. 2004. Violent offenders, moral selves: Constructing identities and accounts in the research interview. *Social Problems* 51 (1), pp. 82–101.

Ralphs, R., Williams, L., Askew, R., and Norton, A. 2017. Adding spice to the porridge: The development of a synthetic cannabinoid market in an English prison. *International Journal of Drug Policy* 40, pp. 57–69.

Regeringen [The Government]. 2003. *Kampen mod narko – handlingsplan mod narkotikamisbrug* [Fight Against Drugs – Action Plan on Drug Misuse]. Regeringen.

Rein, M., and Schon, D. 1993. Reframing policy discourse. In: Fischer, F., and Forester, J. (Eds.), *The Argumentative Turn in Policy Analysis and Planning*. London: UCL Press.

Rhodes, T. 2009. Risk environments and drug harms: A social science for harm reduction approach. *International Journal of Drug Policy* 20 (3), pp. 193–201.

Ritter, A., Hughes, C., and Hull, P. 2017. Drug policy. In: Kolind, T., Thom, B., and Hunt, G. (Eds.), *The Sage Handbook of Drug and Alcohol Studies*. London: Sage.

Ritter, C., Broers, B., and Elger, B.S. 2013. Cannabis use in a Swiss male prison: Qualitative study exploring detainees' and staffs' perspectives. *International Journal of Drug Policy* 24, pp. 573–8.

Rochefort, D.A., and Cobb, R.W. 1993. Problem definition, agenda access, and policy choice. *Policy Studies Journal* 21 (1), pp. 56–71.

Sandberg, S. 2008. Street capital: Ethnicity and violence on the streets of Oslo. *Theoretical Criminology* 12 (2), pp. 153–71.

Schwaebe, C. 2003. *Playing the Game: A Qualitative Study of Sex Offenders in a Prison-Based Treatment Program*. Cincinnati, OH: Union Institute and University.

Shore, C., and Wright, S. (Eds.) 1997. *Anthropology of Policy. Critical Perspectives on Governance and Power*. London: Routledge.

Sparks, J.R., and Bottoms, A.E. 1995. Legitimacy and order in prisons. *The British Journal of Sociology* 46 (1), pp. 45–62.

Stone, K. 2016. *The Global State of Harm Reduction 2016*. London: Harm Reduction International.

Stöver, H., and Hariga, F. 2016. Prison-based needle and syringe programmes (PNSP) – Still highly controversial after all these years. *Drugs: Education, Prevention and Policy* 23 (2), pp. 103–12.

Stöver, H., Hennebel, L.C., and Casselman, J. 2004. *Substitution Treatment in European Prisons: A Study of Policies and Practices of Substitution Treatment in 18 European Countries*. London: European Network of Drug Services in Prisons.

Stöver, H., and Weilandt, C. 2007. Drug use and drug services in prison. In: Moller, L., Stover, H., Jurgens, R., Gatherer, A., and Nikogosian, H. (Eds.), *Health in Prisons: A WHO Guide to the Essentials in Prison Health*. Copenhagen: WHO Regional Office for Europe pp. 85–111.

Strang, J., Gossop, M., Heuston, J., Green, J., Whitely, C., and Maden, A. 2006. Persistence of drug use during imprisonment: Relationship of drug type, recency of use, and severity of dependence to heroin, cocaine, and amphetamine in prison. *Addiction* 10 (8), pp. 1125–32.

Sturop-Toft, S., O'Moore, E.J., and Plugge, E.H. 2018. Looking behind bars: Emerging health issues for people in prisons. *British Medical Bulletin* 125, pp. 15–23.

Swann, R., and James, P. 1998. The effect of the prison environment upon prisoner drug taking. *The Howard Journal of Criminal Justice* 37 (3), pp. 252–65.

Sykes, G. 1958. *The Society of Captives: A Study of a Maximum Security Prison*. Princeton: Princeton University Press.

Tompkins, C. 2016. 'There's that many people selling it': Exploring the nature, organisation and maintenance of prison drug markets in England. *Drugs: Education, Prevention and Policy* 23 (2), pp. 144–53.

Ugelvik, T. 2011. *Fangens friheter. Makt og modstand i et norsk fengsel*. Oslo: Universitetsforlaget.

UNODC. 2009. *Principles of Drug Dependence Treatment: Discussion Paper*. New York: UNODC.

UNODC. 2013. *Contribution of the Executive Director of the United Nations Office on Drugs and Crime to the High-Level Review of the Implementation of the Political Declaration and Plan of Action on International Cooperation towards an Integrated and Balanced Strategy to Counter the World Drug Problem*. Vienna: UNODC.

UNODC. 2017a. *Roadmap for the Development of Prison-based Rehabilitation Programmes*. Vienna: UNODC.

UNODC. 2017b. *Doha Declaration: Prisoner Rehabilitation: Fostering Rehabilitation and Social Reintegration of Prisoners to Provide a New Chance at Life*. Available at: www.unodc.org/prisoner-rehabilitation.

UNODC. 2018. *Treatment and Care for People with Drug use Disorders in Contact with the Criminal Justice System: Alternatives to Conviction or Punishment*. Vienna: UNODC/WHO.

User Voice. 2016. *Spice: The Bird Killer*. Available at: www.uservoice.org/wp-content/uploads/2016/05/User-Voice-Spice-The-Bird-Killer-Report-Low-Res.pdf.

User Voice. 2018. *Nitty Drugs and Broken Trust*. Available at: www.uservoice.org/wp-content/uploads/2018/11/Young_spice_report_v12-screen-pages.pdf.

Van Hulst, M., and Yanow, D. 2016. From policy 'frames' to 'framing': Theorizing a more dynamic, political approach. *American Review of Public Administration* 46 (1), pp. 92–112.

Walker, S., Lancaster, K., Stoove, M., Higgs, P., and Wilson, M. 2018. "I Lost Me Visits": A critical examination of prison drug policy and its effects on connection to family for incarcerated young men with histories of injecting drug use. *Contemporary Drug Problems*, early online.

Watson, T.M. 2016. The elusive goal of drug-free prisons. *Substance Use & Misuse* 51 (1), pp. 91–103.

WHO. 2014. *Prisons and Health*. Copenhagen: WHO Regional Office for Europe.

WHO. 2015. *Prison and Health Fact Sheet*. Copenhagen: WHO Regional Office for Europe. Available at: www.euro.who.int/__data/assets/pdf_file/0020/250283/Fact-Sheet-Prison-and-Health-Eng.pdf?ua=1.

Williams, A., May, D., and Wood, P. 2008. The lesser of two evils? A qualitative study of offenders' preferences for prison compared to alternatives. *Probation and Parole, Current Issues* 6 (3), pp. 71–90.

Zurhold, H., and Stöver, H. 2016. Provision of harm reduction and drug treatment services in custodial settings – Findings from the European ACCESS study. *Drugs: Education, Prevention and Policy* 23 (2), pp. 127–34.

11 Deviant and dangerous

Queer adults, smoker-related stigma and tobacco de-normalisation

Emile Sanders, Tamar M.J. Antin and Geoffrey Hunt

Introduction

Due to our interest in the inequitable impacts of health policies, this chapter explores the experiences and perceptions of queer smokers and former smokers in California as they relate to a tobacco control strategy called 'de-normalisation'. Tobacco de-normalisation includes 'all the programs and actions undertaken to reinforce the fact that tobacco use is not a mainstream or normal activity in our society' (Lavack, 1999, p. 82) and has become a global tobacco control strategy.[1] Throughout the United States (and in other parts of the world as well), tobacco use – and especially smoking – has become significantly less socially acceptable and less prevalent over the past several decades, largely due to the de-normalisation of smoking through the regulation of consumption spaces, increased sales restrictions and taxes and media campaigns. Tobacco de-normalisation depends upon the creation and promotion of stigma as a means of changing societal norms so that smoking becomes undesirable, unacceptable, abnormal (California Department of Health Services, 1998; Bell et al., 2010; Ritchie et al., 2010) and therefore discouraged and reduced (Alamar and Glantz, 2006; Al-Delaimy et al., 2010). These efforts are designed to promote negative societal attitudes towards tobacco, tobacco companies and tobacco use (Chapman and Freeman, 2008; Malone et al., 2012), yet some of these efforts arguably also result in the stigmatisation of smokers themselves (Stuber et al., 2008; Bell et al., 2010; Voigt, 2013).

The state of California helped pioneer tobacco de-normalisation strategies and is considered a leader in US tobacco control because of its success in reducing the prevalence of tobacco use in the general population (Gilpin et al., 2004; Al-Delaimy et al., 2010). Californians purchase about half the number of cigarettes per person compared to national averages, and smoking prevalence in the state declined by nearly 40 per cent between 1990 and 2008 (Al-Delaimy et al., 2010, pp. 5–6). California has banned smoking in all government and private workplaces, childcare facilities and public schools; requires restrictions on smoking in all restaurants, bars, non-tribal gaming establishments, retail stores and recreational facilities and it was the second state to raise the minimum age of purchase to 21 (Truth Initiative, 2018). Furthermore, San Francisco and surrounding Bay

Area counties have their own additional restrictions and taxes, with some localities declaring themselves 'smoke free' and banning smoking in all public places including sidewalks and parks.

However, in California and much of the United States, certain groups of people – many of whom have been historically marginalised by institutional, political and social structures – continue to smoke at higher rates within this policy environment (CDC, 2018; Drope et al., 2018). These groups include people with mental health diagnoses (Warner, 2009), people experiencing homelessness (Baggett and Rigotti, 2010), people in socio-economically and/or educationally disadvantaged positions (Hill et al., 2014; Hefler and Chapman, 2015), some ethnic minorities (Jamal et al., 2014) and queer people (Bye et al., 2005; Gruskin et al., 2007; Cochran et al., 2013; Buchting et al., 2017), a group on whose experiences with tobacco use and regulation this chapter will focus.

This chapter is concerned with the ways that smoker-related stigma, a consequence of tobacco de-normalisation efforts, intersects with other forms of health-based stigma affecting queer bodies that have been historically constructed as pathological, risky and deviant within the dominant health establishment. To understand these intersections, we will present some of the findings from our analysis of 201 in-person interviews with queer adults living in California (primarily the San Francisco Bay Area), who have smoked at least 100 cigarettes in their lifetime.

A note on representation and terminology

Certainly not all people who identify as LGBTQ+ are equally impacted by the historical stigmatisation and marginalisation of non-heterosexual and gender-variant bodies, practices and identities. For many people, the relevance of pathological and criminal queerness is far in the past, many may be protected by their whiteness or their wealth and still others see their sexual and gendered behaviour as inconsequential: they are 'just like everyone else'. For some queer people, though, this legacy of pathology and the corrective force of medical authority applied to bodies like theirs persists; it continues to shape their lives, the meanings ascribed to those lives and the possibilities for a 'viable life' that those meanings create or foreclose (Butler, 2004, p. 2). This is especially true for many who are fat or defined as overweight, who struggle with mental health or have chronic illnesses or other disabilities, whose bodies are black or brown, who present their genders in ways that deviate from heteronormative, biomedical birth-assignments, who have non-monogamous relationships and/or kinky sex, whose freedom in health-related decision making is economically restricted and/or whose bodies are recognised as belonging to the highly scrutinised (medically and otherwise) realm of femininity. Writing about lesbian, gay, bisexual, transgender, queer, non-binary, genderqueer, genderfluid, gender non-conforming, transsexual, pansexual, demisexual, agender, intersex, asexual and other non-heterosexual and/or non-cisgender people as if they are one cohesive group is impossible – these groups are not the same, and the people within these groups are not the same. However, certain structural conditions – primarily sexual prejudice, heteronormativity and sexism (Herek, 2004) – do make these identities and the lives of people whose experiences and bodies can be labelled with these terms somewhat related, at least structurally, and often politically and personally as well. This is why we will refer largely to 'queer' people and 'queerness' – not only in reference to individuals who self-identify as 'queer' but also inclusive of people who use different labels in their self-identification outside of heterosexuality and cisgenderism. 'Queer' – which explicitly names a positionality structured in contradistinction to norma-tivity – underscores the elements of deviance, stigma, otherness and normative health that emerged from perspectives quoted and considered here in relation to smoking in a de-normalised tobacco control policy environment.

Methods

This analysis is based on the narratives of adults living in California who par-ticipated in an ethnographically informed study exploring their perceptions and experiences surrounding tobacco, stigma and identity. We conducted 2.5-hour open-ended interviews with both current and former smokers who qualified as 'sexual and gender minorities' based on participants' self-identification of their sexuality or gender as anything other than straight or cisgender. Participants were recruited on the street, through community-based organisations, social media and classified websites and by referral. Before being interviewed, participants were screened to determine eligibility and once eligible, they completed a close-ended questionnaire designed to collect basic demographic information, tobacco use frequencies and quantities and perceptions of multiple forms of stigma. In-depth interviews included questions about topics such as smoking and other tobacco use, perceptions of tobacco laws and policies, background information about participants' core intersectional identities and experiences with stigma and dis-crimination. To thank participants for their time, they received a $55 honorarium. All interviews were professionally transcribed and cleaned of information com-promising confidentiality. Participants were asked to create their own pseudo-nyms to be used for publication, and these are included in the identifiers attached to each quotation included in the following findings. All study procedures were approved by the Institutional Review Board of the Pacific Institute for Research and Evaluation.

The research team coded transcripts using ATLAS.ti, a qualitative data man-agement software, to process and organise the data into manageable, analytically meaningful segments. The substantial code list included codes such as agency, health, stress, identity, reasons for smoking, cigarettes, perceptions of policies and stigma. Once transcripts were coded, the lead author used a thematic approach to analysis to identify emergent themes from the narrative data (Bernard and Ryan, 2010; LeCompte and Schensul, 2013). Using this approach, we organised related quotation segments from participants' narratives into higher-order themes that established the foundation for depicting the relationships between smoking, health and queer identity (LeCompte and Schensul, 2013). The research team also conducted searches for disconfirming evidence, divergent patterns between interviews and contradictory or conflicting data within interviews to refine and refute our interpretations of the narratives (Antin et al., 2015).

Sample

Our study and its sample were not designed to be representative of California's queer populations. Instead, we sought inclusivity to identify a range of perspectives from California queer adults from which we could ultimately analyse in the aggregate to produce analytically generalisable theory (Bernard and Ryan, 2010). For this project, inclusivity may be defined by gender identity, sexual identity, racial identity, ethnicity, age and social class variation, differences in smoking trajectories, various perceptions of smoking-related stigma and diversity in beliefs related to the main topics of interest for the study.

Descriptive analysis of the brief closed-ended questionnaire illustrates the basic demographic characteristics of the sample and provides some contextualisation of participants' narratives by highlighting the range of experiences within this sample. Seventy per cent of participants indicated that they were a sexual minority only, 7 per cent indicated being only a gender minority and 23 per cent indicated both sexual and gender minority status. Participants varied in age from 19 to 65 years old, with an average age of 38.5, and 35 per cent were under 30 years old. A narrow majority (*n* = 62) of participants identified as 'White', 55 participants identified as 'Black or African American', 21 participants reported other ethnicities (i.e. Asian, Latinx, Native Hawaiian/Pacific Islander and American Indian/Alaskan Native) and 32 participants reported more than one racial or ethnic identity. Thirty-one participants chose not to answer the quantitative question on race and ethnicity. Economic disadvantage was prominent in our sample, with nearly 57 per cent (*n* = 114) of participants reporting yearly household incomes below $20,000 and only 9 per cent (*n* = 18) making $75,000 or more, which in the San Francisco Bay Area may suggest widespread economic disadvantage across the sample due to the high cost of living. Over 57 per cent of participants were unemployed at the time of the study. Twenty-four per cent of participants reported experiencing housing instability in the past 30 days, and notably, narrative data suggest that many more had experienced periods of homelessness at some point in their lives. These results, corroborated by the narrative data, suggest that the experiences and life conditions of the participants in this sample are also shaped by social and material disadvantages resulting from interlocking systems of oppression such as classism, racism, sexism and heterosexism (Collins, 1991; Crenshaw, 1991).

Findings

Narratives from this study indicate that anti-queer stereotypes concerning health are linked to the experience of smoker-related stigma for some participants. We will first demonstrate the connections participants made between the stigmatisation of smokers and of queer people, focusing on significant overlaps in the realm of health-based stigma. Next, we highlight the harmful, interrelated meanings of contamination and disgust that emerged from participant narratives as enfolded within the overlapping health-related stereotypes attached to smoking bodies and to queer bodies. Finally, we conclude with a more in-depth discussion of the implications of these findings within the context of tobacco de-normalisation policies.

Unhealthy smokers, unhealthy queers

In this section, we demonstrate some of the connections participants made between smoking, being perceived as unhealthy and being queer. While these connections are complicated, contested and manifold, we focus specifically on the role of normative notions of health to understand the influence of health-based stigma in participants' experiences of both queer stigma and smoker-related stigma.

The vast majority of participants were well aware of the ubiquitous and stigmatising societal and institutional perception of smokers as unhealthy people (Farrimond and Joffe, 2006; Chapman and Freeman, 2008; Ritchie et al., 2010; Roberts and Weeks, 2017). As Jane, a 19-year-old current smoker who identifies as a trans lesbian put it: 'like, obviously, cigarettes are bad for you'. Obsidian, a 46-year-old current smoker and cis woman who identifies as gay, pointed out structural aspects of smokers' perceived unhealthiness: 'A company won't hire you or they'll charge you more for your insurance, you know, if you smoke'. And Doc, a 20-year-old current smoker who identifies as genderqueer and asexual, underscored the connection between health and stigma even more explicitly: 'ever since people figured out that cigarettes are actually really bad for you, there's been a social stigma'.

However, participant narratives suggest that perceived unhealthiness is not just a source of stigma affecting smokers; it is also highly consequential in stigmatising sexual and gender variance. Deviance from sexual and/or gender norms is positioned within a long history of medicalisation that has served to erroneously and pejoratively associate queerness with poor health. Within this history, deviation from sexual and gender norms has become associated with meanings of disease, mental illness, genetic defects and risk behaviours that variously position queerness as both cause and effect of unhealthiness (Fausto-Sterling, 2000; McGann and Conrad, 2007; Eckhert, 2016; Valdiserri et al., 2018). Some participant narratives referred explicitly to this history in contextualising the stigma queer people (including queer smokers) face. For example, Cody, a 27-year-old current smoker and cis man who identifies as queer, noted how stigma is a particularly pressing issue facing queer communities. He specifically invoked the legacy and lasting impact of the early AIDS epidemic, citing

the perception that AIDS is like a gay male disease, and the long term association that it has had with some kind of moral failing, or moral weakness or character insufficiency. I think that stigma from the late '80s or early '90s continues its legacy.

Cody is not just explaining that the impact of this historically emergent, pathological stereotype (queerness as the origin of disease and disease as the origin of queerness) is ongoing but also, importantly for this analysis, he highlights the power of perceived unhealthiness to stigmatise people, primarily by conflating biomedically defined physiological health with moral and social worth. Though Cody isn't talking here about smoking, his perspective is significant for this analysis because tobacco de-normalisation depends upon and extends this same kind of conflation. Interpreting his specific example of health-based queer stigma within a larger context of normative constructions of health, Cody explains further:

> I think that there is a notion of what it means to be healthy. That there is like a quote unquote 'normal' state of being for the body, and anything outside of that norm is not healthy. . . . [L]ike larger people face this, that if being bigger is considered not normal or not healthy, then there's a lot of stigma around that, as like trying to explain what's wrong with this person. So I imagine that to the extent that LGBTQ is considered not normal, that could also be mapped as not healthy, if somebody holds that view of health, which is very common in our world.

Here Cody gets to the heart of what many critical health scholars argue are the often-obfuscated political and moral dimensions of health and medicine: health has become a powerful logic, language and set of practices through which what is 'wrong' with a body that is defined as 'not normal' (often that which is socially or politically undesirable) can be identified, explained and (in some cases) corrected (Lupton, 1995; Metzl and Kirkland, 2010; Bell et al., 2011). Critically, Cody explains that queerness isn't actually or inherently abnormal or unhealthy, but rather gets 'mapped' as such because it violates power-laden social norms. Working in the opposite direction but along very similar lines, tobacco de-normalisation also depends on the institutional power and social salience of this slippage between health, normativity and morality that Cody framed as particularly important in the construction of queer stigma. By explicitly seeking to make smoking socially unacceptable because it is unhealthy, social de-normalisation strategies may not only reinforce and play into the negative social meanings attached to perceived unhealthiness, they also potentially create a new source of health-based stigma that uniquely impacts queer smokers given this larger historical context.

Other participants didn't use the word 'health' at all but spoke about their perceptions of stereotypes associating queer people with *behaviours* that are framed variously in different contexts as deviant, risky and/or dangerous – things like smoking, drug use and certain sexual practices that in the epidemiological and public health arenas are considered 'health risk behaviors'. For example, Glamis, a 29-year-old current smoker and transgender woman who identifies as straight, perceived overlapping societal assumptions about the behaviours associated with smoking and with being queer. Responding to a question about how society views LGBTQ smokers, she explained that 'They feel like smoking is associated with drugs, sex and promiscuity, and that is how they view LGBTQ. So, they will probably perceive it [smoking and queerness] as going hand in hand'. Glamis perceives that drug use (including cigarettes), promiscuous sex (considered sexually deviant behaviour) and queer people (sexual and gender 'deviants') are all associated with each other from the perspective of the larger society. Non-heteronormative sexual and gender expressions, illicit or excessive drug use and – within the context of tobacco de-normalisation – smoking have all been implicated as forms of medicalised deviance (McGann and Conrad, 2007) in part due to their discursive positioning as dangerous threats to normative morality (Rozin and Singh, 1999; Bancroft, 2009; De Block and Adriaens, 2013).

Similarly, a 38-year-old current smoker who is a gay cis man, Crayola said that in addition to being regarded as 'dirty and dangerous', for queer people specifically smoking is perceived as

> just another vice that we've added to . . . our long list of vices that never *(laughs)* end, because there's the original vice and then, on top of it, *he smokes. On top of it*, you know, it's always *on top of it*. Whereas if it was a straight person, they would probably just say *oh, he just happens to smoke*, you know. . . . In the wider population . . . cigarette smokers are perceived as people who have no control over their addiction, have succumbed to [it]. There's a powerlessness to stop the behavior. Hence, a lot of them also perceive being gay is some sort of disease. So it's a continuum for them, you know. It's part of that inability to change behavior. That's how it's perceived.

Crayola's narrative illustrates how smoker-related stigma has added significance when the smoker in question is already illegitimately marked by deviance, disease and a fundamental lack of 'proper' control for other reasons. In other words, smoker-related stigma looks different on a queer body than a straight body because it does not stand in isolation but instead interacts with other existing and pervasive negative stereotypes ('on top of it') that, at least here, are related to the perception that queerness is equated with poor health ('gay is some sort of disease'). Within a de-normalisation-focused tobacco control policy environment, therefore, smoking while queer represents a particularly potent form of double deviancy, where smoking as a socially and structurally devalued sign of poor health places the weight of this putative 'moral failure' more heavily on the shoulders of those whose bodies have borne this burden before, an association not lost on our participants. That social de-normalisation strategies have unintended and inequitable impacts on queer smokers is not surprising; they're carving their messages into a palimpsest, not a clean slate.

Even participants who didn't frame smoker-related stigma as *exacerbating* queer stigma brought up the ways smoking can be perceived as *confirmation* of harmful stereotypes about queer people. Tabatha, a 27-year-old femme cis woman and current smoker who identifies as queer, at first seemed to doubt whether smoking was viewed with any unique significance when it was done by queer people:

> I don't really know per se that they're viewed – that the intersection of LGBTQ and smoker adds anything. . . . I think, people discriminate against both of those things. But, I think that if they're going to do something shitty, they were going to do something shitty anyway already. And that it's probably not intensified, aside from maybe confirming like, *Queer people are unhealthy*, or something, you know?

Tabatha frames both smokers and queer people as stigmatised (both potential targets of 'discrimination') but rejects the idea that smoker-related stigma is a source or aggravator of queer stigma, especially in actualising experiences of anti-queer harassment or discrimination. However, she does suggest that it is not just smoking that makes a queer smoker seem unhealthy but that poor health is already associated with queerness, and smoking can serve as 'confirmation' of this existing negative stereotype. Participants' worries that smoking would contribute to harmful narratives of queerness as unhealthy and self-destructive are balanced, albeit in politically charged and highly nuanced tension, with their experiences and perspectives indicating that smoking can also serve as a way to cope with and resist the harm experienced from structural conditions that have helped construct and reify these very narratives (Sanders et al., 2019).

Susan, a 23-year-old queer former smoker who identifies as genderfluid or as a woman depending on the context, expressed a similar perspective on queerness, health and normativity as that introduced by Cody, but she also explicitly situates smoking within these normative constructions of health. Susan brings up what she calls 'health agendas', or 'what we're supposed to do with our bodies', pointing out that 'smoking has never been on the list (*laughs*) of what we're supposed to do, or what is healthy. But so are a lot of things, (*laughs*) like being queer. That's also not on that list'. Punctuated by critical laughter, Susan's narrative indicates that from her perspective, the exclusion of certain forms of life (e.g. queer lives, her life) from the official 'list' of 'what is healthy' undermines the relevance of this list's other exclusions, priorities and authority over her consumption practices. Such overlapping exclusions from normative health agendas and mainstream priorities must be considered if we are to fully understand and attempt to mitigate the unintended consequences of tobacco de-normalisation's inequitable impact on queer people as a historically marginalised group of people facing multiple forms of structural disadvantage, including not least in health and medical institutions.

Physical contamination, moral contamination and disgust

The threat of contamination and its relationship to disgust were prominent themes to emerge when participants described their own experiences of stigmatisation.

For instance, after talking about both smoking and queerness being excluded from health agendas, Susan argued it is 'obviously not as bad as it was a few decades ago. But', she added:

> I don't think queer communities have forgotten. We still feel that, even people as young as me. We feel the paranoia and the stigma of our sex lives and our sexualities. . . . [As a pre-teen] I was feeling the kind of shame or this fear of contracting something. . . . I heard the things that people said about queer people being at risk of things or spreading things.

This expectation and fear about 'being at risk of things or spreading things' that Susan felt in shameful relation to her queerness bears a striking resemblance to the narratives participants shared about the general perception of cigarette smokers, especially in regard to spreading disease and harming 'innocent others' (Bayer and Colgrove, 2002; Larsen, 2010; Bell, 2014).

For example, Mac, a 31-year-old current smoker who is a bisexual cis woman, perceived that

> all smokers are viewed as bad. . . . [L]ike a harmful bad. Not like a predator, but like . . . *you're causing harm. You're harmful to this place*, like toxicness, like radioactive waves harmful. *Get away from us* harmful.

Mac's narrative suggests that smokers are perceived as an insidious threat to the environment at large ('harmful to this place'), including other bodies to which they are in proximity ('Get away from us'). She emphasises that smokers are not malevolently *trying* to harm others ('Not like a predator') but nevertheless pose a threat of contamination simply by their presence. This indictment of the smoker is in part due to the diffuse nature of smoke and its ability to transcend important social and physical boundaries, like those between bodies or between 'inside' and 'outside' (Bell, 2014; Dennis, 2016; Tan, 2016b). Moreover, the lack of control associated with the substance user through the medicalised discourse of addiction, where smokers are pathologised as addicts, also plays a part in framing smokers as not only deviant and sick but dangerously ruled by bodily impulses (Keane, 2002; Bancroft, 2009; Bell and Keane, 2012; Bell and Dennis, 2013). As Crayola's narrative in the preceding section illustrated, perceived lack of control is an important part of the stigma and pathology that both queer folks and smokers experience on a 'continuum' related to perceptions about their 'powerlessness to stop' and 'inability to change' behaviours considered socially unacceptable because they have been constructed as both deviant and dangerous.

As we have argued, themes of contamination and contagion emerged frequently when participants described experiences with smoker-related stigma, where the source of those experiences refers abstractly to a society-at-large. However, some participants' narratives emphasised how anti-tobacco messaging cultivated these meanings of contagion and contamination to promote a tobacco de-normalisation strategy. For example, Mike, a 35-year-old gay cis man and current smoker, remarked that

> [I]n the last 20 years, last 15 years, it's gotten harder and harder to really be a smoker. . . . It is just, we are demonized as polluters, poison, death dealers. . . . [W]e've been taught by marketing, by the Truth[2] and all these companies basically saying that, *Yeah. You are smoking poison. There are 6,000 chemicals in cigarettes. You get all these diseases. You are killing people.*

Though predicated upon and often making recourse to the physical health consequences of smoking (for the smoker and for others), anti-tobacco efforts frequently utilise graphic, shocking and/or visceral narratives and imagery intended to elicit disgust from viewers (Lacobucci, 2012; Keane, 2014; Haines-Saah et al., 2015; Lupton, 2015), as strong affective responses are understood to be instrumental in getting the public's attention (Gagnon et al., 2010; Lupton, 2015).

Disgust, which 'evokes repulsion and notions of dirtiness, contamination and decay' (Lupton, 2015, p. 12), was a common reaction participants perceived to their smoking. For instance, as Leroy, a 24-year-old former smoker and bisexual cis man, explicitly stated, 'The perception of your being disgusting comes with cigarette smoking'. He elaborated further on the logic that underlies this perception of smokers as 'disgusting', noting that others think

> That we have a lot of issues, I'm sure. That we are disgusting people, that we are about to die any time. We might get cancer. So, there must be something wrong with that person because he is smoking. . . . *Oh, you smoke. You're a bad person.* Or *you're just a grimy, dirty person. . . . [w]ith issues.*

Leroy's narrative suggests that smokers are considered disgusting because their bodies are perceived to be contaminated ('dirty', potentially/eventually diseased) and decaying ('about to die'). However, this supposed physical contamination is also considered evidence of a corrupted morality ('You're a bad person').[3] This is precisely the kind of social stigma that scholars warned would emerge from social tobacco de-normalisation strategies, which are designed to increase the social unacceptability of smoking in the name of improved health and to justify the increasingly strict regulation of smoking bodies.

For some participants, the anger, contempt and disgust with which others regard them for smoking could not be disentangled from the negative stereotypes and treatment they experience for their non-normatively positioned sexual and/or gender identities or expressions. Indeed, because queer people are 'already going against the norm', Leroy, for example, 'fe[lt] like maybe it's more of an intense thing when people look at that [queer people smoking . . .] *Not only do they smoke! Oh, but, he fucks dudes*'. Disgust reactions to the sexual and gender norm violations of queer sex, represented by the figure of a man 'fuck[ing] dudes', are perceived by Leroy as related to and potentially 'intens[ifying]' negative moral judgements about deviancy, transgression and 'improper' bodily comportment that also influence reactions to smokers as disgusting.

Similarly, Marisol, a 22-year-old cis woman who identifies as queer, described how the connection between disgust and smoking can serve to justify or motivate the physical and social exclusion of a non-dominant social group through the logic of contamination:

> [M]ost of society thinks that smoking is gross . . . and just really bad for your health and it's nasty and *why would you do that*. . . . [W]hen I think of my parents, they think smoking is gross, smokers are gross, but if they are queer or trans and they are smoking, then it's just perceived as like, *that is why you shouldn't hang out with them. They are a bad crowd* or *they are just bad people. They are bad influences*. It just adds on to the stereotype of queer people are bad people or unhealthy or social – what is the word? Like, they are excluded from society.

As other aforementioned narratives have also highlighted, perceived transgressions against important norms about health and contamination, such as smoking, are entangled with negative judgements about other practices considered deviant, such as men 'fuck[ing] dudes' (Leroy), 'promiscuous sex and drug use' (Glamis) and a 'long list of [other] vices' (Crayola). To Marisol's parents, social deviance in the form of smoking confirms the presence and contaminating 'bad influence' of social deviance and otherness in the form of sexual or gender norm transgression. Thus, deviance itself becomes regarded as a form of social contagion to be guarded against. Marisol explains how the ideas of disgust, contamination and social deviance relate not only to each other but also back to our earlier discussion wherein participants perceived smoking stigma to reinforce harmful and alienating stereotypes of queer people being unhealthy. That de-normalisation strategies purposefully invoke disgust, contamination and negative stereotypes about poor health to cultivate the social unacceptability of smoking for the purpose of manipulating individual health behaviours seems especially harmful to queer people in its structurally incompetent ignorance of the highly moralised, historical medicalisation of queerness (Bayer, 1981; Fausto-Sterling, 2000; Drescher, 2010; De Block and Adriaens, 2013; Eckhert, 2016) and widespread oppression and stigmatisation of queer people.

Discussion

The smoker-related stigma perceived by participants in this study supports existing literature on the specific stereotypes attached to smoking bodies (e.g. Farrimond and Joffe, 2006; Chapman and Freeman, 2008; Bell et al., 2010; Ritchie et al., 2010; Voigt, 2013). Researchers have argued that negative meanings of smoking centre around significations of 'dirt, pollution, addiction and disease' (Keane, 2014, p. 3) and that smokers are considered 'a perilous threat to the dominant socio-spatial order' (Tan, 2016a, p. 2) who are 'blamed if they' or those around them 'experience poor health' (Roberts and Weeks, 2017, p. 486). The smoking body has come to be viewed, treated and governed as a dangerous body, marked as a bearer of death and disease, of health risks and of poor health (Keane, 2002, 2014; Bancroft, 2009; Dennis, 2013, 2016; Mair, 2011; Bell and Dennis, 2013; Lewis and Russell, 2013; Tan, 2016a). The narratives of participants in this study further emphasised how these negative meanings and stereotypes about smokers were understood in the larger context of stereotypes about queer people, especially in relation to health and contamination, illustrating how smoker-related stigma is compounded for queer people who smoke.

Roberts and Weeks discuss smoker-related stigma – and the social de-normalisation policies which foster it – as a form of 'healthism' in which the association of smoking with poor health makes it such that smokers are socially and structurally 'devalued' because they are 'deemed unhealthy' (2017, p. 484). Similar effects of healthism have long been leveraged against queer people, and queer stigma is deeply embedded in the medicalisation of non-heteronormative bodies, desires and practices as pathological (Bayer, 1981; McGann and Conrad, 2007; Aguinaldo, 2008; Drescher, 2010; De Block and Adriaens, 2013; Eckhert, 2016). This historical legacy of power-laden pathology can be observed, for instance, in the classification of non-heteronormativity as disease and disorder (Bayer, 1981; Fausto-Sterling, 2000; Drescher, 2010; De Block and Adriaens, 2013), in the discursive construction of HIV/AIDS as a gay disease (Herek and Capitanio, 1999) and in the positioning of queer people as a high-risk minority group(s) in some public health efforts targeting certain behaviours or practices (e.g. substance use, sexual practices, food choice) understood to be 'irresponsible' or self-destructive (Lupton, 1995; Aguinaldo, 2008; Bell et al., 2011; Mair, 2011; McPhail and Bombak, 2015; Valdiserri et al., 2018).

The justification for tobacco de-normalisation efforts, and the stigma they engender, purposefully or not, centres around the health risks associated with tobacco use; that is, the dangers its use poses to not only the user but (and of increasing discursive importance) also those non-users who come into contact with tobacco and nicotine through second- and third-hand smoke (Keane, 2002, 2014; Bayer and Bachynski, 2013; Bell and Dennis, 2013; Bell, 2014; Dennis, 2016). As discussed earlier, smoking represents the threat of contamination within the smoker's own body and to the bodies of the proximate non-smoking public because of the way smoke itself and perceived addiction threaten the integrity of both bodily and social boundaries around health and control. In these ways, smoking has become framed as an environmental contagion that threatens non-users and society at large, and smokers (who are assumed to be or inevitably become addicts) are positioned as the dangerous, careless source of this threat and the health risks with which it is associated (Keane, 2002, 2014; Bancroft, 2009; Dennis, 2013, 2016; Tan, 2016a, 2016b).

Thus, smoking bodies are – within the context of tobacco de-normalisation – dangerous bodies (Dennis, 2016), and because of the predominance of addiction discourse as the medico-authoritative, rational explanation of all substance use (Keane, 2002; Bancroft, 2009), smokers are often only discursively legible to health professionals as pathologically at-risk and to society as immoral, risky, lacking willpower, driven by bodily urges and culpable for not only their own suffering but also the suffering of 'innocent' others. These discursive constructions of smoking bodies as dangerous, pathological, at-risk, and in need of regulation for the utilitarian sake of the general population's health (Bancroft, 2009; Bell et al., 2011; Dennis, 2013, 2016) mirror and intersect with constructions of queer bodies as risky, at-risk and in need of regulation and correction (Dwyer, 2012, 2014; Tan, 2016a; Valdiserri et al., 2018). The stigma now attached to smokers as dangerous, risky and deviant does not 'mark' all smoking bodies in the same way (Goffman, 1959, p. 3). While de-normalisation policies are arguably not intended to target queer populations, there are special and especially serious consequences to mobilising health-based stigma for groups of people whose very alterity to the status quo has been constructed, reconstructed and/or reified by the history of health sciences as power-laden disciplines. Participants' narratives highlight the ways that de-normalisation strategies may put queer and other medically marginalised people at compounded risk of experiencing harmful effects from stigma because of the ways that smoker-related stigma interacts with anti-queer stereotypes that are part of an ongoing legacy of health-based stigma. Given these findings, as well as research demonstrating the disproportionately high prevalence of smoking among queer people, de-normalisation is not just inequitable because it may be less effective for this population but may also be causing undue and inequitable harm.

We intend this chapter to demonstrate not how smoking is exceptionally 'bad' for queer people or how to make social de-normalisation more effective for a particular 'high risk' or 'health disparity' population. Rather, we intend both to demonstrate the ways in which *de-normalisation* may be particularly 'bad' for queer people and illustrate the extent to which health policies – especially those concerned with regulating consumption and individual behaviours – are socially and politically consequential in ways that can reproduce existing inequities and perpetuate harm for those already most endangered by power structures (Lupton, 1995; Race, 2009; Warner, 2009; Bell et al., 2010; Metzl and Kirkland, 2010; Voigt, 2010).

Acknowledgements

This research and preparation of this chapter were supported by grant #R01CA190238 (Antin, PI) from the National Cancer Institute (NCI) of the National Institutes of Health (NIH). The content is solely the responsibility of the authors and does not necessarily represent the official views of the NCI or NIH. Also, sincere appreciation is due to the 201 participants who willing gave their valuable time to this study. Without them, this research would not have been possible.

Notes

1 Though there are important distinctions to be made between 'social denormalisation' aimed at the behavior of individual smokers and 'industry denormalisation' targeting tobacco companies, a full account of these differences is beyond the scope of this chapter, and the former is our primary concern here (for more on these distinctions, see Lavack, 1999; Malone et al., 2012; Voigt, 2013).

2 'Truth' here refers to a prominent youth-focused anti-tobacco ad campaign that began in the late 1990s in Florida and was eventually expanded into a national campaign by the American Legacy Foundation, which is now the Truth Initiative (Truth Initiative, no date).
3 For more on the morally imbued social and cultural significance of contamination, as well as its relationship to disgust, see Douglas (1966), Haidt et al. (1997), Taylor (2007), and Lupton (2015).

References

Aguinaldo, J.P. 2008. The social construction of gay oppression as a determinant of gay men's health: "Homophobia is killing us". *Critical Public Health* 18 (1), pp. 87–96. doi:10.1080/09581590801958255.

Alamar, B., and Glantz, S.A. 2006. Effect of increased social unacceptability of cigarette smoking on reduction in cigarette consumption. *American Journal of Public Health* 96 (8), pp. 1359–63. doi:10.2105/AJPH.2005.069617.

Al-Delaimy, W., White, M., Mills, A., Pierce, J., Emory, K., Boman, M., Smith, J., and Edland, S. 2010. *Two Decades of the California Tobacco Control Program: California Tobacco Survey, 1990–2008*. Final Summary Report. La Jolla, CA: University of California, San Diego.

Antin, T.M.J., Constantine, N.A., and Hunt, G. 2015. Conflicting discourses in qualitative research: The search for divergent data within cases. *Field Methods* 27 (3), pp. 211–22. doi:10.1177/1525822X14549926.

Baggett, T.P., and Rigotti, N.A. 2010. Cigarette smoking and advice to quit in a national sample of homeless adults. *American Journal of Preventive Medicine* 39 (2), pp. 164–72. doi:10.1016/j.amepre.2010.03.024.

Bancroft, A. 2009. *Drugs, Intoxication, and Society*. Cambridge: Polity Press.

Bayer, R. 1981. *Homosexuality and American Psychiatry: The Politics of Diagnosis*. Princeton: University Press.

Bayer, R., and Bachynski, K.E. 2013. Banning smoking in parks and on beaches: Science, policy, and the politics of denormalization. *Health Affairs* 32 (7), pp. 1291–8. doi:10.1377/hlthaff.2012.1022.

Bayer, R., and Colgrove, J. 2002. Science, politics, and ideology in the campaign against environmental tobacco smoke. *American Journal of Public Health* 92 (6), pp. 949–54.

Bell, K. 2014. Science, policy and the rise of 'thirdhand smoke' as a public health issue. *Health, Risk & Society* 16 (2), pp. 154–70. doi:10.1080/13698575.2014.884214.

Bell, K., and Dennis, S. 2013. Towards a critical anthropology of smoking: Exploring the consequences of tobacco control. *Contemporary Drug Problems* 40 (1), pp. 3–19. doi:10.1177/009145091304000102.

Bell, K., and Keane, H. 2012. Nicotine control: E-cigarettes, smoking and addiction. *International Journal of Drug Policy* 23 (3), pp. 242–7. doi:10.1016/j.drugpo.2012.01.006.

Bell, K., McCullough, L., Salmon, A., and Bell, J. 2010. 'Every space is claimed': Smokers' experiences of tobacco denormalisation. *Sociology of Health & Illness* 32 (6), pp. 914–29. doi:10.1111/j.1467-9566.2010.01251.x.

Bell, K., Salmon, A., Bowers, M., Bell, J., and McCullough, L. 2010. Smoking, stigma and tobacco 'denormalization': Further reflections on the use of stigma as a public health tool. A commentary on Social Science & Medicine's Stigma, Prejudice, Discrimination and Health Special Issue (67: 3). *Social Science & Medicine* 70 (6), pp. 795–9. doi:10.1016/j.socscimed.2009.09.060.

Bell, K., Salmon, A., and McNaughton, D. 2011. Alcohol, tobacco, obesity and the new public health. *Critical Public Health* 21 (1), pp. 1–8. doi:10.1080/09581596.2010. 530642.

Bernard, H.R., and Ryan, G.W. 2010. *Analyzing Qualitative Data: Systematic Approaches*. Los Angeles: SAGE Publications Ltd.

Buchting, F.O., Emory, K.T., Scout, Kim, Y., Fagan, P., Vera, L.E., and Emery, S. 2017. Transgender use of cigarettes, cigars, and E-cigarettes in a national study. *American Journal of Preventive Medicine* 53 (1), pp. e1–e7. doi:10.1016/j.amepre.2016.11.022.

Butler, J. 2004. *Undoing Gender*. New York: Routledge.

Bye, L., Gruskin, E., Greenwood, G., Albright, V., and Krotki, K. 2005. *California Lesbians, Gays, Bisexuals, and Transgender (LGBT) Tobacco Use Survey – 2004*. Sacramento, CA: California Department of Health Services.

California Department of Health Services. 1998. *A Model for Change: The California Experience in Tobacco Control*. Sacramento, CA: California Department of Health Services, Tobacco Control Section.

CDC, US Office Smoking and Health. 2018. *Tobacco-Related Health Disparities, Smoking and Tobacco Use*. Available at: www.cdc.gov/tobacco/disparities/index.htm (Accessed October 30, 2018).

Chapman, S., and Freeman, B. 2008. Markers of the denormalisation of smoking and the tobacco industry. *Tobacco Control* 17 (1), pp. 25–31. doi:10.1136/tc.2007.021386.

Cochran, S.D., Bandiera, F.C., and Mays, V.M. 2013. Sexual orientation – related differences in tobacco use and secondhand smoke exposure among us adults aged 20 to 59 years: 2003–2010 National Health and Nutrition Examination Surveys. *American Journal of Public Health* 103 (10), pp. 1837–44. doi:10.2105/AJPH.2013.301423.

Collins, P.H. 1991. *Black Feminist Thought: Knowledge, Consciousness, and the Politics of Empowerment*, New York: Routledge.

Crenshaw, K. 1991. Mapping the margins: Intersectionality, identity politics, and violence against women of color. *Stanford Law Review* 43 (6), pp. 1241–99. doi:10.2307/1229039.

De Block, A., and Adriaens, P.R. 2013. Pathologizing sexual deviance: A history. *Journal of Sex Research* 50 (3–4), pp. 276–98. doi:10.1080/00224499.2012.738259.

Dennis, S. 2013. Researching smoking in the new smokefree: Good anthropological reasons for unsettling the public health grip. *Health Sociology Review* 22 (3), pp. 282–90. doi:10.5172/hesr.2013.22.3.282.

Dennis, S. 2016. *Smokefree: A Social, Moral and Political Atmosphere*. London: Bloomsbury.

Douglas, M. 1966. *Purity and Danger: An Analysis of Concepts of Pollution and Taboo*. New York: Praeger.

Drescher, J. 2010. Queer diagnoses: Parallels and contrasts in the history of homosexuality, gender variance, and the diagnostic and statistical manual. *Archives of Sexual Behavior* 39 (2), pp. 427–60. doi:10.1007/s10508-009-9531-5.

Drope, J., Liber, A., Cahn, Z., Stoklosa, M., Kennedy, R., Douglas, C., Henson, R., and Drope, J. 2018. Who's still smoking? Disparities in adult cigarette smoking prevalence in the United States. *CA: A Cancer Journal for Clinicians* 68 (2), pp. 106–15. doi:10.3322/caac.21444.

Dwyer, A. 2012. Policing visible sexual/gender diversity as a program of governance. *International Journal for Crime, Justice and Social Democracy* 1 (1), pp. 14–26. doi:10.5204/ijcjsd.v1i1.65.

Dwyer, A. 2014. 'We're not like these weird feather Boa-covered AIDS-spreading monsters': How LGBT young people and service providers think riskiness informs LGBT youth – police interactions. *Critical Criminology* 22 (1), pp. 65–79. doi:10.1007/ s10612-013-9226-z.

Eckhert, E. 2016. A case for the demedicalization of queer bodies. *The Yale Journal of Biology and Medicine* 89 (2), pp. 239–46.

Farrimond, H.R., and Joffe, H. 2006. Pollution, peril and poverty: A British study of the stigmatization of smokers. *Journal of Community & Applied Social Psychology* 16 (6), pp. 481–91. doi:10.1002/casp.896.

Fausto-Sterling, A. 2000. *Sexing the Body: Gender Politics and the Construction of Sexuality*. New York: Basic Books.

Gagnon, M., Jacob, J., and Holmes, D. 2010. Governing through (in)security: A critical analysis of a fear-based public health campaign. *Critical Public Health* 20 (2), pp. 245–56. doi:10.1080/09581590903314092.

Gilpin, E.A., Lee, L., and Pierce, J.P. 2004. Changes in population attitudes about where smoking should not be allowed: California versus the rest of the USA. *Tobacco Control* 13 (1), pp. 38–44. doi:10.1136/tc.2003.004739.

Goffman, E. 1959. *The Presentation of Self in Everyday Life*. New York: Doubleday Anchor Books.

Gruskin, E.P., Greenwood, G.L., Matevia, M., Pollack, L.M., and Bye, L.L. 2007. Disparities in smoking between the lesbian, gay, and bisexual population and the general population in California. *American Journal of Public Health* 97 (8), pp. 1496–502. doi:10.2105/ajph.2006.090258.

Haidt, J., Rozin, P., McCauley, C., and Imada, S. 1997. Body, psyche, and culture: The relationship between disgust and morality. *Psychology and Developing Societies* 9 (1), pp. 107–31. doi:10.1177/097133369700900105.

Haines-Saah, R.J., Bell, K., and Dennis, S. 2015. A qualitative content analysis of cigarette health warning labels in Australia, Canada, the United Kingdom, and the United States. *American Journal of Public Health* 105 (2), pp. e61–e69. doi:10.2105/ AJPH.2014.302362.

Hefler, M., and Chapman, S. 2015. Disadvantaged youth and smoking in mature tobacco control contexts: A systematic review and synthesis of qualitative research. *Tobacco Control* 24 (5), pp. 429–35. doi:10.1136/tobaccocontrol-2014-051756.

Herek, G.M. 2004. Beyond 'Homophobia': Thinking about sexual prejudice and stigma in the twenty-first century. *Sexuality Research & Social Policy* 1 (2), pp. 6–24. doi:10.1525/ srsp.2004.1.2.6.

Herek, G.M., and Capitanio, J.P. 1999. AIDS stigma and sexual prejudice. *American Behavioral Scientist* 42 (7), pp. 1130–47. doi:10.1177/00027642990420070006.

Hill, S., Amos, A., Clifford, D., and Platt, S. 2014. Impact of tobacco control interventions on socioeconomic inequalities in smoking: Review of the evidence. *Tobacco Control* 23 (e2), pp. e89–e97. doi:10.1136/tobaccocontrol-2013-051110.

Jamal, A., Agaku, I., O'Connor, E., King, B., Kenemer, J., and Neff, L. 2014. Current cigarette smoking among adults – United States, 2005–2013. *MMWR. Morbidity and Mortality Weekly Report* 63 (47), pp. 1108–12.

Keane, H. 2002. *What's Wrong with Addiction?* Victoria: Melbourne University Press.

Keane, H. 2014. Cigarettes are no longer sublime. *Australian Humanities Review* 57, pp. 1–20.

Lacobucci, G. 2012. New anti-smoking campaign adopts shock tactics. *BMJ* 345, p. e8697. doi:10.1136/bmj.e8697.

Larsen, L.T. 2010. Framing knowledge and innocent victims. Europe bans smoking in public places. *Critical Discourse Studies* 7 (1), pp. 1–17. doi:10.1080/17405900903453914.

Lavack, A.M. 1999. De-normalization of tobacco in Canada. *Social Marketing Quarterly* 5 (3), pp. 82–5. doi:10.1080/15245004.1999.9961068.

LeCompte, M.D., and Schensul, J.J. 2013. *Analysis & Interpretation of Ethnographic Data: A Mixed-Methods Approach* (2nd ed.). Lanham, MD: Altamira Press.

Lewis, S., and Russell, A. 2013. Young smokers' narratives: Public health, disadvantage and structural violence. *Sociology of Health & Illness* 35 (5), pp. 746–60. doi:10.1111/j.1467-9566.2012.01527.x.

Lupton, D. 1995. *The Imperative of Health: Public Health and the Regulated Body*. London: Sage Publications.

Lupton, D. 2015. The pedagogy of disgust: The ethical, moral and political implications of using disgust in public health campaigns. *Critical Public Health* 25 (1), pp. 4–14. doi:1 0.1080/09581596.2014.885115.

Mair, M. 2011. Deconstructing behavioural classifications: Tobacco control, 'professional vision' and the tobacco user as a site of governmental intervention. *Critical Public Health* 21 (2), pp. 129–40. doi:10.1080/09581596.2010.529423.

Malone, R.E., Grundy, Q., and Bero, L.A. 2012. Tobacco industry denormalisation as a tobacco control intervention: A review. *Tobacco Control* 21 (2), pp. 162–70. doi:10.1136/ tobaccocontrol-2011-050200.

McGann, P.J., and Conrad, P. 2007. Deviance, medicalization of, in *The Blackwell Encyclopedia of Sociology*. American Cancer Society. doi:10.1002/9781405165518.wbeosd049.

McPhail, D., and Bombak, A.E. 2015. Fat, queer and sick? A critical analysis of 'lesbian obesity' in public health discourse. *Critical Public Health* 25 (5), pp. 539–53. doi:10.10 80/09581596.2014.992391.

Metzl, J., and Kirkland, A. 2010. *Against Health: How Health Became the New Morality*. New York University Press. Available at: https://muse.jhu.edu/book/10595 (Accessed September 6, 2017).

Race, K. 2009. *Pleasure Consuming Medicine: The Queer Politics of Drugs*. Durham: Duke University Press.

Ritchie, D., Amos, A., and Martin, C. 2010. 'But it just has that sort of feel about it, a leper' – stigma, smoke-free legislation and public health. *Nicotine & Tobacco Research: Official Journal of the Society for Research on Nicotine and Tobacco* 12 (6), pp. 622–9. doi:10.1093/ntr/ntq058.

Roberts, J.L., and Weeks, E. 2017. Stigmatizing the unhealthy. *The Journal of Law, Medicine & Ethics* 45 (4), pp. 484–91. doi:10.1177/1073110517750582.

Rozin, P., and Singh, L. 1999. The moralization of cigarette smoking in the United States. *Journal of Consumer Psychology* 8 (3), pp. 321–37. doi:10.1207/ s15327663jcp0803_07.

Sanders, E., Antin, T., Hunt, G., and Young, M. 2019. Is smoking queer? Implications of California tobacco denormalization strategies for queer current and former smokers. *Deviant Behavior*, doi:10.1080/01639625.2019.1572095.

Stuber, J., Galea, S., and Link, B.G. 2008. Smoking and the emergence of a stigmatized social status. *Social Science & Medicine*. (Stigma, Prejudice, Discrimination and Health) 67 (3), pp. 420–30. doi:10.1016/j.socscimed.2008.03.010.

Tan, Q.H. 2016a. Feeling/filling closet smoking spaces: Negotiating public – private spheres, traversing emotional terrains. *Asian Geographer* 33 (1), pp. 1–21. doi:10.1080/ 10225706.2015.1137218.

Tan, Q.H. 2016b. Scent-orship and scent-iments on the scent-ual: The relational geographies of smoke/smell between smokers and non-smokers in Singapore. *The Senses and Society* 11 (2), pp. 177–98. doi:10.1080/17458927.2016.1190069.

Taylor, K. 2007. Disgust is a factor in extreme prejudice. *British Journal of Social Psychology* 46 (3), pp. 597–617. doi:10.1348/014466606X156546.

Truth Initiative. n.d. *About Us*. Available at: https://truthinitiative.org/about-us (Accessed October 30, 2018).

Truth Initiative. 2018. *Tobacco Use in California*. Available at: https://truthinitiative.org/tobacco-use-california (Accessed January 10, 2019).

Valdiserri, R., Holtgrave, D., Poteat, T., and Beyrer, C. 2018. Unraveling health disparities among sexual and gender minorities: A commentary on the persistent impact of stigma. *Journal of Homosexuality* 66 (1), pp. 571–89. doi:10.1080/00918369.2017.1422944.

Voigt, K. 2010. Smoking and social justice. *Public Health Ethics* 3 (2), pp. 91–106. doi:10.1093/phe/phq006.

Voigt, K. 2013. 'If You Smoke, You Stink.' Denormalisation strategies for the improvement of health-related behaviours: The case of tobacco. In: Strech, D., Hirschberg, I., and Marckmann, G. (Eds.), *Ethics in Public Health and Health Policy: Concepts, Methods, Case Studies*. Dordrecht: Springer Netherlands, pp. 47–61. doi:10.1007/978-94-007-6374-6_4.

Warner, J. 2009. Smoking, stigma and human rights in mental health: Going up in smoke? *Social Policy and Society* 8 (2), pp. 275–86. doi:10.1017/S1474746408004788.

12 Coming out of the closet

Risk management strategies of illegal cannabis growers

Gary R. Potter and Axel Klein

Introduction

The emergence and expansion of indoor cannabis cultivation has been one of the most significant changes to drug markets of recent decades (Decorte et al., 2011). Mirroring a trend reported in many industrialised countries, domestic production has replaced smuggling as the major source of cannabis in the UK. This process of import substitution has been accompanied by a democratisation of the cannabis market (Potter, 2010; Ancrum and Treadwell, 2017).

In media coverage and policy responses, the shift towards domestic production has been portrayed as harmful to society at large. Cannabis growers are seen primarily as profit-driven drug dealers involved in violence and other serious crime. Grow sites – often called cannabis factories or cannabis farms to emphasise both the technological sophistication and commercial intent of domestic cultivation – are linked to fires and flooding, electricity theft,[1] modern-day slavery and various other harms and nuisances. The product itself is considered dangerous – stronger than imported cannabis, linked to mental health problems and addiction and containing harmful chemicals used to maximise yield. In the public narrative, 'skunk' (the term used generically to refer to premium cannabis varieties grown in optimal conditions) is different to the imported cannabis of yesteryear: more dangerous and hence even more worthy of strict prohibitionist responses (Stevens, 2007).

Some of this narrative is legitimate. Links between serious crime and the upper levels of drug markets remain even as large-scale growing replaces importation at the top of the distribution pyramid. High demand and the risk premium associated with illegal commodities make for a lucrative market attractive to professional criminals. There is violence and people-trafficking. Petty crime and nuisance do blight neighbourhoods. Fires and floods occur. The potency and purity of domestically grown cannabis can make for a qualitatively different drug with implications for the health and well-being of consumers (Potter and Chatwin, 2012).

However, while large-scale cultivation may account for a significant share of the market, most cases of cannabis growing do not fit these media stereotypes or policy assumptions. Most growers operate on a small scale, in their own homes. Some of these still seek to make money but they are rarely involved in more serious criminality. Others supply cannabis only to friends on a not-for-profit basis or grow primarily or exclusively for themselves. Increasing numbers are involved in growing cannabis for medical rather than recreational use (Hakkarainen et al., 2015). Many growers, whether growing for medical or recreational consumption, regulate the potency of the cannabis they produce, are proud of the quality and purity of their product and escalate their criminal involvement from possession to cultivation precisely because they do not want to be supporting the 'real' criminals involved in drug dealing (Potter, 2010; Potter et al., 2015).

Regardless of reasons for growing or scale of operation, cannabis cultivation is illegal and growers risk prosecution. Alongside the threat of arrest is the risk of (other) criminals targeting the grower with theft, violence or coercion. For these reasons, cannabis growers seek to remain undetected by the police or those who may report their crimes. This includes hiding activities from family, friends and neighbours to protect both them and the grower from potentially dangerous 'guilty knowledge'. For a significant subset of growers, there is a secondary challenge – to dispel the stereotypes that they are bad people and that their activities are harmful to society.

This chapter explores the ways in which growers manage the risk of detection against the background discourse of cannabis growing as a harmful activity. Growers take practical steps to reduce the chance of being discovered and manage social relationships to reduce the likelihood that their activities are reported by people who do know about them. Many also engage in forms of activism aimed at changing the way their activities are perceived by society, promoting home-grown cannabis as undermining the 'real criminals' who profit from prohibition and reducing the harms associated with the illegal cannabis market.

Cannabis cultivation in the UK

Historically, nearly all the cannabis consumed in the UK has been imported. Most cannabis resin, and a minority of herbal cannabis, continues to originate overseas. Some home-growing of cannabis has likely occurred in the UK for as long as cannabis has been used in this country but the trend towards domestic production utilising more technically advanced methods began in earnest in the 1990s and accelerated in the early 2000s (Potter, 2010). In 1997, Independent Drug Monitoring Unit (IDMU) data showed 'a substantial increase in consumption of domestically-produced cannabis . . . at the expense of imported herbal cannabis [compared to 1994]' but noted that 'resin remains the most common form of the drug' (Atha et al., 1999, p. 2). They estimated that around 30 per cent of cannabis consumed in the UK in 1997 was grown here (p. 16). By 2012 this figure was over 80 per cent (Atha, 2012).

Official data show similar trends. From 1994 to 2000, resin made up around 70 per cent of all cannabis seized in England and Wales (Mwenda et al., 2005). By 2016–2017, herbal cannabis featured in 88 per cent of all cannabis-related drug seizures (Hargreaves and Smith, 2015). The number of seizures involving cannabis plants increased from under 2,000 in 2001 (Mulchandani et al., 2010) to 16,590 in 2011/2012 (ONS, 2018). The total number of cannabis plants seized peaked at over 750,000 in 2009/2010, more than double what it was three years previously (ONS, 2018). While both the number of seizures involving plants and the number of plants seized have declined since, they remain significantly higher than they were at the turn of the century. (The recent reduction likely reflects policing priorities rather than a decline in domestic cultivation; the decline in seizures cuts across all types of cannabis, not just plants.)

The explosion in domestic cannabis cultivation has been fuelled by advances in horticultural science and easy access to information and expertise via the Internet (Bouchard et al., 2011; Potter, 2010). Selective breeding to produce varieties with particularly desirable characteristics has been established for a while, but the spread of the use of indoor growing technology since the 1990s is noteworthy. In 1997, the IDMU reported that 43 per cent of growers in their survey were using 'pedigree' seeds while 70 per cent were only using natural light. Two decades later, 89.7 per cent of UK respondents in an international survey reported using artificial lights (Lenton et al., 2018).

These technologically advanced aspects of cannabis cultivation have contributed to the portrayal of skunk as dangerous. Of key concern is the relationship (often exaggerated in the media) between high-potency cannabis and mental health problems, including psychosis and schizophrenia (ACMD, 2008). Domestically cultivated cannabis has been specifically linked to an increased risk of such conditions (Di Forti et al., 2009) and a reported increase in cannabis addiction (Hall, 2009). Premium cannabis varieties grown in optimal conditions have significantly higher levels of THC and lower levels of CBD than 'traditional' herbal cannabis or cannabis resin (Potter et al., 2017). THC is the main active ingredient in cannabis. CBD, on the other hand, has anti-psychotic properties, offsetting some of the psychoactive effects of THC (Englund et al., 2014; Fakhoury, 2016). High levels of THC, and a higher ratio of THC to CBD, are potentially more harmful to consumers than lower potency strains produced under natural conditions (Morgan and Curran, 2008). It is concerns about the strength of home-grown cannabis and its potential effects on the mental health of users that underpin a decade of newspaper headlines from 'Deadly Skunk Floods City' (Bentham, 2007) to 'Children Aged Nine Damaged By Cannabis' (Borland, 2019).

Further health risks relate to the use of additives (fertilisers, pesticides and plant growth regulators, etc.) to improve yield. In the UK, 61 per cent of cannabis growers reported using chemicals of some kind in the growing process. Some commonly used additives are carcinogenic or have been linked to other health risks. Lack of regulation means that growers are poorly informed about exactly what they are adding to their plants and the effects these chemicals may have on cannabis consumers (Lenton et al., 2018). There are also reports of commercial growers adulterating harvested cannabis with substances including hairspray and glass beads to make it appear of a higher quality or weight (Knodt, 2017; Randerson, 2007; Pawlik and Mahler, 2011). Given the number of people using cannabis and the dominance of domestic cultivation, unregulated additives and adulterants are a potentially serious public health concern (Lenton et al., 2018).

Indoor cultivation methods are also associated with various environmental risks. Automated irrigation systems can cause flooding, and fires can result from the heat generated by grow-lights or from poorly wired electrical equipment or attempts to bypass electricity meters (Potter, 2011). UK local news media regularly report on cannabis farms discovered by emergency services responding to domestic floods or fires – often emphasising the danger to life and damage to neighbouring property. Meanwhile, up to £70 million of electricity is stolen each year to power cannabis farms (OFGEM, 2014).

Police concerns focus not just on cultivation as a criminal offence[2] but also on the links between 'commercial cultivation' (defined here as growing 25 or more plants or having a 'farm'-type set-up, in turn defined by technological sophistication or evidence of ongoing cultivation) and organised crime, violence (including murder; e.g. Surrey Live, 2009) and the supply of other drugs (NPCC, 2014). A serious concern is with victims of people trafficking – often children – being forced to work in cannabis farms[3] (Anti-Slavery International, 2014). The link with other types of crime is also recognised:

> The threat from the domestic commercial cultivation of cannabis in the UK is increasing. There has been an increase in robberies, burglaries and violence (including the use of firearms) linked to cannabis farms. There is an increase in small-scale grow sites. . . . There is evidence of 'taxing' (stealing) of crops and debt bondage being used to control local individuals.
>
> (ACPO, 2012)

Much of the cannabis grown in the UK is undoubtedly done so by 'professional' criminals. The police (ACPO, 2009), NGOs (Anti-Slavery International, 2014) and academic researchers (Savage and Silverstone, 2010) have all emphasised the involvement of Vietnamese OCGs. However, while such groups play a significant role, they do not dominate. The National Police Chiefs' Council (NPCC) report 'a decline in activity among South East Asian offenders and OCGs' with 'a new trend of cultivation sites being controlled by white British OCGs, which employ Vietnamese nationals who are forced to work in cultivation' (NPCC, 2014, p. 4). A rise in Albanian OCG involvement in commercial cannabis cultivation has also been observed (Anti-Slavery International, 2014).

Kirby and Peale describe a shift 'away from large-scale commercial cultivation, at times coordinated by Southeast Asian organized crime groups, to increased cultivation within residential premises by British citizens' (Kirby and Peale, 2015, p. 279). Police data show that white British men aged 25–34 are most commonly involved in commercial cultivation (NPCC, 2014). Ancrum and Treadwell (2017) highlight 'the usual suspects; enterprising, working class males', home-grown criminals motivated by money and willing to engage in whatever 'limited illicit opportunities around them'. Potter (2010, 2011) identifies different organisational approaches to profit-oriented growing including individual operations, partnerships, 'co-operative' and 'franchising' arrangements alongside 'corporate' criminal organisations. Potter's growers were also predominantly younger white men but people from different socio-economic backgrounds – and with differing levels of involvement in other crime – were found across all types.

Many growers are neither involved in other types of crime nor seeking to profit from growing cannabis (Potter et al., 2015). An early UK study identified those who grow only for their own use, those who engage in 'social supply' (i.e. providing cannabis for friends on a not-for-profit basis; see e.g. Potter, 2009) and 'social/commercial growers' (supplying their social networks 'at least in part to supplement their income') as well as 'commercial growers' (defined here as 'growing to make money, and selling to any potential customer') (Hough et al., 2003). Potter (2010) identifies similar categories of sole-use, non-profit and social-supply growers, emphasising the absence of any profit motivation for large numbers of cannabis growers. However, he also describes how some examples of these types progress to commercially oriented cultivation as they recognise – and embrace – the opportunity to make profit.

Both Hough et al. (2003) and Potter (2010) also include medical growers in their typologies – 'motivated mainly by the perceived therapeutic values of cannabis' (Hough et al., 2003, p. ix) and growing to supply themselves or others to treat medical conditions. It has been estimated that up to a million people in the UK could be using cannabis, illegally, for medical purposes (APPG, 2016). Regardless of whether cannabis does provide objective medical benefits in any given case, many thousands of users do believe that cannabis is an effective medicine for a range of different conditions (Hakkarainen et al., 2015). Although some growers may use medical necessity as a justification for what is essentially recreational cannabis use, research shows genuine differences in the profiles of growers who claim medical reasons compared to growers who do not (Hakkarainen et al., 2019). This sub-population of cannabis growers seems to have grown rapidly – or at least become more visible – in recent years, seemingly encouraged by the expanding scientific evidence for the efficacy of medical cannabis and the legalisation of medical cannabis in a number of countries around the world (Klein and Potter, 2018). Growing for medical use is not a legal defence in the UK – the crimes of cultivation, supply and possession remain the same (except in the very few cases where these activities have been licensed by the government). For most medical growers, criminal participation is motivated by desperation or altruism rather than financial reward.

Medical use is not the only motivation behind non-commercial cultivation. An online survey of smaller-scale growers found that 53 per cent of UK respondents reported growing 'to provide myself with cannabis for medical reasons' and 18 per cent reported growing 'to provide others with cannabis for medical reasons'. Other widely cited motives for home-growing relate to avoiding the harms associated with buying cannabis: many home-growers want to avoid both the super-strength, psychosis-inducing, chemically adulterated skunk *and* the criminal dealers that the media reports as dominating the illicit market. Intangible benefits also play a part with growers citing motives like 'pleasure' and 'because the plant is beautiful', but the two most important motivations were to provide 'cannabis for personal use' (93 per cent) and because growing is 'cheaper than buying cannabis' (84 per cent). Only 9 per cent indicated 'so I can sell it' as a motivation for growing (Potter et al., 2015).

It is impossible to know what proportion of growers are driven by different degrees of profit or are involved in other types of crime. While smaller-scale operations can still generate sizeable incomes (Potter, 2010) and larger operations do not necessarily imply other criminal involvement, both academic and police sources suggest the link to serious and organised crime is greater for larger-scale operations aimed at generating higher levels of profit. Applying the 80/20 rule (the 'Pareto principle') suggests that larger-scale commercial growers likely dominate the market in terms of total amount of cannabis produced but that smaller-scale growers exist in much larger numbers. This assumption gains some support from police data showing that 60 per cent of seizures of cannabis plants involved 10 plants or fewer (with 18 per cent involving a single plant) (ONS, 2018).

Some of these smaller growers do make money or are involved in other crime, but there is a clear discrepancy between the image conjured by the idea of commercial, criminal supply and the banal reality of home-based, small-scale production. However, regardless of motivation, scale of operation or other criminal involvement, all cannabis growers are engaged in an activity deemed a serious criminal offence under the law and portrayed in a predominantly negative light by the media. The offence of cultivation carries heavy penalties and although there is a presumption against imprisonment for small-scale, first-time offenders, lengthy sentences can follow where there is evidence of commercial intent or criminal organisation (Sentencing Council, 2012). In the public eye, the associations of skunk as a powerful drug, indoor cultivation as a dangerous activity and cannabis growers as serious criminals increase the stigma associated with growing – and the likelihood of witnesses informing the police. As became apparent during our research, growers also face the threat of victimisation from (other) criminals emboldened by the knowledge that growers – themselves criminals – may be unlikely to go to the police. Yet despite potentially severe sanctions, negative public perceptions and the threat of criminal victimisation, growing persists on a huge scale in the UK.

In the remainder of this chapter, we present data from interviews with cannabis growers in the UK. We describe the strategies used to stay under the radar of law enforcement and criminal groups, of managing social relationships and of countering the negative associations of cannabis growing encountered in the press – thus resisting the framing of themselves and their 'spaces' as 'dangerous'.

Methods

In order to get a better understanding of the diverse practices and cultures associated with cannabis cultivation in the UK, we conducted research with 48 active cannabis growers. We drew on participatory and action research traditions to help overcome the difficulties researching 'active offenders' who may otherwise be reluctant to discuss their illegal activities. We utilised an inductive, ethnographic approach with observations of real-life situations accompanying in-depth qualitative interviews. We worked from a loose interview schedule that ensured we covered certain core topics but allowed conversation to flow unhindered. By employing a qualitative, inductive research framework, we could follow the data as it emerged from the fieldwork and observe the phenomenon take shape.

In the actual research process, from the theoretical frame-setting through informant recruitment to the face-to-face interviewing, researcher and informant are building social capital that serves the interests of all parties and spans several registers. The recording of responses and observations are instrumental for data gathering but also for enacting the researcher's role and consolidating their scientific detachment. At the same time, the empathetic understanding for the informant's position creates a shared understanding of the individual situation and the broader social and political context. In this project, the researchers agreed with their informants that cannabis prohibition was a political fallacy and that it was the law that was wrong, not the grower.

This shared outlook was a prerequisite for establishing trust and getting access to informants. It also provided a situational presence from which conversation could flow back and forth. Informants were given time to expand on issues and to critically reflect on their own actions. With interviews lasting up to three hours, there was ample scope for elaboration, in-depth analysis and sometimes critical appraisal. For some informants the disclosure of sensitive information to a stranger can have a quasi-therapeutic quality. Without training or mandate to expand on this, the researchers did appreciate that their very interest and empathy helped informants to present the normalcy of their actions. Both the research process itself and the subsequent communication through publications and conference presentations are important for de-stigmatising cannabis cultivation and for constructing the cannabis grower as having a moral personhood despite the illegality of this practice.

Our research has then an 'action' dimension in so far as pressing home the case for lifting criminal sanctions and normalising domestic cannabis cultivation. On the one hand, we are hoping to humanise the growers themselves and demonstrate the roles played by opportunity and need. On the other hand, we also seek to expose some of the damage that is inflicted by prohibitionist cannabis policies and that apologists, including government spokespersons, tend to deny, ignore or trivialise.

Findings

With our recruitment process and the extra risk of serious penalties associated with their activities, we never expected to get many respondents who operated as part of OCGs, those involved in high levels of (other) serious crime or those involved in the most profitable levels of commercial cultivation. However, these types were not our target – such growers are the most associated with the cultivation-related harms portrayed in the media and underpinning policy and the most likely to be seen (by themselves and others) as rightful targets of the criminal justice system. Nevertheless, our sample covered a broad spectrum of growers including those growing for personal use, social supply and varying degrees of commercial intent. Many respondents did not fit neatly into any one category or had occupied different roles at different times (cf. Potter, 2010).

Twenty-two of our respondents admitted growing for commercial reasons at some point in their careers, with 12 describing experiences that suggested they had been involved with gangs or OCGs. Twenty-four respondents were mostly restricted to personal and social or social/commercial cultivation (cf. Hough et al., 2003) throughout their growing careers (few growers resist the urge to occasionally share their produce with friends – and most are happy to accept money or something else in return when recipients insist).

> Maria and her husband grow primarily to provide cannabis for their own use. She uses cannabis to manage her 'complex post-traumatic stress disorder, bipolar disorder and . . . psychosis' and he smokes to help with his depression. 'We need it to balance out those symptoms' she says, while also admitting to enjoying the non-medical benefits. Consuming over an ounce (28g) of cannabis a week between them, 'we were spending 140 quid a week on weed. . . . We wanted to be self-sufficient but for medical reasons as well as recreational'. Personal supply is their main motivation but if they have cannabis to spare after meeting their own requirements then 'I have a couple of people who you know, they'll come round. . . . I've got somebody who cuts my hair and they get three grams for cutting my hair, sort of got a barter system. If mates want an ounce it's 140 quid'.

Most of our respondents were primarily producing cannabis for recreational use but 21 were growing at least partly for medical purposes. The difference between medical and recreational use is not always clear-cut (Hakkarainen et al., 2019) – Maria used the term 'mecreational' to describe her and her husband's cultivation. We identified 16 respondents as having a primarily or exclusively medical narrative when we interviewed them (although some had been involved in cultivation for recreational use at earlier points in time), discussed in depth elsewhere (Klein and Potter, 2018).

Five of our respondents had previous involvement in commercial cultivation but were growing primarily for medical purposes when we interviewed them. Colin, for example, has over 20 years' experience of growing cannabis, was 'involved in crime related circles in [his] earlier days, but no more' and now grows only for medicinal use. Lee also had previous involvement in 'organised crime and the criminal milieu' but now grows cannabis for his sick wife and 'for reconstructing [his] spoiled self'. Dale, on the other hand, started growing to provide cannabis for his sick friend but reports that cultivation is now his main source of income.

Respondents included professionals, manual workers and the unemployed as well as students, retirees and those unable to work for health reasons. Ages ranged from those in their early 20s to senior citizens. The sample included 13 women, 8 of whom fitted a predominantly medical narrative and only one of whom was growing commercially (although three others reported previous involvement in or links to commercial cultivation). Our respondents were exclusively white British (with one Portuguese/British dual-national). Discussion of the reasons for and implications of the absence of BME representatives in our sample are beyond the scope of this chapter, but we acknowledge the limitations on generalising our findings beyond white British growers.

Most of our respondents grew indoors using a range of specialist equipment, although some preferred to grow in their gardens or greenhouses. Regardless of scale or technical set-up, all our growers were knowledgeable about the cannabis plant itself, the varieties they grew, their preferred growing conditions and how to harvest and prepare their crops. Many, particularly the medical growers, also demonstrated knowledge and expertise in more advanced processing of their produce – including the manufacture of more concentrated preparations of cannabis (e.g. resins, 'pollen' and 'shatter'), extracts and tinctures tailored to treating specific medical conditions and cannabis-based food and drink (cf. Klein and Potter, 2018).

Identifying threats

All our participants were aware of the threat of arrest and prosecution stemming from their involvement in growing. Cultivation even of a small number of plants for personal use carries heavier penalties under UK law than simple possession of cannabis. Growing on a larger scale or to supply other people is more serious again with an increased likelihood of a custodial sentence (Sentencing Council, 2012). Even those growing primarily for personal use often grew enough plants or employed cultivation methods to be considered 'commercial' under law enforcement definitions such as that set out by the NPCC (2014). Those involved in social or medical supply were generally aware that supply is a more serious offence and carries more severe penalties than possession regardless of motivation or whether the supplier receives financial gain. This extra risk is no deterrent to those who see their criminality as justified. As Emma, who supplies other medical users with a range of oils, capsules and other preparations she makes, says: 'Yes, I'm going to be bang to rights for supplying. I'm going to be done in every aspect. It scares me, of course'.

There is an irony here for those who cite avoiding contact with drug dealers or contributing to the criminal economy as reasons for their growing – they commit more serious crimes themselves in order to avoid supporting 'real' criminals. This situation is particularly poignant for those growing for medical purposes – caught between the debilitation of their health problems, an illicit drug market run by criminals and a legal environment that criminalises their own efforts to produce an effective medicine for themselves or others (Klein and Potter, 2018). However, those involved in overt commercial cultivation accepted that they were committing a more serious criminal offence, although many still took pains to point out how their own involvement in growing was substantively different from that of the stereotypical, organised-crime type growers.

Roger runs a sophisticated operation with two friends. Although they see themselves as connoisseurs and like to experiment with growing different varieties of cannabis to 'keep things interesting' profit is the central motivation and their set-up would fit most definitions of organised crime. Nevertheless, Roger and his mates see themselves as different from the 'real criminals' they see as dominating the UK cannabis market. 'Yes, I know there's a criminal element that comes with cannabis. There's money involved and of course, yes, they're going to be like that, but that's where I'd rather be involved with other people and seeing my kind of people where we're looking out for each other. We're just trying to be healthy and happy rather than being greedy and buying a new BMW or something.'

The risk of arrest and prosecution is real. Thirteen of our subjects discussed being arrested for cultivation-related activities, with three serving prison time (two of whom were commercial growers), two receiving suspended sentences (one commercial and one medical grower) and one more awaiting trial at time of interview (medical and commercial). But while the police are an obvious threat, they are neither the only nor the most serious risk to the illicit cannabis grower. For most growers, other criminals were feared more than the police. Almost everybody we spoke to had heard stories of growers falling victim to theft, violence or extortion as local gangs sought to take advantage of the fact that growers are themselves committing criminal offences and are therefore less likely to report their own victimisation to the police. Six of our respondents had personal experience of such crimes, with a similar number having first-hand knowledge of other growers' victimisation – including three cases where (female) partners of (male) growers had also been recipients of violence or threats of violence, one while heavily pregnant. Two of the victims we spoke to did go to the police – and both were prosecuted for cultivation because of this. The risks attached to contacting the police in cases where the growers have been the victims of crime are discussed further in the following section.

Managing risk

Like the police, criminals can only target growers when they know about their activities. For most growers, therefore, the primary defence against either law enforcement or other criminals is minimising the chance of their activities being discovered. While growing usually take place indoors with the plants and equipment hidden from sight, there are many aspects of cultivation that leave the grower vulnerable to detection. Growing takes place over an extended period (many weeks or months for a single crop, with most indoor growers tending to grow continuously or in recurring cycles) significantly increasing the opportunity for the crime to be detected compared to time-limited offences like thefts or violence – or individual acts of drug dealing. High-intensity grow-lamps can shine brightly through windows – with blacked-out windows also potentially arousing suspicion. Grow-lights in enclosed spaces also generate heat, with growers aware that the police have access to infrared cameras mounted on helicopters. Water pumps and fans can be noisy. High levels of electricity or water consumption at residential properties can lead to investigation by utility companies and referral to the police. Waste material from growing and suspicious activities such as night-time comings and goings (e.g. when passing cannabis on to customers or disposing of residual plant material after harvest) can be noted by neighbours and reported.

Growers employ various techniques to reduce the chance of detection. Carbon filters are used to minimise smell emanation and fans to control heat. Growers use cupboards and curtains to keep plants and lights out of sight – and some construct secret rooms in basements or roof spaces. Many of these techniques have been reported before (Potter, 2010, 2011) but we came across some new approaches. Most notably, the use of specialist 'grow-tents' was widespread. Legally available online or in hydroponic shops, grow-tents are designed to keep the light, heat and smell associated with cannabis cultivation under some control. On multiple occasions, we were surprised to be shown cannabis growing in tents – the familiar pungent smell of mature plants hits full-force once the tent is unzipped but had been undetectable while conducting interviews in adjacent rooms. Other approaches new to us included the use of infrared blocking plastic on windows and the selection of 'tall plants like sweetcorn and sunflowers to hide the cannabis plants . . . tobacco plants to mask the smell' (Jolly) by those growing outdoors.

Growers also seek to minimise the severity of sanctions if they are detected. These approaches are particularly important to those involved in commercial cultivation and include keeping equipment related to supply (e.g. scales, plastic bags or other materials used for packaging cannabis being sold to others, records of transactions) away from grow-sites and using lower-tech cultivation methods to mitigate claims of 'farming', professionalism or ongoing production. Another technique for commercial growers is to spread cultivation over multiple smaller sites so that if any one location gets discovered, there is less chance that the authorities will have evidence of the overall scale of operation. The spreading of cultivation over different properties – with different individuals overseeing each – also minimises the chances that a given site will be traced back to whoever is ultimately behind the growing. Again, these approaches are not new (Potter, 2010, 2011; NPCC, 2014; Kirby and Peale, 2015) but our research suggests they are more widespread than previous work has implied, and that such arrangements are not the preserve of gangs or OCGs.

Hugh is a successful English teacher who now runs his own small language school. He has been growing for many years to supplement his legitimate income but never been involved in any crime other than that related to cultivation, supply and use of cannabis (including revenue offences relating to his illegal income). He has helped 'dozens of others' set up their own growing operations for a share of the crop or profits in a franchising arrangement (Potter, 2010, 2011) but now finds it safer and easier, if 'a bit less lucrative', to operate as a 'consultant' – paid to advise on particular issues encountered by other growers.

Another innovation aimed at lessening the likely severity of punishment if the grower were to be caught came from another long-term commercial grower. Mark described the use of 'sacrificial plants', easy for the police (or criminals) to find should they raid and intended to distract them from looking for the larger-scale operation hidden behind the intricately constructed secret wall in the cellar. Having been arrested before, and previously threatened by criminal gangs, Mark argues that it is better to 'let them find something' if they do come to the house expecting to catch him growing. The easy-to-find plants would explain smells and other evidence of cultivation, hopefully satisfying the curiosity of the police, but should not be enough to result in a prison sentence even if the police deemed the find worthy of prosecution. 'Sacrificial crops' have been reported elsewhere in the context of large-scale outdoor cultivation but not previously encountered in the context of indoor production in the UK (Potter, 2011).

The risk of detection goes beyond the grow-site itself. Many growers were wary of being identified through purchasing equipment and nutrients from grow shops. Some expressed a preference for using cash rather than credit cards (although as Maria said, 'it must have looked very dodgy, us bringing 1200 quid into a grow shop in cash') and about avoiding discussing cannabis explicitly in conversations with shop staff (cf. Potter, 2011). Another concern expressed was with criminals monitoring grow shop customers and tracking them back to their premises. (Maria again: 'You watch out to make sure you're not being followed out the carpark by cars because that's actually one of the biggest indicators that somebody will use that you're growing and I have heard of trackers being put on cars'.)

Growers also seek to control who else knows about their cultivation. Neighbours, passers-by and doorstep callers can become witnesses who might report cultivation directly or become a source of gossip leading to the police, criminals or others becoming aware; the situational techniques described previously also mitigate these indirect threats. Visitors with an expectation of coming into the home (e.g. landlords, utility meter readers, carers) are more of a problem, and even friends and family need to be treated cautiously. Growers in family situations must also manage home life, hiding the grow room from young children and trying to ensure silence from older children and other family members. The problem here is not just that children may talk, increasing the chance of police action (or victimisation by criminals). Children also need to be protected. Parents do not want their children (at least when they are young) consuming their cannabis or harming themselves (or the cannabis plants) by coming into direct contact with the cultivation set-up. A further concern is that growing in the family home could lead to increased sentences or the involvement of social services (with the ultimate threat of having children taken into care) should it come to the attention of the authorities.

All this secrecy can cause problems in the personal and domestic spheres. Growers report persistent anxiety over the threats of law enforcement activity or being targeted by other criminals. This anxiety can be very intense at times and permeates into all areas of daily life. Maria tells us about when she is 'really,

really afraid and the walls are red hot and the helicopter is flying overhead and it's 37 degrees in the bloody tent' and how

> 'it does affect your relationships, it affects the fact that if one of my friends really upsets me and they know what we're doing, that causes an imbalance in the friendship . . . because there's always that risk that you could fall out with somebody and they just think well you know, sod it I'll ring the police on you.'

Interpersonal relationships can be negatively affected not just when friends and family are party to guilty knowledge but also when growers find themselves keeping secrets from loved ones. Sometimes other growers come to be more trusted than family and friends. Those who have been arrested or victimised talk about the trauma, often with long-lasting effect, of those experiences.

Responses to the threat or reality of being targeted by other criminals brings the grower's precarious legal position – and self-perception – to the fore. Some respond with counter-threats or criminal activity of their own, demonstrating a degree of acceptance that they are part of the criminal community against which they also stand in opposition.

> Harriet grows to supplement her income as a cleaner, selling small amounts to friends and the remainder to a dealer she has known for years – after keeping what she needs for her own use. Part of her motivation is to cover the cost of her son's university education – he has Asperger's syndrome and she wants to be able to pay for extra support for him. But she does not argue that her cultivation is a necessity in the way that medical users do, nor deny that she is a criminal 'I do make some money off it, yes I do. . . . I like doing it as well because I like thumbing my nose up at authority.' When she was threatened by local criminals she responded in kind: 'I had a visit one night from somebody who told me that I was to pay rent because he heard what I was growing and . . . if I wanted to grow in the area I had to clear it with him and I had to pay him a rent . . . And I turned around and I said I'm not paying you any fucking rent, he says well I'll come back here with the boys. I says really, come back with the boys. Grabbed my son, my son is 6ft 2, built like a brick shithouse and I called him, baseball bat, I said now do you want to start? I said in fact no fucking better sort him, I went out in the street and I smashed his car and never got him back . . . ' As a single woman, Harriet was aware of her potential vulnerability 'I thought no, I have to stop this now, I have to stop it in its tracks. So I did and I smashed. . . . as I said I went out and I smashed his headlights so he just thought I was a fucking crazy bitch and I've never had any trouble since.'

Others do go to the police, either confident in the sympathy they will receive as medical or non-commercial growers or in recognition that their own risk of prosecution is a price worth paying to see justice against the more serious crimes they have been victims of.

> Nick is a commercial grower who has grown in numerous residential proper-
> ties with 'a guy I knew who was dodgy, who had links to estate agents who
> would happily sign us a gaff out in a fake name, we were doing that for about a
> year and a half. We just rented flats in and around [city], filled them with weed.
> He'd paid for all the equipment, I just got to help him look after it and feed it
> and he knew that I knew what I was talking about and we'd just split it down
> the middle and we earned quite a lot of money off it.' One evening the house
> he was living in was broken into and he and his girlfriend were threatened by
> 'two guys in balaclavas with machetes' who stole his current crop ('thousands
> of pounds worth') saying 'if you call the police, we're coming back'. Nick did
> call the police, explaining that 'I'm a student that grows my own weed and
> I've just been armed robbed' but knowing that 'they can obviously clock I'm
> not just a student that grows weed' because of the size and sophistication of his
> operation. He was charged with cultivation and supply: 'the prosecution were
> looking for two years inside and [my barrister] managed to get me 500 hours
> community service and no fine because I was a student on no income'. Although
> Nick recognised how close he was to getting a custodial sentence he thinks that
> calling the police was the right thing to do. He was frustrated that 'they were
> not in any way interested in catching what I called the real criminals' and that
> he – and his girlfriend – were treated as serious criminals (they were arrested
> by armed police) despite calling the police as victims of violent crime.

> James demonstrated an interesting combination of approaches. He started
> growing for his own medical use (for fibromyalgia and chronic pain), esca-
> lated to supplying other medical users (accepting payment from 'those who
> can', but donating cannabis to others in need) and now also sells to some
> non-medical users to cover some of his overheads. Discussing the threat from
> other criminals (he tells vivid stories of such events happening to other grow-
> ers he knows), he highlights his own contacts in the local criminal under-
> world: 'if you come near my crop and steal it or threaten me in any way
> you will find out that I've got some nice friends . . . including one guy that
> will gladly come and relieve you of any debts you owe, and he won't knock
> at your front door.' He has also contacted the local police to tell them that
> he grows cannabis for his own medical use and inviting them to come and
> discuss this with him although they have not taken him up on this invitation.
> This, he felt, would give him some defence against arrest in the future ('Why
> now?' he will ask, 'you have known about this for two years') but also make
> it easier to report any criminal activity targeted against him.

There were many other examples of growers seeking to reduce risk by engaging with those who might be perceived as a threat rather than relying solely on secrecy. For those involved in medical cultivation, winning over loved ones, carers and medical practitioners was particularly important (see Klein and Potter, 2018) but non-medical growers also sought to change the views of people they come into contact with, explaining – and demonstrating – how home-growing can actually reduce the harms related to domestic cultivation as portrayed in the media. Others go further, overtly campaigning for a change in the law. For example, Brian, a social/commercial grower, tries 'to explain . . . through these letters in the paper and that . . . about how . . . we should have this legal'.

Breaking down stereotypes and reframing the narrative

We have written elsewhere about how medical growers come to redefine themselves as victims, altruistic 'apomedicators'[4] and activists rather than criminals (Klein and Potter, 2018). But it is not just medical-use growers who seek to reframe the narrative around domestic cannabis cultivation.

Growers of all types also seek to dispel the 'skunk myth' that home-grown cannabis is particularly harmful due to its potency or the use of additives and adulterants.

> 'I don't agree with commercial gangster operations because . . . I'm a purist and the dope is actually really bad when it's grown for money.'
>
> (Simon)

> 'It was organic . . . that's why we ended up growing it mostly ourselves because the other growers were crap.'
>
> (Mary)

Personal use, social supply and medical growers are particularly keen to distinguish their own activities from 'real' crimes by emphasising their altruistic motivations. But many overtly commercial growers also seek to distance themselves from the harm-focused stereotypes discussed earlier in the chapter.

> 'I think I'm being a public servant really. . . . I think I'm giving people quality, something that they want. . . . Why buy some shit stuffed with gunk from criminals that don't give a shit about it?'
>
> (Mark)

There is an obvious tension here for those who are profiting from their cultivation or involved in wider criminality relating to their growing activities. But such growers often point out that it is the prohibition of cannabis that pushes them into such behaviours.

> 'We're not bloody criminals. You know, it's prohibition that has caused the black market and has caused the Vietnamese child slaves living in basements making money for gangsters. That's caused by prohibition, you know, and by stepping out of that model and keeping it all under your own roof, as the

cannabis club model encourages, you're taking control away from the gang-sters and away from the law as well because the law is wrong.'

(Lucy)

Although less vociferous than medical growers, some commercial growers also engage in overt activism – joining cannabis social clubs (cf. Decorte and Pardal, 2017) and campaign groups, for example. Not everybody who makes money from cultivation wants cannabis legalised as they recognise that this would undermine their own profit-making enterprises. For others, however, profit (though welcome) is incidental and secondary to ideological views. For example, both Hugh and Mark have made substantial amounts of money through growing themselves and through helping other people become growers. Both recognise that setting up other growers undermines their own potential income; both argue that encouraging more people to grow their own is important as it undermines the more criminogenic aspects of the cannabis market. While happy to make money under prohibition, both are still committed to the ideological aim of legalisation. Other growers do not see legalisation and profit as incompatible, planning instead to become legiti-mate players in a legal cannabis economy should the opportunity arise.

> Alan is in his 30s and has now served two prison sentences for cultivation and supply. Operating at a sizable scale, you might expect Alan to have avoided drawing attention to himself. However, between his prison terms, Alan ran a local cannabis club and pursued a judicial review case against the govern-ment for not considering the possibility of licensing him to grow and supply cannabis under the Misuse of Drugs Act. His campaigning received a lot of local media attention but he continued to grow cannabis on a commercial scale during this period, leading to his arrest and second prison term. His aim, throughout, was to campaign for legalisation thus legitimising his own commercial growing and he saw his willingness to break the law and pay the consequences as an important part of his political activism.

Conclusions

One of our aims in this project was to see how the domestic cannabis cultivation situation in the UK had changed since Potter's research in the early years of the new millennium (Potter, 2010). Broadly speaking, the range of people involved in cannabis cultivation, the methods they employed and their levels of involve-ment in cannabis dealing were similar to those found in this earlier work. The same types and subtypes of personal use, social supply and commercially oriented cultivators were still represented, driven by different combinations of ideology, altruism, medical necessity and financial incentives. More interviewees this time around reported on overlaps with serious and organised crime – whether as par-ticipants or victims – and more people discussed growing for medical purposes. Technological sophistication seemed to have increased – while some growers still resort to soil and sunlight approaches, the use of specialist equipment and techniques to increase yield, to improve security and to process harvested cannabis was widespread. Whether these differences reflect genuine changes, our approach to sampling and recruitment or a greater willingness for growers to discuss their activities with researchers is hard to be sure. However, it is clear that cannabis cultivation in the UK is fragmented and heterogeneous, with serious criminals, opportunistic entrepreneurs, idealistic activists and hobbyists all filling their own niches.

Changes in cannabis policy around the world and the emergence of a legal cannabis industry have influenced the domestic scene. The development of growing technologies has accelerated in the context of legal markets in a number of jurisdictions (particularly in North America) and decriminalisation or tolerance of domestic cultivation in others (including many European countries). The Internet provides easy access to knowledge of growing techniques, the burgeoning scientific evidence of the efficacy of medical cannabis and the tactics and outcomes of legalisation campaigns in those countries adopting more liberal cannabis laws. Policy change elsewhere fuels legalisation arguments and inspires UK activists. Social media enables growers to communicate, exchanging tips and advice but also coordinating political campaigns.

In terms of resisting the negative stereotypes associated with domestic cannabis cultivation, these factors have manifested in two main ways. Growers across the spectrum are generally aware of both the need and the techniques available to minimise the risk of detection through primary prevention methods, with even personal-use growers using technology like grow-tents, carbon-filters and infra-red absorbing film. Many of those involved in cultivation for non-commercial reasons – and even some that are primarily motivated by profit – engage in broader efforts to change the narrative, seeking to distance themselves from the image associated with the 'real' criminal element and supporting changes to cannabis policy that, they argue, would reduce the skunk-related harms that are caused by prohibition rather than inherent in cannabis itself.

There has been some shift in the narrative in the UK. Self-supply[5] and medical use (ACPO, 1999) have long been mitigating factors in sentencing and police decisions on whether to pursue prosecution. Since the 1980s, the police have had an increasing array of disposals to deal with cannabis-related crimes outside of the courts (e.g. cautioning and compounding, PNDs (Penalty Notices for Disorder), fiscal fines and cannabis warnings), although these are primarily used for possession offenses rather than cultivation or supply (Lloyd and McKeganey, 2010). The current sentencing guidelines for drug offences (Sentencing Council, 2012) formalise recognition of social and medical supply, with a presumption towards non-custodial sentences for those involved in such practices. Recent media coverage of some high-profile cases of medical cannabis users (especially the epileptic boys Alfie Dingley and Billy Caldwell; BBC, 2018a; Busby and Bowman, 2018) reflects growing public support for medical use. Changes to the UK law in this area in November 2018 may have been minimal in terms of widening legal access to medical cannabis but show some political willingness to at least consider change. Elsewhere, a number of UK police forces have effectively enacted *de facto* decriminalisation policies with regard to cannabis possession, small-scale cultivation and social supply (Hitchens, 2016). Sixty-three cannabis social clubs (CSCs) registered under the umbrella group UKCSC are open about their existence and their members' involvement in cultivation, but so far none of these have been raided by the police or taken to court. Calls for more wide-reaching reform of cannabis law include many respectable supporters, with former Conservative Party leader William Hague recently becoming the latest big-name politician calling for change (Busby, 2018).

The relationship between the change in narrative and the activist tendencies of growers is a bilateral one – growers sensing a change in public mood are encouraged to be more vociferous campaigners which, in turn, provides momentum to the legalisation movement. There is clearly more support for medical than recreational users. There is also more activism among medical growers than those involved in commercial supply. But many of those involved in cultivation for non-medical reasons, including a number of growers who profit from their activities, also seek to change the narrative around domestic cultivation – emphasising how their activities are not only different from the criminals who dominate the illicit market but actually undermine those criminals by taking custom away from them. Many growers not only make but also embody the argument that cultivation is not inherently linked to the harms highlighted in the media. Examples like Colin and Lee, Mark and Alan show that even those commercial criminal growers who have been involved in serious and organised crime can come back to both support and embody this.

Acknowledgements

This research was funded by the British Academy/Leverhulme Trust small grant scheme (ref. SG132364). Ethical clearance was granted by Lancaster University Faculty of Arts and Social Sciences Research Ethics Committee (ref. FL16005). For further discussion of our methods, see Klein and Potter (2018).

Notes

1 Technically the crime here is abstraction of electricity under s. 13 of the Theft Act 1968.
2 The offence of cannabis cultivation is punishable under s. 6(2) of the Misuse of Drugs Act 1971 (MDA). However, s. 4(2) MDA creates the offence of production, which includes cultivation. The maximum penalty for both on indictment is 14 years' imprisonment. However, offences under s. 4(2) fall within the list of 'lifestyle offences' under the Proceeds of Crime Act 2002 and this allows the sentencing court to make a confiscation order in cases where the defendant(s) has benefited from their criminal conduct (CPS, 2019).
3 The problem of people trafficking and exploitation of child labour is particularly, but not exclusively, associated with Vietnamese groups involved in commercial cultivation (BBC, 2018b; Gentleman, 2018; South China Morning Post, 2018).
4 Apomedication is a portmanteau of apomediation and medication and refers to the sharing of knowledge, beliefs and experiences relating to medical cannabis use between and among users outside of the medical establishment. See Klein and Potter (2018).
5 R. v Brown [1973] Crim. L.R. 62

References

ACMD [Advisory Council on the Misuse of Drugs]. 2008. *Cannabis: Classification and Public Health*. London: ACMD.

ACPO [Association of Chief Police Officers]. 1999. *A Guide to Case Disposal Options for Drug Offenders*. Cumbria: Cumbria Constabulary.

ACPO [Association of Chief Police Officers]. 2009. *Practice Advice on Tackling Commercial Cannabis Cultivation and Head Shops*. London: ACPO.

ACPO [Association of Chief Police Officers]. 2012. *UK National Problem Profile: Commercial Cultivation of Cannabis 2012*. London: ACPO.

Ancrum, C., and Treadwell, J. 2017. Beyond ghosts, gangs and good sorts: Commercial cannabis cultivation and illicit enterprise in England's disadvantaged inner cities. *Crime, Media, Culture* 13 (1), pp. 69–84.

Anti-Slavery International. 2014. *Trafficking for Forced Criminal Activities and Begging in Europe Exploratory Study and Good Practice Examples*. London: Anti-Slavery International. Available at: www.antislavery.org/wp-content/uploads/2017/01/trafficking_for_forced_criminal_activities_and_begging_in_europe.pdf.

APPG [All Party Parliamentary Group for Drug Policy Reform]. 2016. *Access to Medicinal Cannabis: Meeting Patient Needs*. London: APPG. Available at: https://drive.google.com/file/d/1mx0Q33DCm4OsGnw3L3GDYpMHvwOq7nVw/view?usp=sharing.

Atha, M.J. 2012. *Cannabis – An Introduction*. Presented at HIT Seminar. Wigan: IDMU.

Atha, M.J., Blanchard, S., and Davis, S. 1999. *Regular Users II: UK Drugs Market Analysis, Purchasing Patterns & Prices 1997*. Wigan: IDMU.

BBC. 2018a. Alfie Dingley to get medicinal cannabis. *BBC News*, 19 June 2018. Available at: www.bbc.co.uk/news/av/uk-politics-44538100/alfie-dingley-to-get-medicinal-cannabis-aujid-javld.

BBC. 2018b. Police uncover £3m Fleetwood cannabis farm. *BBC News*, 17 December 2018. Available at: www.bbc.co.uk/news/uk-england-lancashire-46598125.

Bentham, M. 2007. Deadly skunk floods city. *Evening Standard*, 15 October 2007. Available at: www.standard.co.uk/news/deadly-skunk-floods-city-6678202.html.

Borland, S. 2019. Children aged nine damaged by cannabis. *Daily Mail*, 25 March 2019. http://mailonline.newspaperdirect.com/epaper/viewer.aspx?issue=10482019032500000000001001&page=1&article=0c41088a-c63c-4b9c-b8a2-6f4a29fbbc08&key=ArDNPTOpjjwwrFzNwv%2B8yA%3D%3D&feed=rss.

Bouchard, M., Potter, G., and Decorte, T. 2011. Emerging trends in Cannabis cultivation – and the way forward. In: Decorte, Tom, Potter, Gary, and Bouchard, Martin (Eds.), *World Wide Weed: Global Trends in Cannabis Cultivation and Its Control*. Aldershot: Ashgate.

Busby, M. 2018. William Hague calls for Theresa May to legalise cannabis. *The Guardian*, 19 June 2018. Available at: www.theguardian.com/society/2018/jun/19/william-hague-theresa-may-legalise-cannabis.

Busby, M., and Bowman, V. 2018. Home office returns cannabis oil for boy's epilepsy treatment. *The Observer*, 16 June 2018. Available at: www.theguardian.com/society/2018/jun/16/billy-caldwells-mother-hopeful-of-cannabis-medicine-licence.

CPS [Crown Prosecution Service]. 2019. *Drug Offences*. London: CPS. Available at: www.cps.gov.uk/legal-guidance/drug-offences.

Decorte, T., and Pardal, M. 2017. Cannabis social clubs in Europe: Prospects and limits. In: Colson, R., and Bergeron, H. (Eds.), *European Drug Policies: The Ways of Reform*. London: Routledge.

Decorte, T., Potter, G., and Bouchard, M. (Eds.) 2011. *World Wide Weed: Global Trends in Cannabis Cultivation and Control*. Ashgate: Aldershot.

Di Forti, M., Morgan, C., Dazzan, P., Pariante, C., Mondelli, V., Marques, T.R., . . . Murray, R.M. 2009. High-potency cannabis and the risk of psychosis. *British Journal of Psychiatry* 195 (6), pp. 488–91.

Englund, A., Morrison, P., Atakan, Z., and Kralj, A. 2014. 'The Good, the Bad, the Ugly': Experimental human studies of CBD, THC, and THCV. *Schizophrenia Research* 153 (1), p. S32.

Fakhoury, M. 2016. Could cannabidiol be used as an alternative to antipsychotics. *Journal of Psychiatric Research* 80, pp. 14–21.

Gentleman, A. 2018. Trafficked, beaten, enslaved: The life of a Vietnamese cannabis farmer. *The Guardian,* 31 January 2018. Available at: www.theguardian.com/world/2018/jan/31/trafficked-beaten-ensaved-life-of-cannabis-farmer-vietnam.

Hakkarainen, P., Asmussen Frank, V., Barratt, M.J., Dahl, H.V., Decorte, T., Karjalainen, K., . . . Werse, B. 2015. Growing medicine: Small-scale cannabis cultivation for medical purposes in six countries. *International Journal of Drug Policy* 26 (3), pp. 250–6.

Hakkarainen, P., Decorte, T., Sznitman, S., Karjalainen, K., Barratt, M., Frank, V., . . . Wilkinson, C. 2019. Examining the blurred boundaries between medical and recreational cannabis – Results from an international study of small-scale cannabis cultivation. *Drugs: Education, Prevention and Policy* 26 (3), pp. 250–8. doi:10.1080/09687637.2017.1411888.

Hall, W. 2009. The adverse health effects of cannabis use: What are they, and what are their implications for policy? *International Journal of Drug Policy* 20, pp. 458–66.

Hargreaves, J., and Smith, K. (Eds.) 2015. *Seizures of Drugs in England and Wales, 2014/15 (Statistical Bulletin 06/15).* London: Home Office.

Hitchens, P. 2016. Top Politician Admits it – There is de facto decriminalisation of Cannabis *Hitchens Blog, Mail on Sunday,* 28 April 2016. Available at: http://hitchensblog.mailonsunday.co.uk/2016/04/top-politician-admits-it-there-is-de-facto-decriminalisation-of-cannabis.html.

Hough, M., Warburton, H., Few, B., May, T., Man, L.H., Witton, J., and Turnbull, P.J. 2003. *A Growing Market: The Domestic Cultivation of Cannabis.* York: Joseph Rowntree Foundation.

Kirby, S., and Peale, K. 2015. The Changing pattern of domestic Cannabis cultivation in the United Kingdom and its impact on the cannabis market. *Journal of Drug Issues* 45 (3), pp. 279–92.

Klein, A., and Potter, G. 2018. The three betrayals of the medical cannabis growing activist: From multiple victimhood to reconstruction, redemption and activism. *International Journal of Drug Policy* 53, pp. 65–72.

Knodt, M. 2017. Contaminated Cannabis – The unavoidable consequence of prohibition. *Marijuana.com,* 27 January 2017. Available at: www.marijuana.com/news/2017/01/contaminated-cannabis-the-unavoidable-consequence-of-prohibition/.

Lenton, S., Asmussen Frank, V., Barratt, M.J., Potter, G., and Decorte, T. 2018. Growing practices and the use of chemical additives among a sample of small scale cannabis growers in three countries. *Drug and Alcohol Dependence* 192, pp. 250–6.

Lloyd, C., and McKeganey, N. 2010. *Drugs Research: An Overview of Evidence and Questions for Policy.* London: Joseph Rowntree Foundation.

Morgan, C.J.A., and Curran, H.V. 2008. Effects of cannabidiol on schizophrenia-like symptoms in people who use cannabis. *British Journal of Psychiatry* 192, pp. 306–7.

Mulchandani, R., Hand, T., and Panesar, L.K. 2010. *Seizures of Drugs in England and Wales, 2009/10.* London: Home Office.

Mwenda, L., Ahmad, M., and Kumari, K. 2005. *Seizures of Drugs in England and Wales, 2003*. London: Home Office.

NPCC [National Police Chiefs' Council]. 2014. *UK National Problem Profile: Commercial Cultivation of Cannabis*. London: NPCC.

OFGEM [Office of Gas and Electricity Markets]. 2014. *Tackling Electricity Theft: The Way Forward*. London: OFGEM.

ONS [Office for National Statistics]. 2018. *Seizures of Drugs in England and Wales, Financial Year Ending 2018: Data Tables*. London: ONS. Available at: https://assets.publishing.service.gov.uk/government/uploads/system/uploads/attachment_data/file/754678/seizures-drugs-mar2018-hosb2618-tables.ods.

Pawlik, E., and Mahler, H. 2011. Smoke analysis of adulterated drug preparations. *Toxichem Krimtech* 78, pp. 200–10.

Potter, D.J., Hammond, K., Tuffnell, S., Walker, C., and Di Forti, M. 2017. Potency of Δ^9 – tetrahydrocannabinol and other cannabinoids in cannabis in England in 2016: Implications for public health and pharmacology. *Drug Testing and Analysis* 10 (4), pp. 628–35.

Potter, G. 2009. Exploring retail-level drug distribution: Social supply, 'real' dealers and the user/dealer interface. In: Demetrovics, Z., Fountain, J., and Kraus, L. (Eds.), *Old and New Policies, Theories, Research Methods and Drug Users Across Europe*. Lengerich: PABST Science Publishers.

Potter, G. 2010. *Weed, Need and Greed: A Study of Domestic Cannabis Cultivation*. London: Free Association Books.

Potter, G. 2011. Keeping down the weeds: Cannabis eradication in the developed world. In: Decorte, Tom, Potter, Gary, and Bouchard, Martin (Eds.), *World Wide Weed: Global Trends in Cannabis Cultivation and Its Control*. Aldershot: Ashgate.

Potter, G., Barratt, M.J., Malm, A., Bouchard, M., Blok, T., Christensen, A.S., . . . Wouters, M. 2015. Global patterns of domestic cannabis cultivation: Sample characteristics and patterns of growing across eleven countries. *International Journal of Drug Policy* 26 (3), pp. 226–37.

Potter, G., and Chatwin, C. 2012. The Problem with Skunk. *Drugs and Alcohol Today* 12 (4), pp. 232–40.

Randerson, J. 2007. Warning issued over cannabis adulterated with glass beads. *The Guardian*, 12 January 2007. Available at: www.theguardian.com/society/2007/jan/12/drugsandalcohol.drugs.

Savage, S., and Silverstone, D. 2010. Farmers, factories and funds: Organised crime and illicit drugs cultivation within the British Vietnamese community. *Global Crime* 11 (1), pp. 16–33.

Sentencing Council. 2012. *Drug Offences Definitive Guidelines*. London: Sentencing Council.

South China Morning Post. 2018. Vietnamese child slaves toil in secret UK cannabis farms. *South China Morning Post*, 21 August 2018. Available at: www.scmp.com/news/world/europe/article/2160653/vietnamese-child-slaves-toil-secret-uk-cannabis-farms.

Stevens, A. 2007. My cannabis, your Skunk: Reader's response to 'the cannabis potency question'. *Drugs and Alcohol Today* 7 (3), pp. 13–17.

Surrey Live. 2009. Vietnamese man 'murdered over botched drug deal'. *Surrey Live*, 28 October 2009. Available at: www.getsurrey.co.uk/news/local-news/vietnamese-man-murdered-over-botched-4822539.

13 Framing substance use problems

Influence on key concepts, methods of research and policy orientation

Alfred Uhl

Introduction

Basic convictions related to specific worldviews shape the way facts are selected or omitted to frame lines of argumentation. The choice of a research project is commonly based on ideas of the importance of a topic and thus at least unconsciously may be shaped to support certain convictions and values. Thus, there is a risk that readiness to scrutinise methods and interpretations may be low if results support convictions while this may be much higher if results challenge these convictions.

This chapter aims to expose some questionable forms of framing in connection with the international discourse on alcohol policy. The focus is not on evidence emphasised or omitted to direct the recipients' thought, which may be criticised as well, but on popular but flawed interpretations of research findings. The examples chosen appear to be widely accepted because they are cited and repeated so often that they are almost turned into 'common sense dogmas'. The topics addressed are, firstly, approaches used to quantify 'harm to others due to alcohol' and, secondly, convictions concerning 'drinking alcohol while lactating'.

Proportionality as a central element of human rights legislation

A central question in modern democracies is how far law-making bodies and administrations, representing a majority of voters, are entitled to interfere with individual behaviours and lifestyles. From a modern human rights perspective, it is clear that minority rights must be respected and that majorities are not entitled to blindly impose their convictions. In democratic institutions, these principles are laid down in constitutions which usually relate explicitly to declarations of human rights. A central element of human rights legislation is proportionality (Greer, 2000). According to Barak (2012, p. 3, cited in Huscroft, 2014), proportionality analysis rests on four central pillars, for which the burden of justification is usually placed on the state:

1   Legitimacy: Are the intended restrictions established for a proper purpose?
2   Rationality: Are the intended restrictive measures rationally connected to the achievement of this purpose?

3   Necessity: Are there no less restrictive measures available to achieve the same purpose?
4   Proportionality *stricto sensu*: Do the advantages of implementing restrictive measures outweigh the disadvantages induced for those who are restricted?

The first point, legitimacy, demands that there should not be any arbitrary restriction enacted as an end in itself. Traditional aspirations to outlaw and sanction behaviours that do not really harm anybody but may alienate some people, like not adhering to certain dress codes, are hard to defend as legitimate. There should be a clearly defined and sensible goal to be achieved with any restrictive measure. The judgement as to whether restrictive measures are legitimate in the light of human rights issues depends primarily on theoretical and ethical considerations.

In order to be able to deal adequately with the second and third points (rationality and necessity), scientific evidence is indispensable. Popular measures may be ineffective and less restrictive measures may be equally successful in yielding the desired results.

The fourth point – to attain 'proportionality in the literal sense' (proportionality *stricto sensu*) – depends on both scientific evidence and basic value judgements. How much does the right to chat with friends in the evening outweigh the right of neighbours to sleep in silence? Or more precisely: how often do neighbours have to tolerate what amount of noise at what time of day before one can legitimately demand that the state intervenes? Rules concerning this question cannot be derived from simply assessing the level of noise and studying the impact of noise on sleep quality, even though this information is doubtless of relevance for the decision.

The issue of proportionality arises only if the interests of third parties are seriously violated or if actors endanger themselves. From a human rights perspective, if behaviours are only detrimental for the actors themselves, the risk must be very high to justify restrictive measures. Societies are obliged to inform and support individuals in health matters and should try to convince them to choose a healthy lifestyle but mature and informed individuals should be entitled to decide for themselves how to behave, even if public health experts and decision-makers do not perceive their behaviour as a good choice.

How far to go with regulations and restrictions is not a simple task. Restrictive measures experienced as unreasonable may be rejected as coercive paternalism from a libertarian point of view. Sometimes even stronger terminologies, like 'Nanny State' or 'Health Fascism', are used to express disapproval of public actions to fight smoking, alcohol consumption, drinking sweet beverages and other behaviours considered to be detrimental to health (e.g. DeMaria, 2013, Lefever, 2012) and to frame restrictive interventions as undemocratic and unacceptable.

The libertarian conviction that the state must not interfere if adults choose a more pleasurable life over a longer, healthier one is not undisputed however. Wiley et al. (2013), for example, have criticised the negative framing of state interventions on behalf of unwilling individuals (as in the aforementioned manner): they defend a certain amount of paternalism in order to solve problems collectively that, they believe, apparently cannot be solved individually. Instead of 'reaffirming the language of personal responsibility', the authors suggest to 'utilize the language of a democratic process'. The idea here is to frame democracy as a system where the majority is entitled to interfere against the will of minorities for the sake of their health with restrictive measures.

Somewhere in the middle between welcoming and rejecting coercive paternalism is the notion of libertarian paternalism, in the sense of nudging as Thaler and Sunstein (2008) proposed. The basic idea of nudging is to create environments and exposures that softly lead individuals to behave in a certain way, openly admitting the intention to make certain choices more likely. The idea is not to force behaviour change on individuals and to accept if these choices are rejected by the target persons.

An unambiguous statement against coercive paternalism for the sake of public health can be found in the Ottawa Charter, an important document advocating health promotion (WHO, 1986a). The explicit goal of health promotion, as defined in this document, is to empower individuals in the sense of 'enabling people to increase control over, and to improve, their health'. What needs to be provided is 'a supportive environment, access to information, life skills and opportunities for making healthy choices'. The focus is clearly on 'providing information, education for health, and enhancing life skills', even though changes in legislation and taxation to 'make the healthier choice the easier choice' are mentioned as well. The latter concession must not be interpreted as justification of paternalism though, as a discussion paper written by the authors of the Charter published in the same year (WHO, 1986b) demonstrates. The authors state:

> There is a possibility with health promotion that health will be viewed as the ultimate goal incorporating all life. This ideology, sometimes called healthism, could lead to others prescribing what individuals should do for themselves and how they should behave, which is contrary to the principles of health promotion.

The idea of the WHO Ottawa Charter quite obviously is to promote public health primarily through informing and empowering the population and not through coercing people into choosing a healthy lifestyle. For example, the official Austrian Addiction Prevention Strategy passed by the Austrian government (BMG, 2015) explicitly expresses concordance with the emancipatory approach of the Ottawa Charter, and there are many other examples elsewhere: publications by government-funded structures in Austria, Germany and Switzerland (BMG, 2015; BZgA, 2018, Gesundheitsförderung Schweiz, 2018).

Regardless as to whether a person's worldview rejects coercive paternalism, is convinced that democratically justified paternalism is legitimate or tends towards a compromise in the sense of libertarian paternalism, a strategy to make it acceptable from all three perspectives is to frame restrictive measures as necessary to protect third party interests (legitimacy) and to demonstrate that they are proportionate (rationality, necessity and proportionality *stricto sensu*).

Different perspectives and frames in the alcohol field

In the alcohol field, there is a long tradition of alcohol epidemiologists and anti-alcohol activists being in favour of a dedicated alcohol control policy. They frame their approach as 'evidence-based alcohol policy' (Bruun et al., 1975; Edwards et al., 1994; Babor et al., 2003). A systematic analysis of the scientific literature backing up this claim reveals that central conclusions are far less convincingly derived from empirical evidence than usually implied (Uhl, 2015). The control approach is persuasively framed as cheap and effective without any adequate alternative. To support this framing with a catchy slogan, the term 'three best buys' was coined (Bloom et al., 2011). The expression 'three best buys' is an umbrella term incorporating 'tax increases', 'restricting access to retailed alcohol' and 'bans on alcohol advertising'.

Framing policy as 'evidence-based' suggests that policy can be derived from empirical facts alone. But this camouflages the role value decisions actually play (Uhl, 2007). Modern literature on research methodology almost unanimously declares that the attempt to derive what should happen (policy) from what there is (empirical evidence) is logically flawed. This problem is commonly referred to as 'is–ought problem'. The inherent logical error in reasoning was labelled 'naturalistic fallacy' by Moore (1960). That practical decisions in the alcohol policy field cannot be solely derived from empirical evidence was even supported by Baumberg (2008), one of the two authors of a very influential book supporting a determinedly evidence-based alcohol control policy (Anderson and Baumberg, 2006). The 'control approach' in the alcohol policy field is particularly popular in the Protestant-dominated world. It is commonly referred to as 'population approach', whereby alcohol is generally and indiscriminately framed as a dangerous substance.

In the Catholic-dominated world, a different perspective is popular – to discriminate strictly between moderate alcohol use and harmful use. Moderate alcohol consumption is perceived as positive or neutral and only harmful alcohol use is problematised. This perspective is a 'liberal problem focused approach' and frames alcohol as an ambiguous substance, giving pleasure if used moderately and harm if used immoderately. A popular slogan frame for the control perspective is 'Less is better!', an expression Anderson (1996) chose as the title for his book. A popular slogan frame for the problem-focused perspective is 'Consume in moderation!' (e.g. ODPHP, 2019).

Framing the context in a specific way to enhance certain conclusions is a common mechanism when people try to convince others and an important tool for activists to promote their ideas. Framing according to Entman (1993) works via selecting 'some aspects of perceived reality' and making 'them more salient in the communicating text, in such a way as to promote a particular problem definition, causal interpretation, moral evaluation and/or treatment recommendation'. Selecting supportive information and omitting other information works to influence others, because, as Kahneman (2011) pointed out, recipients of information usually do not realise if the information presented to them is incomplete and in fact does not allow them to draw sensible conclusions. Kahneman called this shortcoming of human thinking 'WYSIATI' (an acronym for 'What You See Is All There Is'). If the information presented to frame the context stems from renowned scientists or influential decision-makers, the likelihood that recipients trust the information instead of critically questioning its validity and completeness is particularly high. Chabris and Simons (2011) called this phenomenon 'illusion of confidence'.

Researchers and policy advocates who want to convey a certain perspective systematically search for evidence to support their view and frame the research question in a way which sustains their position. Scientific conclusions useful to support a particular position are welcomed as 'advocacy tools' and seldom critically scrutinised. At the same time, the motivation to critically question the validity of results favouring the opposite position is usually high. Because there are currently strong tendencies in the field of scientific alcohol epidemiology, prevention and therapy to frame alcohol in general as a 'dangerous substance', in the remainder of this chapter I focus on conclusions and assertions made to support this position, which I argue are factually untenable.[1] My criticism of framing alcohol as a 'dangerous substance' by misinterpreting empirical research findings should not be seen as a way to define alcohol as a 'harmless substance' but as an attempt to weigh positive aspects and negative aspects of alcohol use against each other as accurately and critically as possible to arrive at a balanced view.

Harm to others caused by alcohol use

As has already been mentioned, it is hard to justify restrictive measures to prevent adverse behaviours of individuals if their behaviours do not impact on third parties but only endanger their own health. In contrast, it is relatively easy to justify measures against behaviours that impact negatively on bystanders, like drunk driving, being drunk at the workplace while handling dangerous machinery or harming partners while intoxicated. BAC limits when driving, alcohol bans at workplaces and expelling violent partners from the shared home are commonly accepted.

In many countries, alcohol use was traditionally and is still perceived as harmless and enjoyable behaviour as long as alcohol is not consumed excessively. Most people are aware that excessive consumption induces severe problems for consumers and for third parties, but they oppose dedicated alcohol control policy measures designed to impact on moderate users and excessive users alike (the 'population approach' in contrast to the 'liberal problem-focused approach'). Efforts of temperance activists and health professionals to uphold an alcohol policy characterised by high prices and reduced alcohol availability in Northern Europe came under pressure in the wake of moves towards European integration and some elements had to be modified. Ideas to reinstall a stricter alcohol control policy seemed quite unrealistic when Northern Europe countries became members of the European Union.

This situation changed as the public perception of cigarette smoking gradually altered in the Western world, giving rise to the hope that a similar change in perception is feasible regarding alcohol as well. As long as smoking cigarettes was primarily seen as a behaviour only impacting negatively on smokers themselves, smoking was widely tolerated. With an increasing awareness that smoking does not only annoy non-smokers but may affect the health of bystanders significantly, a radical change of perspective took place, that is, there was a frame shift. Smoking was no longer perceived as an innocuous pastime. More and more people started to perceive smoking near them as an unacceptable risk to their health and started to insist on breathing clean air. Smokers more and more accepted the new situation and smoking bans in public places were enacted and are now widely accepted.

When health professionals and temperance activists in the alcohol field saw this development, the idea to try a similar approach by reframing the alcohol issue accordingly was tempting. In analogy to 'passive smoking', the term 'passive drinking' was coined, suggesting that drinking alcohol inflicts harms on third parties as well (Burgess, 2009). But this attempt to reframe drinking as a behaviour impacting negatively on others did not succeed. This framing was intuitively not plausible. Passive smokers inhale smoke, but victims of alcohol users are not harmed by involuntarily ingesting alcohol. They may be harmed by the consequences of drinkers' behaviours. The term 'passive drinking' lost popularity and the expression 'Harm to Others because of Somebody's Drinking' or shorter 'Harm to Others' or even shorter 'H2O' was coined.

Attempts to frame drinking alcohol as a behaviour that commonly harms others led to an increase of research activities to support this view. More and more projects were started by researchers already convinced that alcohol commonly induced massive problems for bystanders. The basic idea was to initiate projects in a way to support this conviction and not to emphasise the complex relationship between alcohol consumption and adverse outcomes. A simple way to achieve a high percentage of negatively affected bystanders is to aggregate anything from minor nuisance to severe problems inflicted by somebody who apparently had drunk alcohol and to choose a long period of time. If data are generated in this way and presented without any attempt to relativise the results – by comparing them to nuisance and problems inflicted in situations where no alcohol is used – the results are misleading.

One of the instruments developed to assess harm to others because of somebody else's drinking in the above sense is the 'Harm at Community Level' module of the SEAS questionnaire (Standardised European Alcohol Survey Instrument) developed within the RARHA (Reducing Alcohol-Related Harm) project (Moskalewicz et al., 2016). This project was funded by the Second EU Health Program, involving all 28 EU Member States plus Iceland, Norway and Switzerland and additionally 29 collaborating partners, such as the EMCDDA, WHO, the Pompidou Group and OECD between 2014 and 2016. A similar instrument at the European level is the 'harm to others module' used within the international ESPAD project (ESPAD Group, 2015).

The SEAS module on harm to others targets eight areas of harm. The introductory statement to this module is 'Now let me ask you some questions about various problems that can occur because of somebody else's drinking', followed by a notice that the reference time for the following eight items is the last 12 months. The items are as follows:

1   Because of someone else drinking, have you been woken up at night?
2   Because of someone else drinking, have you been verbally abused, that is, called names or otherwise insulted?
3   Because of someone else drinking, have you been harmed physically?
4   Because of someone else drinking, have you been involved in a serious argument?
5   Have you been a passenger with a driver who had had too much to drink?
6   Have you been involved in a traffic accident because of someone's drinking?
7   Because of someone else drinking, have you felt unsafe in public places, including public transportation?
8   Have you been annoyed by people vomiting, urinating or littering when they have been drinking?

For each of these questions, the interviewees were asked to additionally add if they were affected 'a lot', 'a little' or 'not at all' by this event.

The overall result across all involved countries in the RARHA context (except Greece and Italy, where these variables were not assessed) was that 63 per cent of the respondents had experienced some negative effects because of somebody else's drinking over the last 12 months (Moskalewicz et al., 2016). Being confronted with the fact that drinking alcohol is harming almost two-thirds of the population within one year is alarming at first sight. A critical look at the items puts the initial impression into perspective though.

The item 'Being woken up at night in the last 12 months' includes anything from 'being woken up just once in the last 12 months without any relevant disruption of sleep' to 'continuous regular sleep disturbances over a long time period'. Being verbally abused ranges from 'a friend laughing and saying "You're stupid"' to 'being in a situation generating massive fear of being physically assaulted'. Being harmed physically ranges from somebody 'dropping a glass and someone scratching his finger minimally' through 'being attacked and seriously injured'. Feeling unsafe in public places ranges from 'a mild unjustified insecurity' to 'an extremely threatening situation'. To be in a serious argument ranges from 'minor disagreement' to 'a very serious conflict with long-lasting consequences'. The additional question 'Were you affected a lot?' adds a bit of sense to the endeavour but does not really resolve the inherent problem of arbitrarily aggregating irrelevant and highly relevant adverse situations within one variable. This approach presents minor nuisance implicitly as a relevant problem by counting it in one category along with highly serious problems.

Another aspect to consider is that the interviewees have to judge whether the events they remember are causally related to alcohol consumption and not only associated. For individuals highly critical of alcohol use and convinced that alcohol is a major cause of various problems, when they experience problematic behaviour, they may attribute all problems to alcohol use, even if the attribution is groundless.

All humans, regardless of whether they drank alcohol or were completely sober, regularly cause situations that inflict negatively on others. For example, if someone makes a barbecue in his garden, his neighbours may be bothered by the smell of smoke and grilled meat. In such situations, a compromise, acceptable to both parties, has to be sought. It is absurd to create a fuss about minor nuisance and non-dramatic problems that everybody experiences occasionally and normally hardly minds. Because people barbecuing in the garden very likely drink a beer or glass of wine as well, all negative effects associated with barbecuing can be directly framed as problems due to alcohol consumption.

If problems are described for a specific group only, like for people who drank alcohol, the impression is suggested that these problems are specific to drinkers of alcohol and that comparable groups are not characterised by those problems (intuitive zero assumption). In order to put things into perspective, it is important to apply instruments, like the 'Harm to Others' module of the SEAS questionnaire, to other groups as well – and particularly to people who have not consumed alcohol. The intuitive zero assumption results from the usual way humans deal with incomplete information (Kahneman, 2011). Information actually needed for sensible conclusions but not available at the moment is usually substituted intuitively in the simplest possible manner. A good example is the usual interpretation of alcohol-associated traffic accidents as 100 per cent caused by alcohol, even though roughly a third of alcohol-associated accidents would have happened without alcohol influence as well (Krüger et al., 1995). Everyone knows that sober people cause traffic accidents as well – most accidents are caused by sober people – but being confronted with the number of alcohol-associated accidents, virtually everyone spontaneously treats these figures as accidents caused by the effects of alcohol.

Not to be misunderstood. Nobody can doubt that excessive alcohol use causes serious problems for the drinkers themselves and for third parties as well. It is undeniable that engaged research on this issue is justified and necessary. Sensible research could help to understand the processes behind these phenomena and their impact. This requires qualitative research focusing on ways to design and implement countermeasures to reduce relevant alcohol-induced harm. Only if these problems and their practical relevance are well understood would it make sense to assess these problems with adequate instruments quantitatively. Superficial and undifferentiated questionnaire approaches – like the 'Harm at Community Level' module of the RARHA SEAS questionnaire – should therefore be handled with great caution as research tools.

Drinking alcohol while lactating

In many cases, heavy alcohol consumption during pregnancy causes serious damage to the unborn child (Foetal Alcohol Syndrome = FAS or Foetal Alcohol Effects = FAE). The prevalence of FASD in Europe is estimated around

0.2 per cent (Lange et al., 2017). There is no conclusive scientific evidence that occasional moderate alcohol consumption during pregnancy can cause relevant damage to the unborn child, but it is nevertheless advisable, in view of the current state of knowledge, to advise pregnant women to completely avoid alcohol during pregnancy as a measure of precaution (RCOG, 2006).

The situation is totally different if 'alcohol consumption and breastfeeding' is the issue, even though both situations seem analogous at first glance: both situations involve mothers, babies and alcohol. During pregnancy, if the mother drinks alcohol, this alcohol reaches the mother's and the baby's organism only diluted once. If the baby drinks this mother's milk, the alcohol is diluted a second time and only reaches irrelevant levels in the baby. This can be illustrated with a simple back-of-the-envelope calculation yielding somewhat higher results than must be realistically expected.

If alcoholic beverages are consumed, the alcohol disperses quite rapidly through the watery parts of the body (Koob and Moal, 2006). Around two-thirds of the human body consists of water (Watson et al., 1980). A woman with 75 kg body weight thus has around 50 L body water. If she drinks half a litre of an alcoholic beverage, the dilution ratio is 1:100. More specifically, if the beverage is half a litre of beer with an alcohol concentration of 5 vol%, the 'theoretical alcohol content' in the woman's body water amounts to 0.05 vol% alcohol. The volume of breast milk normally consumed by a baby is around 2 per cent of the baby's body water volume – or expressed differently, the dilution ratio is 1:50. If the mother's milk contains 0.05 vol% alcohol, the theoretical alcohol content to be reached in the baby's body water thus is 0.001 vol% alcohol.

In the aforementioned calculation, the 'theoretical alcohol' content was calculated, which is the alcohol content that could be reached if there were no alcohol metabolism while the alcohol is absorbed from stomach and intestines and if there were no first-pass metabolism in the liver before alcohol reaches the circulatory system. In reality, this theoretical alcohol concentration can never be reached. The actual level is always considerably lower.

The aforementioned back-of-the-envelope calculation assumed that the mother lactates her baby exactly when the maximum alcohol level is reached in her mother's milk – which is rarely ever the case. On average, the level is much lower.

In the aforementioned calculation, the theoretical alcohol content was expressed in vol% alcohol in the body water. The usual measure of alcohol blood concentration (BAC) is in gram (g) per litre (L) blood. In order to translate volume (millilitre) into gram, the density of alcohol must be considered (0.789 g/mL) and in order to translate body water into blood – respectively mother's milk – it has to be considered that both fluids contain roughly 20 per cent non-aqueous constituents. Because of these two factors, 0.05 vol% alcohol in body water translates roughly into a BAC of 0.03 g/L – respectively 0.03 g/L alcohol concentration in mother's milk. Furthermore, 0.001 vol% alcohol in body water of a baby translates into a BAC of 0.00064 g/L. To illustrate this: if an adult would drink 1 L of mother's milk with 0.03 g/L alcohol, the amount of alcohol he ingests would be equivalent to the same adult drinking two thimbles of beer with 5 vol% alcohol.[2]

There are two popular myths commonly referred to in the context of alcohol consumption and breastfeeding. In the alcohol literature, it is often claimed that babies may die at very low BAC levels and that their alcohol metabolism is extremely slow (BZgA, 2004). A possible explanation for this conclusion is that ADH activity in humans is not fully developed until the age of 5 years (Feuerlein, 1979). This fact was very likely intuitively equated with reduced alcohol metabolism by authors warning that the alcohol metabolism in babies is extremely slow. But Feuerlein explained that the ADH activity does not correspond to the alcohol oxidation speed. He did not mention though that alcohol metabolism in children under the age of 5 years is similar to adults in spite of this fact.

One has to concede that research on this question is not easy. Experimental studies concerning the alcohol metabolism in small children are barely conceivable, because hardly any ethics committee would agree to administer alcohol to newborns and infants in order to determine the lethal alcohol level or to determine their alcohol metabolism rate. There are a few scientific articles shedding light on this situation though. The director of an intensive care unit in the United States reviewed all cases of alcohol poisoning in infants over a long period and found that all of them had survived very high blood alcohol levels, whereby not a single child had died. All of them had survived without intensive care treatment and in one case the observed metabolism rate was twice as high as in adults (Ragan et al., 1979). There is another (highly unethical) study on the metabolism rate in small children, done in the former German Democratic Republic (Schippan et al., 1975). The authors argued that an economic situation might come, where it might be necessary to feed children with alcohol, if no other food was available. They administered alcohol to very young babies and infants and studied their metabolism rate. It turned out that the clearing rate was 0,013 g/L per hour, which is only slightly below the average metabolism rate of 0.15 g/L per hour in adults. Other authors described even higher alcohol clearing rates in babies than in adults: Leung (1986) in two babies who had accidentally consumed alcohol and Marek and Kraft (2014) presented further examples.

These results suggest that small children are neither extremely vulnerable to alcohol effects nor that their alcohol metabolism is significantly lower than in adults. This result corresponds with the fact that alcohol is constantly produced naturally in every human body from sugar, starch and lactic acid (Pfannhauser, 2004). If alcohol could not be metabolised in the organism of babies when they are born, they would face lethal alcohol poisoning within a few days.

A comparison of the alcohol content in breast milk after the mother consumed alcohol moderately with normal foods also provides a convincing picture. If a mother drank half a litre of beer, as in the aforementioned example, the maximum alcohol concentration that could be reached in the mother's milk is 0.03 g/L. As Pfannhauser (2004) pointed out,

- a litre of freshly made apple juice contains 2 g of alcohol (7 times as much);
- freshly made apple juice 6 hours after pressing contains 6 g alcohol (20 times as much);

- one kg blended bread contains 2–4 g alcohol (7–14 times as much);
- ripe bananas 8 days after purchase contain 5 g alcohol (17 times as much);
- 1 kg sauerkraut contains 5 g alcohol (17 times as much);
- kefir contains 5 g alcohol (17 times as much).

Although it is unquestionable that breast milk from a mother who consumed moderate amounts of alcohol cannot cause the slightest problem for a breastfed child, for the sake of completeness it should also be mentioned that there is another line of argumentation to discourage breastfeeding mothers from consuming alcohol as well.

This argument is that alcohol consumption by the mother impacts negatively on the amount of mother's milk drunk by the baby. This could be due to a smaller production of mother's milk, due to an inhibition of the 'let-down' reflex related to oxytocin or due to babies rejecting milk with a noticeable alcohol flavour. Some authors (e.g. Menella and Beauchamp, 1991) support the idea that after the mother had drunk alcohol, babies consumed less mother's milk, based on empirical studies: others support that beer consumption increases lactation through prolactine production, but the latter relate this effect not to alcohol but to other ingredients of beer (e.g. Carlson et al., 1985).

We can imagine many situations, like friends coming over for a chat, a telephone call, stress, eating spicy food and many more that may impact on the amount of mother's milk babies consume at single feeding occasions, but normally such a deficit is compensated with the next meals. If the mother's milk production is insufficient at a certain stage, putting the baby on more often increases the amount of milk to the amount needed. To date, there are no experimental studies that have investigated the longer-term influence of occasional alcohol consumption by mothers on their baby's milk intake or on the weight gain of these babies. Only such studies could challenge the assumption that an occasional reduction in the mother's milk consumed is automatically compensated with the next meals.

To advise mothers not to drink any alcohol at all while breastfeeding is not justified. The mother may enjoy an occasional glass of wine or beer without any hesitation. To advise mothers to pump breastmilk before drinking alcohol and then to feed the infant with the bottle or to advise mothers not to lactate for three hours after their last alcohol consumption is not justified either. If the alcohol actually interferes with milk production or 'let-down' reflex, these recommendations would not make any sense anyway. Such claims induce unnecessary restrictions for mothers and problems for babies. Such suggestions may even motivate some mothers to stop lactating, which should not be encouraged of all.

Not to be misunderstood. It is of course perfectly okay if lactating mothers and their partners – or anybody else – decide to totally refrain from drinking alcohol, provided they want to do so. Not to drink any alcohol is a personal decision anybody may take and there is nothing wrong with such a decision. But there is also nothing wrong with a mother drinking alcohol moderately while breastfeeding, whenever the mother desires to do so. To emphasise that there is no scientific justification to demand lactating mothers refrain from moderate alcohol consumption is of course not meant as a carte blanche to engage in excessive alcohol use. Excessive alcohol use – regardless if it is the mother or the father and regardless if the mother is still lactating or not – very likely has adverse effects on the children and should be avoided.

To sum up, to instruct lactating mothers not to drink any alcohol is scientifically not justified. What many people do not realise is that the alcohol the mother drinks is diluted once into the unborn baby's blood before the baby is born but diluted twice if alcohol is ingested via mother's milk in the lactation phase. The alcohol level reached in unborn babies during pregnancy is definitely physiologically relevant: the level in breastfed babies is physiologically irrelevant. Gundert-Remy et al. (2012) came to a similar conclusion based on theoretical model calculations.

Conclusions and discussion

Alcohol policy is a matter of many interests. On the one hand, there are industries involved in the production, distribution or selling of alcohol that benefit from alcohol and consumers who perceive and frame alcohol use as an integral part of their culinary, social and cultural lives. They present alcohol consumption positively and only put excessive alcohol consumption in a negative light (liberal problem–focused approach). On the other hand, there are temperance-oriented associations, which frame alcohol as a dangerous substance, and public health activists, whose explicit duties include curbing harmful alcohol consumption. The latter commonly expect to be successful in curbing alcohol abuse if highly restrictive measures to reduce the availability of alcohol and to prohibit alcohol advertising (control approach) are implemented.

Both sides are convinced that their own perspective is correct and they expect research to support their convictions and frames. This is especially true for adherents of the control approach, who label their position 'evidence-based alcohol policy' and deprecate any deviating positions as supporting industry interests for economic benefit. They commonly expect researchers to advocate for the control approach. Advocacy and research, if understood correctly, have different aims however. The aim of advocacy is to convince others about a given position without scrutinising one's own position while the aim of research should be to challenge any given positions, in order to gain better insights. The basic orientation of research, as suggested by Popper (1935), should be not to support certain convictions and frames but to look at as many alternative perspectives as possible, to draw up various hypotheses, to question all of them critically and to judge unsustainable hypotheses negatively.

The aim of this chapter is not to criticise and obstruct initiatives against problematic alcohol consumption by refuting scientific interpretations serving as frames supporting certain conclusions but to strive for a more meaningful research approach allowing problem areas to be described more precisely, to understand the mechanisms of problem genesis in more detail and to develop appropriate measures to reduce problematic alcohol consumption without unduly demonising moderate alcohol consumption. Science must not aim at supporting existing beliefs and frames but contribute to achieving a balanced and realistic picture of reality. This is only feasible if applied researchers are willing to get more involved in fundamental methodological aspects and limitations, even if this endeavour results in more uncertainty and ambiguity.

Notes

1 I do not focus on equally problematic convictions trivializing alcohol based on public convictions and cultural traditions, since these are not or hardly supported by science anyway. Examining popular myths in the population about positive alcohol effects that are not scientifically substantiated would nevertheless be an interesting task, which, however, requires well-planned systematic assessments of popular convictions and cannot be done by analysing and criticising conclusions conveyed in the existing scientific literature.
2 This example may appear strange at first sight, since adults don't drink mother's milk. The example was chosen to illustrate how little alcohol mother's milk contains, even if the mother initially drank half a litre of beer.

References

Anderson, P. (Ed.) 1996. *Alcohol – Less Is Better*. WHO Regional Publications, European Series, No. 70, Copenhagen.
Anderson, P., and Baumberg, B. 2006. *Alcohol in Europe: A Public Health Perspective*. London: Institute of Alcohol Studies.
Babor, T., Caetano, R., Casswell, S., Edwards, G., Giesbrecht, N., Graham, K., Grube, J., Gruenewald, P., Hill, L., Holder, H., Homel, R., Österberg, E., Rehm, J., Room, R., and Rossow, I. 2003. *Alcohol: No Ordinary Commodity – Research and Public Policy*. New York: Oxford University Press.
Barak, A. 2012. *Proportionality and Pretence – Proportionality: Constitutional Rights and Their Limitations*. New York: Cambridge University Press.
Baumberg, B. 2008. Against evidence-based policy: Over-claiming social research and undermining effective policy. *Paper Presented at the Social Policy Association Conference*, 25 June, Edinburgh.
Bloom, D.E., Chisholm, D., Jané-Llopis, E., Prettner, K., Stein, A., and Feigl, A. 2011. *From Burden to "best buys": Reducing the Economic Impact of Non-communicable Diseases in Low- and Middle-Income Countries*. Geneva: World Economic Forum and WHO.
BMG. 2015. *Österreichische Suchtpräventionsstrategie – Strategie für eine kohärente Präventions- und Suchtpolitik (Austrian Addiction Prevention Strategy – Strategy for a coherent prevention and addiction policy)*. Wien: Bundesministerium für Gesundheit.
Bruun, K., Edwards, G., Lumio, M., Mäkelä, K., Pan, L., Popham, R.E., Room, R., Schmidt, W., Skog, O.J., Sulkunen, P., and Österberg, E. 1975. *Alcohol Control Policies in Public Health Perspectives*. Helsinki: Finish Foundation for Alcohol Studies, Vol. 25.
Burgess, A. 2009. The politics of health risk promotion. 'Passive Drinking': A 'Good Lie' too far? *Health Risk and Society* 11 (6), pp. 527–40.
BZgA. 2004. *Website der Kampagne "Bist du stärker als Alkohol" der Bundeszentrale für gesundheitliche Aufklärung: FAQ – Häufig gestellte Fragen*. Available at: www.bist-du-staerker-als-alkohol. de/daten/gaq. htm#stoff (Accessed June 30, 2004).
BZgA. (Ed.) 2018. *Leitbegriffe der Gesundheitsförderung und Prävention*. Köln: Bundeszentrale für gesundheitliche Aufklärung.

Carlson, H.E., Wasser, H.l., and Reidelberger, R.D. 1985. Beer-induced prolactin secretion: A Clinical and laboratory study of the role of salsolinol. *Journal of Clinical Endocrinology and Metabolism* 60 (4), pp. 673–7.

Chabris, Ch.F., and Simons, D.J. 2011. *The Invisible Gorilla and Other Ways Our Intuition Deceives Us* (EPub Edition). New York: Harper Collins.

DeMaria, A.N. 2013. The Nanny state and 'Coercive Paternalism'. *Journal of the American College of Cardiology* 61 (20), pp. 2108–9.

Edwards, G., Anderson, P., Babor, T.F., Casswell, S., Ferrence, R., Giesbrecht, N., Godfrey, C., Holder, D.H., Lemmens, P., Mäkelä, K., Midanik, L.T., Norström, T., Österberg, E., Romelsjö, A., Room, R., Simpura, J., and Skog, O.J. 1994. *Alcohol Policy and the Public Good*. Oxford: Oxford University Press.

Entman, R.M. 1993. Framing: Toward clarification of a fractured paradigm. *Journal of Communication* 43 (4), pp. 51–8.

ESPAD Group. 2015. *ESPAD Master-Questionnaire 2015*. Lisbon: EMCCDA.

Feuerlein, W. 1979. *Alkoholismus – Missbrauch und Abhängigkeit. 2. überarbeitetet und erweiterte Auflage*. Stuttgart: Thieme.

Gesundheitsförderung Schweiz. 2018. *Strategie 2019–2024*. Schweiz, Bern: Gesundheitsförderung.

Greer, S. 2000. *The Margin of Appreciation: Interpretation and Discretion under the European Convention on Human Rights*. Human Rights Files No. 17, Strasbourg: Council of Europe Publishing.

Gundert-Remy, U., Partosch, F., Mielke, H., and Stahlmann, R. 2012. Alkohol und Stillen. *Suchtmedizin in Forschung und Praxis* 14 (1), pp. 17–25.

Huscroft, G. 2014. Proportionality and pretence. *Constitutional Commentary*. 383, pp. 229–55. Available at: https://scholarship.law.umn.edu/concomm/383.

Kahneman, D. 2011. *Thinking, Fast and Slow*. London: Penguin Books.

Koob, G.F., and Le Moal, M. 2006. *Neurobiology of Addiction*, London: Academic Press.

Krüger, H.P., Kazenwadel, J., and Vollrath, M. 1995. Grand rapids effects revisited: Accidents, alcohol and risk. Alcohol, drugs and traffic safety: *Proceedings of the 13th International Conference on Alcohol, Drugs and Traffic Safety T95*, held under the auspices of the International Committee on Alcohol, Drugs and Traffic Safety ICADTS, Adelaide, 13–18 August 1995, 1, pp. 222–30.

Lange, S., Probst, C., Gmel, G., Rehm, J., Burd, L., and Popova, S. 2017. Global prevalence of fetal alcohol spectrum disorder among children and youth: A systematic review and meta-analysis. *JAMA Pediatrics* 171, pp. 948–56.

Lefever, R. 2012. The health fascists are trying to take over our lives. *Daily Mail Online*, 18 March. Available at: www.dailymail.co.uk/debate/article-2116848/The-health-fascists-trying-lives.html.

Leung, A.K. 1986. Ethyl alcohol ingestion in children. A 15-year review. *Clinical Pediatrics* 25 (12), pp. 617–19.

Marek, E., and Kraft, W.K. 2014. Ethanol pharmacokinetics in neonates and infants. *Current Therapeutic Research* 76, pp. 90–7.

Menella, J., and Beauchamp, G. 1991. The transfer of alcohol to human milk effects on flavor and the infant's behavior. *The New England Journal of Medicine* 325 (14), pp. 981–5.

Moore, G.E. 1960. *Principa Ethica* (Original: First Edition 1903). Cambridge: University Press.

Moskalewicz, J., Room, R., and Thom, B. 2016. *Synthesis Report – Baseline Assessment and Suggestions for Comparative Monitoring of Alcohol Epidemiology Across the EU*. Warsaw: PARPA – The State Agency for Prevention of Alcohol related Problems.

ODPHP. 2019. *Drink Alcohol Only in Moderation, Homepage of the Office of Disease Prevention and Health Promotion of the U.S. Department of Health and Human Services.* Available at: https://healthfinder.gov/HealthTopics/Category/health-conditions-and-diseases/heart-health/drink-alcohol-only-in-moderation (Accessed April 25, 2019).

Pfannhauser, W. 2004. *Alkohol: Freund oder Feind? Aspekte der Lebensmittelchemie, Vortrag* am ÖGE – *Symposium "Alkoholprävention"* am 19. September. Technische Universität Graz, Institut für Lebensmittelchemie und -technologie, Graz.

Popper, K.R. 1935. *The Logic of Scientific Discovery.* London: Taylor and Francis e-Library, 2005.

Ragan, F.A., Samuels, M.S., and Hite, S.A. 1979. Ethanol ingestion in children. A five-year review. *The Journal of the American Medical Association* 242 (25), pp. 2787–8.

RCOG. 2006. *Alcohol and Pregnancy: Information for You.* London: Royal College of Obstetricians and Gynaecologists.

Schippan, R., Wagler, S., and Zschocke, D. 1975. Untersuchungen zur Äthanolelimination bei Kindern. *Kinderärztliche Praxis* 43 (5), pp. 193–201.

Thaler, R.H., and Sunstein, C.R. 2008. *Nudge: Improving Decisions about Health, Wealth, and Happiness.* New Haven: Yale University Press.

Uhl, A. 2007. How to camouflage ethical questions in addiction research. In: Fountain, J., and Korf, D.J. (Eds.), *Drugs in Society European Perspectives.* Oxford: Radcliffe, pp. 116–30.

Uhl, A. 2015. Evidence-based research, epidemiology and alcohol policy: A critique. *Contemporary Social Science* 10 (2), pp. 221–31.

Watson, P.E. Watson, I.D., and Batt, R.D. 1980. Total body water volumes for adult males and females estimated from simple anthropometric measurements. *American Journal of Clinical Nutrition* 33 (1), pp. 27–39.

WHO. 1986a. *Ottawa Charter.* Geneva: World Health Organisation.

WHO. 1986b. Health promotion: A discussion document on the concepts and principles. *Health Promotion* 1, pp. 73–6.

Wiley, L.F., Berman, M.L., and Blanke, D. 2013. Who's your Nanny? Choice, paternalism and public health in the age of personal responsibility. *Journal of Law, Medicine & Ethics* 41 (Suppl 1), pp. 88–91.

14 Conclusion

Risk, danger and policies towards psychoactive substances

Susanne MacGregor and Betsy Thom

Key points and shared themes

The chapters in this collection have looked at the ways in which certain groups of people, spaces or places have been defined as dangerous and the role of risky substance use in this. Nicholls and Berridge (Chapter 2) gave a historical account, drawing mainly on the UK, and showed how attitudes have changed towards alcohol, drugs and tobacco, while Sato (Chapter 3) showed how policy towards methamphetamine use in Japan was influenced by the perception that danger came from outsiders. Hallam demonstrated from his case study of celebrity women in 1930s London (Chapter 4) how the threat of modernity was visualised through exposure of the lives of these women and how their drug-taking was associated with ideas of deviant sexuality and rebellious behaviour. Similarly, in Japan abuse of amphetamines was associated with fears of social unrest (Sato, Chapter 3). Thom, Herring and Milne (Chapter 5) also focused on women, showing how women's reproductive role has been highlighted in advice on drinking and they discussed the growing influence of the precautionary principle in health information and lobbying.

The issue of intersectionality was raised by Stengel (Chapter 6) whose case study demonstrated the overlapping of gender identity with injecting drug use, homelessness, poverty, sex work and ROMA ethnicity in creating a concentration of dangers for a group of women in Budapest, Hungary. The attempt to counter danger through the construction of safe spaces was described. Another minority ethnic group, Turkish drug users in Ghent, Belgium, was discussed by De Kock (Chapter 7) who emphasised the distinctiveness of the European as opposed to the American and British (Anglo-Saxon) broad cultural frames influencing policies. Van Hout (Chapter 8) looked at another minority ethnic group, Irish Travellers, and showed how they suffer discrimination from a range of policies which do not respect their way of life: she argued this could be called structural oppression and discussed how drug and alcohol use has emerged as a micro-level response to these experiences.

In De Kock and Van Hout's chapters (Chapters 7 and 8, respectively), the way in which policies and cultures operating at macro-level impact at meso-level in shaping services and then again affect life at micro-level by influencing social relations and the self-image of individuals was a shared theme. This aspect was taken up by Duke and Kolind (Chapter 10) who focused on a particular dangerous space, the prison, in which especially at-risk populations are concentrated as a result of macro-policies which impact differentially on specific subgroups. The way in which the ascription of a status such as drug user or drinker to some members of a group is then spread out and used to contaminate the whole social group – such as particular ethnic minorities or social classes – formed the core of the chapter from MacGregor and O'Gorman (Chapter 9): they showed how the poor as a social group have been demonised in contemporary Britain by explaining their poverty as due to use of drink and drugs and how this has been used to justify increasingly punitive social policies towards them. Such processes of scapegoating and exclusion are also experienced by queer adults in San Francisco who smoke tobacco, in a context where the de-normalisation of smoking has become a central theme in public health campaigns (Sanders, Antin and Hunt, Chapter 11). Stereotypes themselves are dangerous because they can lead to false responses and blanket sanctions, as Potter and Klein point out in their discussion of people who use and grow cannabis (Chapter 12). Several of the chapters also demonstrate how groups act to protect themselves and develop survival strategies in response to policies which define them as dangerous. For example, the risk management strategies of illegal cannabis growers, discussed by Potter and Klein (Chapter 12), are especially important in a context where policies towards cannabis are changing in a number of countries. Uhl in Chapter 13 considered how the framing of certain behaviours and groups as dangerous affects the ways in which evidence is interpreted, thus potentially biasing the form and content of policies.

What emerges from these in-depth studies is that policies and social responses are not solely nor mainly to do with the actual substance – like opium, alcohol or tobacco, as discussed by Nicholls and Berridge (Chapter 2) – but about who uses it and where. There are debates about how dangerous particular substances are per se – to justify their categorisation in law as dangerous drugs and justify controls on their use. More often, it has been argued that it is the abuse or misuse of drugs or substances which is dangerous, thus giving more attention to identifying the types of people who abuse or misuse drugs and implying that there can be legitimate forms of use (Sato, Chapter 3). As Hallam explained in Chapter 4, in the passing of the UK *1920 Dangerous Drugs Act*, which defined dangerous drugs, attention was mainly on those who used them, who were seen as vicious addicts who used for pleasure (as contrasted with patients who received prescribed drugs from acceptable medical sources to alleviate pain). The worry was about the lifestyle not so much the drug itself. What is acceptable and what is judged deviant or atypical varies with the social status of a category: so that, for example, men are allowed to exhibit behaviours frowned upon if engaged in by women (as indicated in Chapter 5 by Thom, Herring and Milne). The big social divides are, of course, class, race and gender but sexuality, age, citizenship and subdivisions within all classifications also influence perceptions. When people discuss use of substances like alcohol, drugs and tobacco, often these are proxies for worries about deeper social issues, especially social change – mobility, migration and immigration, changing social values, for example around sexuality, threats to identities and changes in power relations. Tolerance seems to depend on a sense of being comfortable, safe and secure: insecurity and a sense of fear and danger breed intolerance.

Certain social groups have been pioneers in encouraging social change, such as artists, painters and poets or bohemians in general. For those who resist change, stigmatisation and stereotyping entrench perceptions of danger and enhance fear and avoidance of these groups. Social distance is maintained between groups by associating specific substances with defined groups – such as opium and the Chinese in nineteenth-century England (Nicholls and Berridge, Chapter 2) or meth-amphetamines with Koreans, Taiwanese and Iranians in Japan (Sato, Chapter 3) or injecting drug use with the ROMA in eastern Europe (Stengel, Chapter 6), drink and the Irish, especially Irish Travellers (Van Hout, Chapter 8), smoking tobacco and the deviant (Sanders, Antin and Hunt, Chapter 11) and tobacco, drink and drugs with the poor and disadvantaged (MacGregor and O'Gorman, Chapter 9).

Two key systems in all societies are those of production and reproduction, and changes in these systems or perceived threats to established ways of social organisation are particularly salient. Fears for the future of the race or nation and for future generations have figured prominently in discussions of the dangers of substance use. Eugenic arguments have often been present in these discourses, with substance use linked to the threat of degeneracy and the decline of a civilisation (Hallam, Chapter 4). Ideas of intergenerational transmission as referenced to the poor in the UK (MacGregor and O'Gorman, Chapter 9), Irish Travellers in Ireland (Van Hout, Chapter 8) or the Roma in Hungary (Stengel, Chapter 6) are forms of eugenic framing of social problems. Here dangerousness is attributed especially to ways of behaving that impact on the role of women, particularly in child-bearing, with arguments about the protection of the unborn child figuring prominently (Thom, Herring and Milne, Chapter 5). Substance use has played a key part in defining broad social arrangements, as with attitudes to drink and control of the poor in England, as Nicholls and Berridge outlined (Chapter 2). These attitudes also helped in the construction of the respectable, organised working class and its institutions and the emergence of a key cleavage between the respectable and the rough, with the disreputable poor being associated with excessive drinking while Methodism and Temperance helped form the British Labour Party. More recently, the disreputable poor have been defined also in terms of drug-taking as MacGregor and O'Gorman showed (Chapter 9). In the United States, the new Jim Crow regime reinforced racial divides and drug laws served a key role in the social control and oppression of African Americans, as Michelle Alexander has argued (Alexander, 2012).

Attitudes and perceptions of behaviours as acceptable or unacceptable, as socially approved or disreputable, as safe or dangerous have changed as a result of organised pressures such as those coming from social movements like the Temperance Movement, anti-smoking campaigns or the Harm Reduction Movement. More recently, a social movement of Cannabis Social Clubs (Potter and Klein, Chapter 12) as well as social movements aiming at acceptance of medicinal cannabis have altered perceptions of the dangers of cannabis by emphasising the potential benefits to be derived from its use. The change in attitudes to cannabis in the United States and Canada in recent years is remarkable and was influenced by organised social movements. In England and elsewhere, as Potter and Klein have shown (Chapter 12), there has been resistance to the perception that cannabis growers are dangerous and engaged in a harmful activity. This has sometimes taken the form of activism. However, there are some real dangers and hazards arising from the fact that production and distribution continue to be illegal in some countries. In response, growers have developed strategies to avoid harm and danger such as keeping your head down and staying below the radar (Potter and Klein, Chapter 12). There are battles of ideas within which alliances and pressure groups play key roles. The outcome of these battles – whose ideas win out – can lead to a reframing of policy. As Duke and Kolind have shown (Chapter 10), framing is a constant power struggle – between health and criminal justice issues and between attention to demand and attention to supply.

Scientific evidence has played a role in these changes in perceptions, especially when combined with campaigns and lobbying. The actions of advocacy organisations have been crucial in influencing the shape of policy and policy priorities; their role has been key in framing and/or problematising and they are key intermediaries with regard to information dissemination. However, questions have been asked about how balanced is their selection of facts. At times they have helped to create panics in the public and possibly excessive feelings of guilt among substance users (Thom, Herring and Milne, Chapter 5).

The harm reduction approach differs from the temperance or abstinence approaches to substance use in aiming to be evidence-based and non-judgemental (Stengel, Chapter 6). Here as much attention is paid to the role of dangerous spaces – the risk environment – as focusing on the characteristics of particular groups. Living in a hostile risk environment such as a prison or being homeless encourages risky ways of using drugs (Duke and Kolind, Chapter 10; Stengel, Chapter 6). As a form of resistance and positive response, activists aim to construct safe spaces – as with Chicks Day in Budapest (Stengel, Chapter 6) or treatment wings in prisons (Duke and Kolind, Chapter 10). A similar idea is that of the provision of safe injecting facilities for drug users found in a number of European cities – or family friendly pubs in England (Nicholls and Berridge, Chapter 2). Different countries have been sympathetic or hostile to ideas of harm reduction at various times, depending on their larger cultural and political frameworks. There have also been clashes or disjunctures between the rhetoric of harm reduction in international guidance and actual practice on the ground, as Duke and Kolind point out in Chapter 10.

The perception of the safety of a place depends on the location of the viewer. O'Gorman in her studies of drug use in Dublin pointed out how areas deemed dangerous by conventional society were seen as safe homes by those who lived there, who felt they could relax when they returned after venturing out into the centre of the town (O'Gorman, 2005). Similarly, gangs feel safe in their own territory but threatened when they venture into another postcode or area. Reactions to the location of services for substance users in an area – from clubs to pubs to half-way houses, rehabilitation services or safe injecting facilities – reflect how far their users are seen as belonging to that area or as threats to a way of life. Historically, the very idea and existence of the asylum as a shelter or an oasis for vulnerable and marginal groups indicated the need for safe spaces where people could be treated differently and with compassion. With the move to deinstitutionalisation, it appears there are now fewer such safe spaces available: it could be argued that increasing rates of imprisonment indicate the replacement of these safe spaces for mentally ill people with the more dangerous prison environments, which exacerbate the threats to those contained therein.

What studies also indicate is the particular danger associated with moving between spaces: for example, particularly dangerous risky moments arise when leaving prison, moving between one regime and one set of social supports to another or none (Duke and Kolind, Chapter 10). Moving between services can similarly present dangers (De Kock, Chapter 7). Those who move around seem to experience specific dangers – the homeless or Travellers, for example – linked to their lack of control of the spaces they occupy and lack of social supports (Van Hout, Chapter 8; Stengel, Chapter 6).

In contemporary societies, the key role of the media stands out in constructing images of dangerousness: a classic example is their frequent presentation of images of excess drinking among young women collapsed in the street to create fear among the general public and calls for something to be done about the problem of drink. Critical incidents and the amplification of these through media attention have played a key part in shifts in the framing of problems and moves towards policy change (Suto, Chapter 3). The media, especially newspapers, exploit these events to increase their circulation – shocks and entertainment are their currency (Hallam, Chapter 4). Stereotypes often appear to have been deliberately constructed by the sensationalist press or groups of politicians with particular agendas (MacGregor and O'Gorman, Chapter 9).

The key distinctions between normal and abnormal, mainstream and undercurrents or conventional society versus subcultures permeate debates on policy and practice. The clearest example of this is in the explicit idea of de-normalisation operating in health promotion strategies in many contemporary societies. The aim to de-normalise the use of tobacco as made explicit in international policy through the Framework Convention on Tobacco Control and thence cascaded down into national and local policies has had a perhaps unanticipated consequence in demonising those who continue to smoke. Sanders, Antin and Hunt (Chapter 11) have described the deliberate creation of stigma as a mode of control in public health policies. Smoking is now concentrated in certain groups, among the poor, the mentally ill, the homeless, ethnic minorities and queer people. Resistance to such stereotyping and shaming can be to wear the label with pride, to smoke defiantly – or use other substances defiantly as among the bohemians referred to elsewhere (Hallam, Chapter 4). Sanders, Antin and Hunt are particularly acute in drawing attention to the contemporary perception of smokers as unhealthy with the implication of moral weakness (Chapter 11). They discuss how healthism as a mode of ideological control is prominent today as the idea has gained ground that lifestyle is the main explanation for ill-health and premature death (see also Uhl, Chapter 13). Those who are obese or have lung or liver disease, for example, have only themselves to blame and it seems to be poor and 'odd' people among whom these behaviours are concentrated. Failure is written on the body. Thus, society can absolve itself of responsibility to care for such people other than by giving them health messages about better ways of living. Policies such as improved access to health services, social care and housing or redistribution of income and wealth are displaced in favour of policies of mere information dissemination.

Policy implications

What emerges from the chapters in this collection is awareness that policies change – none more striking than recent changes in policies on cannabis. A similar seismic change occurred in attitudes towards tobacco. These represent changing views on what substances and whose use, in what ways, are seen as dangerous. Historical studies show changes in attitudes and policies with industrialisation, urbanisation and modernisation: we may ask if there will be changes now in this new twenty-first century period of technological revolution? The current concern around synthetic substances seems to be part of the current phase, with perceptions of dangers lurking in the Internet and policy regimes designed to deal with older substances proving inadequate. (New forms of regulation such as the UK's Novel Psychoactive Substances Act are attempts to respond to this.) As RAND researchers recently commented:

> Much as the synthesis of heroin in the late 19th century displaced morphine and forever changed the opiate landscape, the country may again be standing at the precipice of a new era: Inexpensive, accessible, and mass-produced synthetic opioids might displace heroin, which could have important and hard-to-predict consequences.
>
> (Pardo et al., 2019, p. xvi)

Substance use and especially perceptions of misuse and abuse have often been viewed as social diseases, labels particularly applied to the poor and outsider groups: the central policy aim has been to spread new values, habits and lifestyles through forms of rehabilitation, treatment, resettlement and recovery. Competing policy proposals depend on contrasting definitions of the problem and of stereotyped target groups. A close reading of policies shows that their design and implementation act to control specific groups and behaviour in specific places. It is also clear that policies always involve values – they are never purely evidence-based. Assessment of risk is influenced by whom and where substances are taken. A key distinction within substance-related policies has to do with whether or not the activity is deemed illegal or merely inadvisable. Where use or possession of a substance is deemed illegal, this makes production, marketing and consumption inherently more dangerous, as Potter and Klein point out (Chapter 12). Any compulsion involves the state and the law. In the West, the distinction between illegal drug taking and use of substances like alcohol and tobacco is fundamental, although in other countries use of alcohol is also prohibited. The sanctions associated with illegal drug use involve use of the criminal justice system rather than health and social care systems. Treatment has at times been offered to the compliant and unthreatening, while the full force of the law and use of the justice system is deemed appropriate for those defined as dangerous.

There are variations in how policies have been implemented and chapters in this collection have shown that how harsh the sanctions are has varied between social groups, for example, between men and women or racial or ethnic groups. Even within health care, however, there are distinctions such as between voluntary treatment and mandated or compulsory treatment, as with the cases described by Hallam (Chapter 4). The idea of compulsory treatment has been supported by reference to the disease concept, formulated and applied by the medical profession, with the implication that a disease definition is value free, that is, lacking in moral overtones. Call for an evidence-based approach to problems and policies is often simply a call to rid debate of moral condemnation and blame and adopt a more compassionate approach to those affected – defined as addicts or alcoholics or nicotine dependents.

Who determine responses and policies? The cases examined in this collection have demonstrated that perceptions of problems and policy arrangements are dependent on systems of power: policy-makers are also socially constructed. All policy formations link to sets of interests, as Nicholls and Berridge showed with reference to the brewers' interest in tied pubs (Chapter 2). Any proposals for change threaten some interests and benefit others, so the resolution of debates reflects the balance of power among competing interest groups.

Policies involve the use of state power. Questions arise about the legitimacy of the use of state power and the distinction between the public arena and private space. When and where can and should the state intervene is a key issue, justified by concerns for public health, often involving children or women as the bearers of children. Policy as a form of regulation of people and certain groups and spaces inevitably involves inspection and surveillance whether by the police (Hallam, Chapter 4) or public health agencies (Uhl, Chapter 13). Methods of intervention have ranged from controls on the use of space (licensing controls and public order offences) to controls on behaviour (ways of using certain substances) to fiscal policy (taxes on alcohol and tobacco) to control of adverts (bans on TV ads or association with sports) and an array of health education messages and campaigns (Thom, Herring and Milne, Chapter 5). The protocols and guidance issued to clinicians and practitioners entrench sets of perceptions and framings of the problem, which influence the impact of policies on the ground. The ubiquity of risk assessments in contemporary societies involves many professionals and bureaucrats in constant monitoring of procedures. Within this has emerged the concept of an at-risk population who may be a special target for health interventions, as described by Stengel (Chapter 6). An array of specially designed services has developed to meet specific needs, often run by especially committed and sensitive voluntary sector organisations. A key question thus raised is whether we need specialised services for the numerous, specialised, multiple needs identified by those aware of intersectionality or would it be better to make all mainstream services more sensitive and culturally aware with regard to race, gender, sexuality, language, etc. (De Kock, Chapter 7). Proposals to encourage cultural competence as a skill in service staff aim at equal access and equal quality of treatment but, as De Kock notes, overly stressing cultures has its own problems where training can inadvertently involve stereotyping of ethnic groups and cultures. The experience of users of services has often been one of attack from a hostile environment – for them policy and practice environments can be perceived as themselves presenting dangers. Stigma acts as a deliberate deterrent to claiming or using services – the old principle of the New Poor Law. The entrenchment of stigma within selective services, specific to poor and marginalised groups, is illustrated by the repeated attempts to eliminate stigma by changing the label given to the target group or change to the name of a service. Van Hout (Chapter 8) also points out the existence of low levels of trust in institutions, agencies and authorities, especially among marginalised social groups or those who have experienced discrimination and hostility from external authorities, which presents barriers to knowledge and help seeking and hinders the best laid plans of many public health practitioners and social care services. Duke and Kolind (Chapter 10) also analysed clashes between the rhetoric of harm reduction in international guidance and actual practice on the ground, pointing to difficulties of implementation, especially in spaces like those of the prison. These difficulties may be because of political resistance, austerity, lack of resources, a dominant law and order ethos or represent clashes of cultures, including those of different professions and organisations where trying to work together in partnership.

Related to these observations is the notion of the unintended consequences of policy. Whether or not the effects of prohibitionist policies – such as those leading to the displacement of production to other geographical areas, replacement of substances with those of higher potency and danger, distortion of expenditure towards expensive criminal justice and away from health and social care – are actually unintended has been much debated (MacGregor, 2017). Whether or not the effects of the de-normalisation policies towards tobacco, espoused at international and national levels, in stigmatising and further excluding people who smoke were deliberate or accidental, or policies targeting troubled families in the UK, as described by MacGregor and O'Gorman (Chapter 9), were accidental and unthought through or deliberate, they have functioned to establish public health agencies as part of an interlocking system of oppression as experienced by those on the receiving end of these policies (Sanders, Antin and Hunt, Chapter 11; MacGregor and O'Gorman, Chapter 9; Van Hout, Chapter 8).

The diversity and complexity of many contemporary populations seem to render any simple practice response dubious: some argue these should be replaced by holistic, humane and person-centred responses. However, the presence of violence within some services like Accident and Emergency departments or street agencies is a challenge to any easy adoption of such approaches. In health education and promotion, as Thom, Herring and Milne noted in Chapter 5, simple messages are generally favoured but these can be too simplistic and distort understandings. A key problem is how to construct messages and guidance applicable to large diverse populations. This chapter also raised the question how do professionals and policy-makers come to judgements on risk and what to prioritise or target for attention? Which methods are used for which substances and who are the targets of policy are a matter of political decision-making – that is, the setting of priorities, for example, mass media campaigns with regard to smoking and drinking focusing on pregnant women (Nicholls and Berridge, Chapter 2; Thom, Herring and Milne, Chapter 5: Uhl, Chapter 13). Politics is about priorities, so it is within the political realm that these choices are made and what these choices are depends on the balance of power and sets of values within particular cultures and political arrangements. In justifying their choices, politicians often point to a lack of consensus in the scientific community as one barrier to simple adoption of evidence-based policies.

A key argument of the chapters in this collection is that different policies depend on different framings of the problem. Sato (Chapter 3) stressed that at any one time in any one country, there may be several competing or complementary frames present. This was also argued by Duke and Kolind (Chapter 10). The battles between competing framings – health or criminal justice, for example – are ongoing and it is rare for there to be one universally shared perception. It can also be the case that the perception enshrined in law and policy differs from the framings agreed by majorities of stakeholders and factors, such as competing priorities, inertia and lack of agreement on alternatives, as well as failures of political organisation and communication, can leave laws and policies in place even when many agree they are no longer fit for purpose. Policy changes do occur, however. Evidence in these chapters has pointed to the role of events and publicity around critical incidents in prompting policy change. Celebrity deaths played this role in 1930s England, as Hallam showed in Chapter 4, as they did in Japan, as described by Sato (Chapter 3).

The public health approach and use of the precautionary principle

An expansive notion of public health

Several chapters have raised the issue of the use of the precautionary principle and questioned whether or not this is being used appropriately. Is public health becoming too cautious, as Thom, Herring and Milne implied (Chapter 5), or intervening on the basis of a false understanding of evidence, as argued by Uhl (Chapter 13)? Is it amplifying the exclusion of different or atypical people through de-normalisation policies, as Sanders, Antin and Hunt described (Chapter 11)?

The public health approach is often praised as an alternative to prohibitionist or criminal justice approaches when discussing illicit drugs policies. With regard to alcohol, the public health approach is associated with attempts to limit the overall consumption of alcohol per capita in a population rather than focusing on particular groups who drink excessively or paying attention to the quality of alcohol available in the market. Similarly, with respect to nicotine, harm reduction policies support use of e-cigarettes but this is opposed by those who see attention to the mode of delivery as simply a device by producers to maintain their grip on the market. Understandings of what is a public health approach vary across countries, times and substances (MacGregor, 2016).

One understanding of a public health approach is as disease prevention while another is of health promotion. Yet another is as harm reduction. All involve concepts of risk and threats to health. There is much debate about what are the dangers from which populations should be protected and how far the state should intervene in individual lives to do so. Promotion of a public health approach is now found across a wide area of social problems beyond the traditional arenas of health and social care. For example, ideas of public health are now used in the context of policing, as with policies to deal with knife crime and violence (Slutkin nd; WHO, 2002). A number of bodies in England (covering public health, policing, local government and others) have signed up to a Public Health and Social Care Consensus statement which defines a public health approach in terms of five core elements:

- starting with **populations** (rather than individuals);
- seeking to understand and address the **causes of the causes**;
- championing **prevention**;
- intelligent use of **data and evidence base**;
- organisations working in **partnership** with each other and communities.

It could be asked to what extent is this definition particular to public health or does it not refer to a wider group of social policies in general? While this expansive notion of the role of public health has value, it is also very ambitious and presents a potential challenge of overreach. In this statement, the case is made that

> Key risk factors for poor health align closely with risk factors for offending; and those who are or are at risk of offending as a group are more likely to suffer from multiple and complex health issues, including mental and physical health problems, learning difficulties, *substance misuse* and increased risk of premature mortality. By working together and intervening early to address the common factors that bring people into contact with the police and criminal justice system and lead to poor health we can improve public safety, prevent offending and reoffending, reduce crime and help to improve outcomes for individuals and the wider community (our italics).

Among their priorities are

> To enable the police service, public health teams and other partners to work better together to support families enrolled in the troubled families

programme, domestic abuse victims, children subject to Child Protection Plans and the management of sexual and violent offenders and those with complex dependencies such as drugs, alcohol or mental health.

The focus, it seems, is on a strata of society with complex needs and the well-meaning intention is to identify at-risk groups and intervene early in order to prevent later problems of criminality and ill health. The question is how these priorities will be operationalised and whether policies may in practice act to stigmatise and stereotype without improving lives. How they operate in practice would be influenced by the general political and cultural arrangements in a society, especially whether liberal or authoritarian.

The precautionary principle

Cass Sunstein has criticised the use of the precautionary principle in contemporary societies, asking what is the relation between fear, danger and the law (Sunstein, 2005)? He defines the precautionary principle as the idea that regulators should take steps to protect against potential harms even if causal chains are uncertain and even if we do not know that harms are likely to come to fruition. He points out that risks exist on all sides of social situations and precautionary steps create dangers of their own. Diverse cultures focus on very different risks because social influences and peer pressures accentuate some fears and reduce others. His main argument is that law responds to people's fears. He distinguishes between debates and laws in democratic societies (characterised by deliberation) and in populist societies (at worst tending to demagoguery): the latter are more likely to fall prey to public fears that are baseless – and, we may add, exhibit reactions to fears that have been fomented by political actors in order to entrench their power. On the other hand, he notes that there may exist serious risks of which the public are insufficiently fearful such as perhaps air pollution or climate change where the role of science and expertise is particularly important in educating the public about these dangers and encouraging changes in laws and regulations. Sunstein argues that the contemporary state of affairs is one in which individuals and societies have to make decisions in a context of risk and uncertainty. However, he sees the expansion of the use of the precautionary principle as paralysing – freezing responses rather than encouraging careful analysis of conditions. An example we could think of here would be with regard to medicinal cannabis where the argument currently made in the UK is that there is a lack of evidence to support its prescription and this then acts to inhibit prescriptions in cases such as severe epilepsy in children or chronic pain in adults where evidence is growing of its value in those jurisdictions where it is available such as Canada, the Netherlands and Israel. David Nutt of DrugScience has argued that the current UK Misuse of Drugs Act inhibits legitimate scientific research on a number of substances such as LSD which might prove of value if only hypotheses could be tested.

The reason the precautionary principle works in this paralysing way, Sunstein argues, is because of the human susceptibility to worst-case scenarios: people focus on the worst case and neglect the probability that it will actually occur (2005, p. 6). Here Sunstein's arguments parallel those of Uhl in Chapter 13 in this collection. Sunstein calls this phenomenon 'probability neglect' leading people to focus on the worst case even it if is highly improbable. This is certainly the case with regard to the classification of ecstasy in the UK Misuse of Drugs Act due to the attention given in press and media coverage to the catastrophic deaths of young people without consideration of the actual prevalence of use of this substance. The tendency is also to focus on an identifiable subgroup who then face the burden of restrictions as illustrated in many chapters in this collection: policies go far beyond what is useful or necessary to respond to the threat. Sunstein adds that 'stereotyping of groups significantly increases when people are in a state of fear. . . . [W]hen people are afraid, they are far more likely to tolerate government action that abridges the freedom of members of some "out group"' (2005, p. 209). Thus,

the availability heuristic and probability neglect often lead people to treat risks as much greater than they are in fact and hence to accept risk reduction strategies that do considerable harm and little good [and] . . . when the burdens of government restrictions are faced by an identifiable minority rather than by the majority the risk of unjustified action is significantly increased. . . . [P]recautions can be worse than blunders; they can be both cruel and unjust.

(Sunstein, 2005, p. 222)

A related phenomenon is that of 'system neglect' understood as an inability to see that risks are part of systems and that interventions into those systems can create risks of their own. Sunstein argues for the use of cost-benefit analysis as preferable to that of the precautionary principle in judging the risks, dangers and potential harms of any activity: one needs to calculate the possible benefits as well as any possible risks. Cost-benefit analysis he sees as a partial corrective against both excessive and insufficient fear in the case of health and safety regulation. (An interesting example of the application of this approach can be found in an analysis of drugs policies carried out for the reform advocacy organisation Transform (Rolles, 2009)).

While Sunstein's main focus is on environmental policy, the arguments can be applied equally in public health. He distinguishes between weak and strong versions of the precautionary principle. The weak version is almost a truism and unarguable, that is, that lack of decisive evidence of harm should not be a ground for refusing to regulate. As a strong version of the precautionary principle, he quotes Dr Brent Blackwelder, President of Friends of the Earth, in 2002 (2005, p. 19):

where there is a risk of significant health or environmental damage to others or to future generations and when there is scientific uncertainty as to the nature of that damage or the likelihood of that risk then decisions should be made so as to prevent such activities from being conducted unless and until scientific evidence shows that the damage will not occur.

It is this strong version of the precautionary principle that some like Thom, Herring and Milne (Chapter 5) and Uhl (Chapter 13) have seen being applied especially towards alcohol and which is certainly applied with regard to a number of substances, especially cannabis, controlled under drug laws in some countries but not in others. As Sunstein points out and as demonstrated in the cases described in this collection, people and societies are selective in their fears: 'every nation is precautionary about some risks but not others' (2005, p. 21). Sunstein argues that regulation of one risk may actually increase other risks – as is undoubtedly the case in the implementation of drugs policies in the UK.

Sunstein also says that 'people are far more willing to tolerate familiar risks than unfamiliar ones even if they are statistically equivalent' (2005, p. 43). This is seen to be the case by drug and alcohol campaigners in the UK who argue that the risks and harms related to alcohol consumption are generally underestimated currently (especially compared to cannabis) as alcohol is such a familiar substance. Sir Ian Gilmore, a leading campaigner, has also compared alcohol to tobacco saying, 'there is undoubtedly harm from second-hand smoke but the range and magnitude of harms is likely to be even greater from alcohol'.[1] In a campaign to draw attention to the dangers of second-hand drinking, ten categories of harm were mentioned ranging from harassment to assault: 'second-hand drinking covers such a spectrum of human experience that a wide range of measures is required to confront it'.[2] A number of specific policy areas were then discussed as relevant: support for children with alcoholic parents; drunk driving; diagnosis of FASD; and the attempt to de-normalise second-hand drinking. Policies mentioned by Gilmore as priorities included minimum unit pricing, combined with increasing duty on alcohol; and he added that governments 'need to stop leaving alcohol to the free market like soap powder and treat it as a potentially serious health risk as it has done with tobacco'.[3] Allowing that campaigners need to select and emphasise to get their message across, some of the criticisms made by Uhl in Chapter 13 seem relevant to this illustration. However, health conditions relating to heavy long-term alcohol consumption (as with tobacco or other psychoactive substances) do need to be addressed not only because of the harms caused to individuals and families but also because of the costs and pressures they place on health and other public services. As a letter to the *Lancet* commented, Europe 'has the highest prevalence of drinkers, heavy episodic drinking, alcohol consumption per capita, and the lowest proportion of abstainers, compared with other WHO regions' (Goiana da Silva et al., 2019). There is great variation among countries in the policies adopted and not all policies are adequately enforced. Policy changes have to be culturally acceptable and workable if they are to be effective.

In choosing between policies, Uhl raises the question of the right balance between freedom and paternalism (Chapter 13). Sunstein's answer to this, with his colleague Richard Thaler, is to argue for libertarian paternalism – or nudging as it is more widely known. Where people are not sufficiently fearful (as used to be the case with regard to drinking and driving or use of safety belts in cars, or with regard to smoking and arguably today with respect to use of alcohol in some countries – hard drinking countries perhaps), this approach is said to offer a way forward. Libertarian paternalism is defined as 'an approach that preserves freedom of choice while encouraging both private and public institutions to steer people in directions that will promote their own welfare' (Sunstein, 2005, p. 203). The central empirical claim is that in many domains, people's preferences are labile and ill-formed, so open to persuasion.

Concluding comments

The multidisciplinary approach adopted in this collection, drawing on history, criminology, sociology, social policy and public health and using a range of qualitative research methods, has allowed a multilayered, multifaceted and rich understanding of some of the issues around concepts of safety and dangerousness and how these have fed into problematisations and policy prescriptions regarding risk and substance use in different countries at different times. The studies reported in this collection demonstrate the value of qualitative, fine-grained research to explain the how and why in order to help to design policies to respond to the correlations demonstrated by epidemiological data such as those showing associations between inequalities and ill-health.

It is also the case that although there may be tough regulations if there is only loose enforcement, what happens on the ground may be very different from what is inscribed in laws and policy statements. The interventions of the people working in professions, bureaucracies, street agencies and other arenas and the resistance to top-down policies which come from substance users and from local initiatives, all make for a more complex picture than simple models of policies and interventions sometimes imply.

Underlying all laws and policies are sets of values, norms and habits, and disagreements about values have to be resolved through political processes, ideally forms of deliberative democracy: policies can never be solely based on neutral evidence. In designing and implementing public policies, there is an underlying issue of how much trust and respect populations and social groups have for experts and expertise: it is commonly said today that this is declining and we need to ask why this has come about. As researchers ourselves – as the contributors to this volume mostly are – we would be wise to consider how to improve trust in our research if we are to justify our existence and the time we devote to these activities. Ideas of co-production, for example, are one response to these questions. Scientists and social scientists have a role to play in contributing to democratic dialogue and encouraging understanding of issues and respect for individual and cultural differences. A major social issue such as substance use will always be contentious and where the state becomes involved through criminal justice or public health institutions, discussions will be held about the right degree of interference in individual lives, which can only be legitimated on the grounds of public health and protection of the vulnerable. Those involved have to aim to balance fairness towards individuals with the interests of the public. In these discussions, evidence plays a part: one improvement for social researchers would be to make greater efforts to include and value experiential evidence and user voices. As scientists, we should also aim to adopt a critical approach, challenge conventional wisdom and ensure we give as much attention to thinking as we do to observing. The tactics of the powerful both in the state and among business interests are well known: faced with uncomfortable ideas and evidence, they will challenge the science, add confusion, say we need to see more research, and sow doubt about the extent of expert consensus. Scholars and scientists who enter the public arena have to be prepared to deal with these oppositions and remain independent, be willing to do unconventional research and think critically while challenging the powerful. They also need thick skins.

Notes

1 Quoted in Paula Cocozza, The toll of second hand drinking. *The Guardian*, July 9th, 2019, pp. 6–7.
2 Ibid.
3 Ibid.

References

Alexander, M. 2012. *The New Jim Crow: Mass Incarceration in the Age of Color Blindness.* New York: The New Press.
Association of Directors of Public Health, Association of Police and Crime Commissioners, Clinks, College of Policing, Faculty of Public Health, Local Government Association, Nacro, National Association for Voluntary and Community Action, National Police Chiefs Council, NHS England, Public Health England, and the Royal Society for Public Health. 2018. *Policing, Health and Social Care Consensus: Working Together to Protect and Prevent Harm to Vulnerable People.* London: National Police Chiefs' Council. Available at: https://www.npcc.police.uk.
Goiana da Silva, F., Cruz e Silva, D., Lindeman, M., Hellman, M., Angus, C., Karlsson, T., Renström, M., and Ferreira Borges, C. 2019. Implementing the European action plan on alcohol. *The Lancet,* 3 September 2019. Available at: http://dx.doi.org/10.1016/S2468-2667(19)30174-4.
MacGregor, S. 2016. Public health approaches to substance use: A critique. In: Kolind, T., Thom, B., and Hunt, G. (Eds.), *The Sage Handbook of Drug and Alcohol Studies: Social Science Approaches.* London; California; New Delhi; Singapore: Sage, pp. 628–43.
MacGregor, S. 2017. *The Politics of Drugs: Perceptions Power and Policies.* London: Palgrave Macmillan.
O'Gorman, A. 2005. *Drugs and Social Exclusion.* PhD. Middlesex University, London.
Pardo, B., Taylor, J., Caulkins, J.P., Kilmer, B., Reuter, P., and Stein, B.D. 2019. *The Future of Fentanyl and Other Synthetic Opioids.* Santa Monica, CA: RAND.
Rolles, S. 2009. *A Comparison of the Cost Effectiveness of Prohibition and Regulation of Drugs.* London: Transform.
Slutkin, G. n.d. Violence Is a Contagious Disease. Chicago: Cure Violence.
Sunstein, C.R. 2005. *Laws of Fear: Beyond the Precautionary Principle.* Cambridge: Cambridge University Press.
WHO. 2002. *World Report on Violence and Health.* Geneva: WHO.

Index

Note: page numbers in *italics* indicate figures; page numbers in **bold** indicate tables.